Plato's Press
CHICAGO, ILLINOIS

THE LIBRARY
OF CONGRESS HAS
CATALOGUED THIS TEXT AS FOLLOWS
Registration: TXu002259392 / 2021-05-05
Title: Moral Philosophy: A Theoretical and Practical Approach to Moral Decision-Making
Description: Electronic File (eService)
Copyright: Jeffrey Wallace Bulger
Date of Creation: 2021
Authorship: Jeffrey Wallace Bulger
Rights & Permissions: Jeffrey Wallace Bulger

BulgerDr@gmail.com

ISBN 978-1-62252-010-7 (Paperback)
ISBN: 978-1-62252-011-4 (Ebook)

Moral Philosophy

A Theoretical & Practical Approach To Moral Decision-Making

© 2021 paperback

ISBN 978-1-62252-010-7
9 781622 520107

Moral Philosophy

Moral Philosophy

Table of Contents

I. EPISTEMOLOGY & METAPHYSICS

II. MID-LEVEL PRINCIPLES

III. MORAL THEORY

IV. PRINCIPLISM

Va. INFORMED CONSENT

Vb. INFORMED CONSENT

VIa. CASE ANALYSIS PARADIGM

VIb. Dr.Ethics™ Informed Consent

VII. SEVEN READINGS

1. MORAL DEVELOPMENT

2. HONEYBEE DEMOCRACY

I. EPISTEMOLOGY & METAPHYSICS

I. In The Beginning

A. Big Bang Misnomer

[1:1] In the beginning there was the "Big Bang." However, this event was neither "big" as the universe arose from an infinitesimal point, nor was there a "bang" as there was not only no medium for "sound" but there also were no perceivers to have the subjective experience of "Bang".

[1:2] Despite the "Big Bang" being a pejorative misnomer coined by Fred Hoyle in 1949, there is now broad coherent academic consensus that everything that exists has come into existence through the process of evolution and that the "Big Bang" is now the accepted term for referring to such a beginning. This evolutionary process has resulted in not only all the galaxies, solar systems, and biological life, but also all cognitive experiences of living beings including such experiences as moral values.

[1:3] Since evolution is the acknowledged academic explanatory process for the existence of all that exists, including cognitive experiences, it follows that the process of evolution, as manifested by natural selection, is also the academic explanation that can be provided for the origins of the principles of morality. It makes no difference as to whether or not the existence of something is material or cognitive, the process of evolution is still the agreed upon universal academic explanation.

B. Non-Teleological

[1:4] Because evolution is based on empirical facts, and because empirical facts can only provide deterministic cause and effect relationships, it is academically recognized that it is impossible to empirically observe any evolutionary purposes or ends. Purposes and ends—teleology, are subjective cognitive determinations and since empirical facts can only provide objective facts, it follows that empirical facts cannot provide evidence of not only evolutionary purposes or ends but it also cannot provide any empirical evidence of any moral purposes or ends. This non-teleological account of evolution is not controversial as it would be unreasonable to expect empiricism to provide something that it is not capable of providing, i.e. purposes or ends. As John Stuart Mill said, albeit in the context of happiness: we shouldn't expect more from life than what it is capable of bestowing[1].

[1:5] From this non-teleological evolutionary point of view, the question then arises as to how the principles of morality, which have purposes and ends, have evolved into existence.

[1:6] One academic description is that morality, culture, and worldviews in general are immaterial cognitive developments that are transferred or passed on from one generation to the next by the evolutionary process of natural selection. Richard Dawkins coined the term "meme" to refer to such natural selection or transference of cognitive values[2]. However, if morality is in fact immaterial, then it also follows that morality cannot be established by empirical evidence.

[1:7] Evolution therefore appears to be reductively dualistic with empiricism providing the factual evidence for evolution independent of purposes and ends, and "mematic evolution" providing for the social evolution of cognitive values that have purposes and ends.

C. Natural Selection

1. Survival of the fittest vs natural selection

[1:8] Natural selection is a subcategory of evolution in that it refers to the mechanisms or processes that results in the passing

---

1 Mill, Utilitarianism, Chapter 8, [2:72].

2 Dawkins, Richard (1989). The Selfish Gene (2 ed.). Oxford University Press. p. 192. ISBN 0-19-286092-5. "We need a name for the new replicator, a noun that conveys the idea of a unit of cultural transmission, or a unit of imitation. 'Mimeme' comes from a suitable Greek root, but I want a monosyllable that sounds a bit like 'gene'. I hope my classicist friends will forgive me if I abbreviate mimeme to meme. If it is any consolation, it could alternatively be thought of as being related to 'memory', or to the French word même. It should be pronounced to rhyme with 'cream'."

on of genetic traits by reproduction. Since natural selection is based on empirical facts it follows that there are no teleological purposes or ends that can be discerned outside of subjective cognitive experiences and/or evaluations. The evolution of biological creatures is called natural selection, not "survival of the fittest" as it is sometimes mistakenly referred to.

[1:9] Biological natural selection is the empirical evidence that shows that those beings that are most able to successfully reproduce will predominate and pass on their genetic traits and thus exist. This reproductive ability is necessarily accompanied by adaptation, i.e., the ability to adapt to the ever-changing environment. As a result, natural selection is not "survival of the fittest," as that term would imply that there is an end or purpose that nature is pursuing, i.e., fitness, rather than just reproductive success. Since it is impossible for empirical evidence to observe anything except determined cause and effect relationships, and since "survival of the fittest" generally implies a purpose or end, it follows that "survival of the fittest," like the "Big Bang" is a contradictive misnomer.

[1:10] If "fittest" is defined simply as "survival" in order to make the phrase "survival of the fittest" coherent with "natural selection," then "survival of the fittest" becomes a meaningless term as is shown by replacing the term "fittest" in "survival of the fittest" with "survival" which then results in "survival of the those who survive." It is certainly a capital "T" Truth like an analytic statement, but it is not a statement that provides any additional knowledge: it is a tautology.

[1:11] Biological natural selection is a purely descriptive process of the unfolding of biological nature and therefore it cannot impart any value or purpose.

[1:12] If there is any value, purpose, or meaning in the physical universe it seems that it would be only because cognitive beings are able to subjectively conceive of the universe as valuable, purposive, or meaningful, not because there is any value, purpose, or meaning empirically found in physical nature itself, or independent of subjective cognitive experiences of beings. Therefore, since moral principles exist as cognitive experiences, and since moral principles have purposes and ends, it follows that moral principles cannot be empirically determined, rather the nature of the existence of moral principles must be a purely *a priori* subjective experience.

2. Evolution vs. creationism

[1:13] The distinguishing characteristic between creationism—a purposeful theistic creation of the present world, and evolution is that evolution has independent and verifiable evidence from a broad range of academic disciplines in its support, and creationism does not have a single academic empirical discipline that is able to support its faith-based position. Astronomy, Geology, Paleontology, Biology, Chemistry, Physics, just to name a few academic disciplines, have all independently concluded, using the scientific method, that both empirically and rationally that a non-purposive evolution is the best explanation of the origin and nature of the universe with all its biological beings and with all it's cognitive experiences. This multidisciplinary academic agreement is called coherency. Creationism, on the other hand, is a nonacademic, nonscientific, faith-based conclusion that is incoherent with academics. This observation does not necessarily disprove faith-based creationism, such as for example theistic evolution, as empiricism can only provide evidence for the making of rational conclusions. However, if the faith-based creationism asserts statements of fact that are empirically determined to be false, such as for example, a geocentric worldview, or flat Earth, then empiricism would be able to discredit those so called "factual claims" as being false.

[1:14] Therefore, although empiricism cannot provide evidence for the nonexistence of the tooth fairy or god, it is the case, as mentioned earlier, that academics can provide both empirical and rational proofs that particular factual or rational claims are false, contradictory, and/or logically inconsistent.

[1:15] Since academic education is about academic subjects, and since creationism is not an academic worldview, it would be absurd to conclude that creationism ought to be given equal academic time when dealing with the empirical sciences any more than in faith-based investigations equal time ought to be given to academic empirical science. So also when dealing with morality. Since academics uses empirical and rational evidence for establishing the nature of reality, and since this is an academic text, it follows that the study of the nature and origins of the principles of morality will also have to be presented using the empirical and rational scientific method, not those that are based on faith or some other nonscientific method.

[1:16] On the other hand, if the academic subject were to be Anthropology, Philosophy of Religion, or Sociology and the focus was to address how faith or belief in creationism or theistic evolution—(now often referred to as intelligent design), has arisen independently of academically accepted scientific evidence, then it would be an appropriate subject to address in academia.

3. Representative heuristic errors

[1:17] A heuristic is an intuitive mental shortcut for making decisions quickly. Heuristic decision-making often works quite effectively, yet at other times heuristic decision-making may introduce errors. For example, in judging distance the heuristic use of clarity is often times used. Objects of less clarity are intuitively judged to be further away than objects of more clarity. As a result, on clear days with little humidity distances are often times heuristically underestimated. On hazy days, distances are often times over estimated. Overall the distance heuristic is effective enough for most distance judgments for humans to effectively interact with their environment for survival.

[1:18] One academic explanation of why so many people think of a purposeful universe or a purposeful creation is that those judgments are based on intuitive heuristic errors. For example, the representativeness heuristic is the psychological propensity to evaluate probabilities in such a way that to the degree to which "Y" represents "X" is the degree towards which it is believed that "Y" comes from "X." This may be true for some situations, but not true for other situations, causing errors of intuitive judgments, i.e., a heuristic error. A representative heuristic error, for example, would be the conclusion that an emotional event implies an emotional cause. The heuristic error is that the cause could be something other than emotional. In the discussion of "survival of the fittest" the representative heuristic error would be that since many beings experience purpose, then it follows that the cause of that purpose must have been caused by a purposeful universe or caused by some purposeful god when in fact cause and effect relationships can only determined a series of events, in that one event follows another independent of the determination of a purposeful universe or a purposeful god. More specifically, just because the principles of morality have purposes, it does not logically follow that the causation of those purposes was necessarily purposeful itself, rather it can be scientifically explained by the nonpurposive processes of natural selection.

4. Philosophers Historical Influence

[1:19] Richard Dawkins asks the question, "Why did it take so long for a Darwin to arrive on the scene?"[3] This questions is especially pertinent since evolution and natural selection is such a simple and easy concept to understand as compared to many of the other scientific understandings that preceded it. So why did evolution take so long in becoming scientifically accepted, and why do more than 40% of Americans still deny the scientific empirical evidence that humans evolved from other animals, and think that they were created by God within the last 10,000 years?[4]

[1:20] A significant cause of such a scientific delay is probably because of a combination of both religious and academic indoctrination. Religious indoctrination because of religious revelations such as those found in the book of Genesis but perhaps even more influential and seminal to the scientific delay was the academic indoctrination that was incorporated into religious doctrines. This antievolutionary worldview started with Pythagoras,

---

3 Richard Dawkins, The Greatest Show On Earth: The Evidence For Evolution, (New York: Free Press, 2009), p. 21.

[4] Ibid. p. 7.

then spread to Socrates, Plato, and Aristotle and then ultimately to the entire history of academia. These philosophers were arguably the most important and influential academic contributors the world has ever known. As a result it was philosophical leaders, not religious leaders, who were the most significant contributors to the delay in the scientific advancement of evolution for the past 2000 years.

[1:21] Plato combined Heraclitus's ever-changing flux and Parmenides eternal never-changing one. The Pythagorean ideal perfection of geometry in which perfection only exists independently of the physical world was extended by Plato to be the immutable, nontemporal, and nonspatial forms. These perfect and unchanging forms is what made knowledge possible for Plato.

[1:22] Although Aristotle rejected the apartness of the forms, and therefore Plato's mind body dualism, he was still fundamentally a Platonist. For Aristotle every holistic individual thing has two aspects, matter and form, and either without the other is an abstraction and unreal. As an acorn grows into an oak tree, the oak tree is the form or purpose that the acorn serves. The acorn is the potentiality of there being an oak tree, and the oak tree is the actuality of this potentiality. The acorn is the basis that makes an oak tree possible—potentiality; and the oak tree is the purpose, or end, toward which the acorn grows—actuality.

[1:23] These concepts of Plato's unchanging immutable forms, together with Aristotle's potentiality and actuality created the infertile parking lot environment that evolution and natural selection has had to set its roots in.

[1:24] Perhaps the question, "Why did it take so long for a Darwin to arrive on the scene? is not the right question. Perhaps the question should be "How was it possible that evolution and natural selection was able to grow roots in such an infertile environment?" The answer to this question, as will be further discussed, was greatly influenced by empirical evidence, and rational analysis.

[1:25] Likewise, morality is indistinguishable from evolution and natural selection in that it can be approached as an academic discipline. Such an approach is not an atheistic or anti-religious perspective or worldview, rather the perspective that will be presented is the result of the epistemological justification of empirical evidence and rational analysis.

Summary: In The Beginning

[1:26] All of reality has evolved into existence regardless of whether you are referring to planetary systems or moral principles. Since evolution is based on empirical evidence, and since empirical evidence can only observe cause and effect relationships, it follows that epistemologically there can be no empirical claims of purposes and ends as purposes and ends are subjective claims not empirical claims. However, persons intersubjectively agree that they do have purposes and ends and that needs to be explained.

[1:27] Religion, along with creationism, may be one way of explaining purposes and ends, yet for academic scientific enquiry such epistemological and metaphysical claims of "faith" are not acceptable. It would be inappropriate to give equal time to both evolution and creationism in an academic setting as there is no empirical evidence for creationism and academics is based on empirical evidence and rational analysis.

[1:28] Purposes and ends that are conceived as being part of the evolutionary framework can be explained as heuristic errors of representativeness, in which the purposeful effect is thought to be necessarily caused by a purposeful cause. However, it is known that causes do not necessarily have the characteristics or attributes of the effects and therefore such evaluations may be an intuitional error, hence the name heuristic error.

[1:29] Purposes and ends that are conceived as being part of the evolutionary framework can also be explained as being part of a long history of academic indoctrination based on antievolutionary worldviews starting with Pythagoras, then spreading to Socrates, Plato, Aristotle and then ultimately to the past 2000 years of academia.

[1:30] It is through the continued process of empirical evidence and rational analysis that scientific advancement is prevailing and the same will be the case with the study of moral theory.

II. Historical Moral Issues

[2:1] The following is a list of five historically significant issues that need to be addressed when attempting to use the scientific method for an empirical and rational determination of the metaphysical nature of morality.

[2:2] In summary the issues are: 1) Hume's is-ought problem, 2) Kant's noumenal and phenomenal realm, 3) Mill's proof of means to ends vs ends, 4) Moore's naturalistic fallacy, and 5) Dawkins memetic natural selection.

[2:3] This section briefly presents the issues, then the next section will present the primary and secondary qualities distinction, then there will be the section on determinism and free will. After these sections are completed, establishing holistic dualism, it will then be shown how holistic dualism is able to successfully address each of the five historic issues.

A. David Hume (1711 – 1776) "is-ought problem"

[2:4] David Hume, in his Treatise of Human Nature, 1739, brought attention to the issue of what can and cannot be determined by empirical evidence. Hume's argument states that from descriptive statements of fact, it is impossible to prove or derive any prescriptive statements of "ought.[5]"

[2:5] This was then labeled the "is-ought problem" and sometimes also referred to as "Hume's Guillotine."

---

[5] Hume, David (1739), A Treatise of Human Nature, London: John Noon, book III, part I, section I p. 489.
In every system of morality, which I have hitherto met with, I have always remark'd, that the author proceeds for some time in the ordinary ways of reasoning, and establishes the being of a God, or makes observations concerning human affairs; when all of a sudden I am surpriz'd to find, that instead of the usual copulations of propositions, is, and is not, I meet with no proposition that is not connected with an ought, or an ought not. This change is imperceptible; but is however, of the last consequence. For as this ought, or ought not, expresses some new relation or affirmation, 'tis necessary that it shou'd be observ'd and explain'd; and at the same time that a reason should be given; for what seems altogether inconceivable, how this new relation can be a deduction from others, which are entirely different from it.

B. Immanuel Kant (1724 – 1804) "noumenal and phenomenal realms"

[2:6] Immanuel Kant,[6] in his Groundwork of the Metaphysics of Morals, 1785, also argued that there were limits to the types of knowledge that can be provided by empirical evidence. If knowledge of moral principles can only be based on a pure *a priori* metaphysics, i.e., pure rationality independent of empirical observations, then it follows that empirical knowledge is of no help in the determination of moral principles.[7]

[2:7] Kant made the distinction between the intelligible—the noumenal world of freedom, and the sensory—the phenomenal world that is wholly determined. Kant argued that although the creation of moral principles is an exercise of rational freedom—the noumenal, it was still practically useful and practically permissible to consider those moral principles as if they were empirically determined laws of nature—the phenomenal.[8,9]

---

[6] All page numbers found in brackets after a Kant quote, e.g. [#], are the page numbers of the Konigliche Preussische Akademie der Wissenschaften edition of Kant's works.

[7] Immanuel Kant, The Groundwork for the Metaphysics of Morals, (1785), Translated by James W. Ellington, (Indianapolis: Hackett Publishing Company, 1981). pp. 22-23, [411-412].
All moral concepts have their seat and origin completely *a priori* in reason. ... They cannot be abstracted from anything empirical, which is contingent. Principles should be derived from the universal concept of a rational being in general.

[8] Ibid, p. 54, [453].
If I were solely a member of the intelligible world, then all my actions would perfectly conform to the principle of the autonomy of a pure will—actions resting on the supreme principle of morality. If I were solely a part of the world of sense, then my actions would have to be taken as in complete conformity with the natural law.

[9] Ibid, p. 61, [462].
Reason should not search for a supreme motive of morality that is empirical. Reason should not dwell in empty space, i.e., space of transcendent concepts. The idea of a pure intelligible world regarded as a whole of all intelligences to which we ourselves belong as rational beings, (i.e., universal kingdom of ends in which we conduct ourselves according to maxims of freedom as if they were laws of nature), is a useful and permissible idea.

C. John Stuart Mill (1806 – 1873) "means to ends vs ends"

[2:8] John Stuart Mill, in Utilitarianism, 1861, pointed out that "means to ends" can be proven empirically but that "ultimate ends," are ends in and of themselves, and therefore cannot be proven empirically, as they are not means.[10]

D. G. E. Moore (1873 – 1958) "naturalistic fallacy"

[2:9] G. E. Moore, in his book Principia Ethica, 1903, on a related but distinct point, argued that morality, with regard to the teleological, the end or "good," could not be determined or defined by appealing to one or more natural properties. Moore held that the "good" was in fact indefinable, like the experience of the color yellow, and therefore, if someone were to make a claim about ethics by appealing to one or more natural properties, such as pleasure or preference, and if they were then to claim that the natural properties were entirely the same as goodness, then it would follow that they would be committing the naturalistic fallacy.[11],[12]

---

[10] Mill, Utilitarianism, Chapter 8, [1:33-36].
On the present occasion, I shall, without further discussion of the other theories, attempt to contribute something toward the understanding and appreciation of the "utilitarian" or "happiness" theory, and toward such proof as it is susceptible of. It is evident that this cannot be proof in the ordinary and popular meaning of the term. Questions of ultimate ends are not amenable to direct proof. Whatever can be proved to be good must be so by being shown to be a means to something admitted to be good without proof.

[11] G. E. Moore, Principia Ethica (1903), Chapter10 paragraph 2.
Consider yellow, for example. We may try to define it, by describing its physical equivalent; we may state what kind of light-vibrations must stimulate the normal eye, in order that we may perceive it. But a moment's reflection is sufficient to show that those light-vibrations are not themselves what we mean by yellow. They are not what we perceive.

[12] Ibid, Chapter 10 paragraph 3.
It may be true that all things which are good are also something else, just as it is true that all things which are yellow produce a certain kind of vibration in the light. And it is a fact, that Ethics aims at discovering what are those other properties belonging to all things which are good. But far too many philosophers have thought that when they named those other properties they were actually defining good; that these properties, in fact, were simply not "other," but absolutely and entirely the same with goodness. This view I propose to call the "naturalistic fallacy."

E. Richard Dawkins (1941 – Present) "memes"

[2:10] Richard Dawkins coined the term "meme" (sounds like "gene") to refer to the cognitive or nonphysical process of natural selection. Biological evolution through the process of natural selection results in the transference of physical traits, such as the "color" of a person's hair, eyes, or skin, and is controlled by genes. Mental evolution through the process of natural selection results in the social transference of mental traits such as moral principles and traditions and is controlled by memes.

[2:11] Since the entire cosmos, and biological universe has no purpose or end "in mind," then it follows that moral principles also have no purposes or ends independent of minds.

[2:12] However, moral principles do in fact have purposes, or ends, and they are therefore mind dependent. From this point of view, the existence of moral principles is solely because morality has been naturally selected in a similar manner as the physical process of the passing on of genetic traits by reproduction. However, in the case of morality, instead of physical genes being used to transfer physical traits, cognitive experiences and worldviews are transferred from one generation to the next in the form of cognitive cultural transmission of memes.

[2:13] Since, from this perspective, the origin of moral principles is the result of cognitive beings learning or being imprinted with cognitive memes, with their accompanying purposes and ends, and since it follows that those experiences are in fact real experiences and therefore do exist cognitively, and since all that descriptively exists is the result of evolution, then it follows that the origin of moral principles has come about through the process of evolution or more specifically natural selection.

Summary: Historical Moral Issues

[2:14] Five considerations that must be addressed when dealing with the issue of subjective moral purposes and ends are: Hume's is-ought fallacy, Kant's recognition that moral purposes must be based on a pure *a priori* metaphysics, Mill's analysis that ultimate ends cannot be empirically proven, Moore's naturalistic fallacy, and Dawkins' explanation of memetic natural selection.

III. Primary & Secondary Qualities

[3:1] A scientific approach as to how principles of morality can have purposes and ends can be at least partially explained by making the distinction between primary qualities and secondary qualities, a dualistic reductive framework.

[3:2] Primary qualities are defined as those qualities that exist independently of minds, and secondary qualities are defined as those qualities that exist only because there is a mind that experiences them. In other words, primary qualities are mind independent and exist whether or not minds exist, and secondary qualities are mind dependent and exist only in the experiencing of the mind.

[3:3] The question with regard to the nature of moral principles is whether or not moral principles are primary qualities—independent of the mind, or secondary qualities—an experience dependent on the mind.

[3:4] Historically scientists and philosophers have differed as to the conclusion of whether or not moral principles are primary or secondary qualities. Plato, for example believed that morality, or the "Good" was a form that existed independently of minds and therefore as a primary quality. Most modern and contemporary scientists and philosophers hold to the position that morality is a cognitive activity that does not exist independently of cognition and therefore is a secondary quality.

[3:5] A closer look as to what can be known about these dualistic qualities and the nature of their reality follows.

A. Color

1. Naïve realist

[3:6] With regard to materialism, a "naïve realist" is a person who believes that the mental experience of color or the "experiential quality of green" (secondary qualities) is actually part of the object being perceived, (primary qualities), i.e. committing a form of the naturalistic fallacy as presented by G. E. Moore.

[3:7] Grass, for example, is not physically green as the mind experiences greenness, rather grass is "colorless" in that the grass only absorbs and reflects particular wavelengths of light that ultimately stimulates the brain that causes trichromatic beings, for example, to have the mental experience of "green." The physical causation of "green" is radically different from the cognitive experience of "green."

[3:8] Grass may be reflecting 5,300 angstroms of light that the perceiver's eye then translates into electrical impulses, that stimulate certain parts of the brain, which then causes the perceiver to experience the quality of green, but clearly that subjective cognitive experience is not part of the object. In fact the experience of green has very little physical resemblance, if any at all to 5,300 angstroms of light. There is no quality of green in the world, rather green is a subjective experience in the mind and is therefore indefinable by empirical facts or even by language. The green experience is a real experience, but it would be an error to assume that green exists in the physical world independent of experience. The truism is: without experiencers there are no experiences. In other words, without experiencers the experience of green does not exist.

[3:9] Likewise moral principles are real experiences but it would also be an error to assume that morality exists in the physical world independent of experience. If morality is a pure cognitive experience, and if there were no experiencers to experience morality, then morality would not exist. Morality is mind dependent.

[3:10] The color green is an indefinable experience just as moral feelings are also indefinable experiences. Green is indefinable in that a person can point to grass and say: "this is what I mean by green," realizing that language is distinct from the experience. Language is not a "snapshot" or "picture" of a subjective experience, rather language is more like a pointing towards something to be subjectively observed or a reference to such a subjective experience and therefore the experience of green or the experience of the feelings of morality is also indefinable.

2. Sophisticated realists

[3:11] The "sophisticated realist" are those individuals who recognize that there is an external reality—realists, yet are also able to understand the mental distinction between sense experience caused by sense data—secondary qualities, and the causation of sense data—primary qualities.

[3:12] As mentioned above, the naïve realist is a person who holds to the belief that cognitive experiences—(secondary qualities that are mind dependent), are in fact part of the nature of the object—(primary qualities that are independent of minds). Such naïvety is exemplified by beliefs such as that the grass is literally "green" just as the person subjectively experiences it.

[3:13] Primary qualities are the causation of the sense data itself. Since primary qualities are independent of minds, it follows that primary qualities would continue to exist, even if there were no minds. These are the qualities that would be perfectly consistent with noncognitive evolution and noncognitive natural selection.

[3:14] Secondary qualities are sense-data perceptions or subjective cognitive experiences. It follows that if secondary qualities are defined as subjective cognitive experiences, and if these subjective cognitive experiences are dependent on minds that experience them, then without minds there would be no secondary qualities. Secondary qualities are of course real, but their reality is a subjective reality, and whatever the experiences may be, they only exist when they are being experienced by an experiencer, i.e., they are mind dependent. The nature of morality appears to be of this latter category, i.e., secondary qualities.

[3:15] However, as will be shown later, just because an experience is subjective, it does not follow that the experience is necessarily relative. Rather, experiential beings seem to have more intersubjective agreements than disagreements with regard to their subjective cognitive experiences.

[3:16] It will also be shown, that with regard to moral principles—Principlism, that there are more intersubjective agreements than disagreements on the broad and general principles of autonomy (self-rule), beneficence (do good), nonmaleficence (do no harm), and justice (be fair).

B. Sound: Tree In The Forest

[3:19] Another example of an indefinable subjective experience is that of sound as illustrated by the famous tree in the forest analogy presented by Bishop Berkeley (1685-1753).

[3:20] Question: If a tree falls in a forest and there are no perceivers around to hear it, would it make any sound?

[3:21] Answer: If sound is defined as airwaves then certainly there is sound present when the tree falls. If sound is defined as the experience a person has after their eardrums have been stimulated creating electrical impulses that stimulate the neurons in the brain creating a subjective cognitive experience of sound (say "CRACK!") then of course there is no sound in the forest if there are no cognitive perceivers there to experience the sound of the tree falling, as the sound referred to is the mental subjective experience of "CRACK!".

[3:22] However, the naïve realist will incorrectly think that the subjective cognitive experience of sound, is a factual objective reality and therefore falsely conclude that if a tree falls in the forest and there is no perceiver to perceive it that the subjective cognitive experience of sound would still be present, i.e., the naturalistic fallacy.

[3:23] Notice that the issue has nothing to do with the skepticism of sound existing or the determining of how a person would know whether or not there was sound existing, rather the issue is the distinction between the primary qualities that cause the sense data, (the air waves), and the secondary qualities, (the subjective cognitive experiences caused by the sense data). Since secondary qualities only exists as experiences of perceivers and if there are no perceivers in the forest, then of course it would be impossible for experiential sound to be present as a secondary quality.

[3:24] To make the point even more clear, the physical world independent of perceivers is a silent world, and what most people define as "sound" is actually only the "experience of sound" that only occurs in minds as subjective cognitive experiences. The world independent of experiencers is obviously experientially silent and experientially colorless, and the experiences of perceiving beings is often times noisy and colorful.

[3:25] It is also the case that the subjective cognitive experiences (secondary qualities) have very little resemblance, if any at all, to the air pressure waves that cause the sense data by moving the perceiver's ear drums that then creates electrical impulses that stimulates the neurons in their brains which then create the subjective indefinable cognitive experience of "sound."

C. All Sense Data

[3:26] Like color and sound, the subjective cognitive experiences of taste, smell, touch, and all other sense data experiences, are all secondary qualities. Primary qualities are defined to be the first link of causation that ultimately results in the experience of secondary qualities in the mind.

[3:27] Whether a person can gain knowledge of primary qualities through the use of secondary qualities is another very interesting epistemological question. It can be argued that those qualities that can be described mathematically, i.e., that are not sense dependent, are those qualities that are in fact primary. But mathematics is certainly not the nature of primary qualities, as the Pythagorians believed, rather mathematics is currently understood to be a language of representation, or thought processes, that has been constructed to help people understand more logically and systematically the "nature of reality," and/or logical relationships. However, if mathematics is composed of analytical statements, then it can be argued that mathematics is simply tautological equations or restatements of its own mathematical reality or worldview. Moral principles might also be much like mathematics, an analytic language of statements that simply rephrase in different words the moral reality or worldview of the agent and/or society.

1. Solipsistic states

[3:28] If the only experience a perceiver is capable of having are secondary qualities, then it follows that it would be impossible for perceivers to experience a primary quality, as all experiences are by definition secondary qualities.

[3:29] Descartes, using the process of methodological doubt, doubted the existence of everything that was doubtable. All secondary qualities such as sight, hearing, touch, smell, and taste, are all doubtable. Even being awake is doubtable as everything could be a dream. However, when doubting one's own existence, that oddly ended up being an affirmation of existence as a doubting being. Existence as a thinking substance ended up being an indubitable truth. That is how Descartes came up with his famous aphorism: "I think therefore I am." The difficulty was getting out of this solipsistic state, i.e., isolated within a person's own subjective cognitive experiences.

[3:30] But don't people in fact "know" some primary qualities with regard to the world around them without having any sense data of such experiences, as for example, protons, neutrons, and electrons? However, if they "know" that "knowing" by definition is a secondary quality.

[3:31] In other words, the primary and secondary quality distinctions have the potential of leaving the individual in a solipsistic state, meaning that the experiencer, is not able to know anything other than their own subjective experiences. If so then morality may also have the potential of ending up being a solipsistic state.

a. Rational arguments against solipsism

[3:32] Three rational arguments for the existence of not only the solipsistic "thinking substance" but the external world as well.

1) A person cannot experience another's experiences

[3:33] If all a person can know are their own experiences, yet at the same time they cannot know what it is like to be a bat, cat, or fish, then it seems rational to think that those external entities must in fact exist independently of their thoughts, otherwise they would be able to know what it was a like to be a bat, cat or fish.

2) Languages are communal

[3:34] Languages, at least those that are written or verbal, are not private as they are ways of communicating to others, not just to oneself. Since a person cannot control what other's communicate to them, and since individuals must learn the vocabulary and how to communicate with the vocabulary, it is rational to conclude that individuals in communicating communities are not alone.

3) Most perceptions are determined

[3:35] The fact that people are determined in their perception of sense data, such as "green grass," is evidence that something external must be the cause of the impressions, e.g., a person cannot will to see "pink grass" and then perceive "green" as "pink." Therefore it is rational to conclude that there is an external cause of the determined perceptions.

b. Empirical arguments against solipsism

[3:36] Three empirical arguments for the existence of not only the solipsistic "thinking substance" but the external world as well.

1) Empiricism proves existence not nonexistence

[3:37] Empirically a person cannot prove that something does not exist. Rather evidence can only "give evidence" for existence. Since there are numerous examples of evidence for existence and none for nonexistence the following truism must be the case: existence must exist.

2) Technology interacts with the environment

[3:38] Technology is a means for interacting with the surrounding environment. Without the surrounding environment there would be no technology. There is technology. Therefore the external environment must exist.

3) Natural selection necessitates existence

[3:39] Natural selection is the ultimate empirical evidence of existence. Since all sciences converge on the principles of evolution and natural selection, and since natural selection works on the basis of existence reproducing into other existences while adapting to the changing environments, then it follows that there is the existence of an external reality.

2. Dualistic worldviews are a misperception

[3:40] Another serious issue related to the making of the distinction between primary and secondary qualities is the dualistic worldview that it tends to create. From this dualistic point of view there seems to be primary qualities that are in the physical world of causation, and then there are the secondary qualities that are in the mental world of experience.

[3:41] This dualism may be helpful for discussion and understanding, but it also may be incorrect to separate out the physical world from the mental world if reality is in fact holistic.

[3:42] Holistically a subjective cognitive experience cannot be independent of the physical world because in order to have a subjective cognitive experience there is the necessary condition of having a physical brain with neurons.

[3:43] Since this is the case, then the dualistic divisions that seem to arise because of the primary and secondary distinction is ultimately a misperception, even if it was helpful for cognitive analysis.

[3:44] It is also interesting to note that although the mental world of experience, such as personal identity or morality is totally dependent on the existence of the physical world, i.e. the brain, it is also true that the "physical world" of the universe has no dependence for its existence on the mental world of experience.

[3:45] The divisions related to primary and secondary qualities certainly seems to be helpful in understanding the type of metaphysical existence, or nature of reality, of the experiential world of morality, yet it still must be realized that helpful tools, or conceptions of reality, may not be the complete or correct picture of reality.

Summary: Primary Qualities & Secondary Qualities

[3:46] Metaphysically primary qualities are that which exist even if they are not perceived, and secondary qualities are that which exist only if they are perceived, such as color, taste, touch, sound, and smell.

[3:47] A naïve realist is a person that holds to the belief that secondary qualities are primary qualities. A sophisticated realist is a person who recognizes that there is a distinction between primary and secondary qualities. Both are called realists because they are making metaphysical claims for existence.

[3:48] Several issues arise because of the primary secondary qualities distinction. Three of them are as follows:

1. Idealism

[3:49] Epistemologically, only secondary qualities can be known. If all knowledge is cognitive then all knowledge, is by definition secondary qualities. Therefore it is impossible to come to any knowledge of primary qualities that are independent of secondary qualities. It is not only possible that cognitive experiences could have little if any resemblance at all to the causation of such experiences, but it is also the case that there is no evidence that primary qualities even exist because all experiences are by definition secondary qualities. Idealism is the position that the only knowledge that can be known are secondary qualities.

2. Solipsism

[3:50] Epistemologically, the only experiences that cognitive beings can have are their own subjective experiences—secondary qualities, and therefore the self, is all that a thinking being can know. For humans, this is certainly a type of epistemological anthropocentrism in which all knowledge can in fact only be from the human subject's perspective. Since it is impossible to have any experiences other than what the self experiences, it follows that there is no evidence that can establish anything other than the metaphysical existence of the self. Descartes' "I think therefore I am" exemplifies this because if a person affirms their existence then they exist, and even if they deny their existence the very activity of denying is an affirmation of their existence at least as a thinking substance. However, this still leaves the "thinking substance" in a solipsistic state.

a. Three rational arguments against solipsism

1) Persons cannot experience another's experiences.

[3:51] If all that a person can know are their own experiences, yet at the same time they cannot know what it is like to be a bat, cat, or fish, then it seems rational to think that those external entities must in fact exist independently of their thoughts, otherwise they would be able to know what it was a like to be a bat, cat or fish.

2) Languages are communal.

[3:52] Languages, at least those that are written or verbal, are not private as they are ways of communicating to others, not just to oneself. Since a person cannot control what other's communicate to them, and since individuals must learn the vocabulary and how to communicate with the vocabulary, it is rational to conclude that individuals in communities are not alone.

3) Most Perceptions are determined.

[3:53] The fact that people are determined in their perception of sense data, such as "green grass," is evidence that something external must be the cause of their impressions. Therefore it is rational to conclude that there is an external cause of the determined perceptions.

b. Three empirical arguments against solipsism

1) Empiricism proves existence not nonexistence.

[3:54] Empirically a person cannot prove that something does not exist as the evidence of a nonexistent something would obviously not exist. Rather evidence can only "give evidence" for existence. Since there are numerous examples of evidence for existence and none for nonexistence the following truism must be the case: existence must exist.

2) Technology interacts with the environment.

[3:55] Technology is a means for interacting with the surrounding environment. Without the surrounding environment there would be no technology. There is technology. Therefore the external environment must exist.

3) Natural selection necessitates existence.

[3:56] Natural selection is the ultimate rational evidence of existence. Since all sciences converge on the principles of evolution and natural selection, and since natural selection works on the basis of existence reproducing into other existences while adapting to the ever changing environments, then it follows that there is the existence of an external reality.

3. Dualism

[3:57] Metaphysically there seems to be a mind-body dualism that is created or implied when using the primary and secondary quality distinction. Dualistically the non-cognitive physical world can exist independently of the mind, however, holistically the mind is totally dependent on the physical world of the brain as cognition cannot occur without physical neurons and their activities. This dualistic distinction is a position that has been recognized and presented since Democritus, 2500 years ago, to the present.

IV. Determinism & Freedom

A. Determinism

[4:1] Physical evolution and biological natural selection, with their descriptions of non-purposive processes refer to deterministic cause and effect processes. These cause and effect processes include both the mind independent primary qualities and the mind dependent secondary qualitative experiences since the experiences of the mind seem to be just as empirically determined as primary qualities by the causative influences of sense data, rational thought, language and other types of deterministic causations.

[4:2] Although these secondary qualities are subjective cognitive experiences, in contrast with primary qualities that are mind independent, it is still the case that these secondary qualities are just as causally determined as the mind independent primary qualities as causal determinism is not a matter of degree. Cause effect relationships are either causally determined or they are not causally determined. In contrast, knowledge is a matter of degree as it is impossible to have full knowledge—omniscience, rather a person can only at best have substantial knowledge. If knowledge is gained in discrete amounts, and if it takes time to gain such discrete knowledge, then it would take an infinite amount of time to gain an infinite amount of knowledge and therefore omniscience could never be attained in such a manner, i.e. knowledge is a matter of degree in contrast with determinism which is not a matter of degree.

[4:3] Mind independent causations of sense data, such as wavelengths of light, stimulates the perceiver in such a way that the perceiver does not freely choose to have the experience of say "green," rather the experience of greenness is an involuntary response to the sensory stimulation. In other words, a perceiver cannot look at "green grass" and voluntarily make it look pink.

[4:4] Rational thought such as logic, a mind dependent activity that certainly would not exist without a physical brain, is also determined, but not by what is typically understood as physical cause and effect relationships, rather logic is determined by rationally determined relationships. For example:

1. If p then q
2. p
3. Therefore q

[4:5] Like logic, *a priori* rational truths of mathematics are also deterministic, e.g., 5+7=12. However, if secondary qualities are that which exists only if there are minds then secondary qualities should include not only the deterministic experiences of the mind, but also the nondetermined experiences of freedom so often associated with morality.

B. Freedom

[4:6] Since both primary and secondary qualities are deterministic concepts, and since beings do in fact experience having freedom in the choosing of various purposes and ends, it follows that the primary and secondary quality distinction does not seem to provide the whole picture of reality. On the one hand, if the only categories of existence are the primary and secondary qualities that are both deterministic, then the experience of freedom doesn't really exist and is at best just an illusion. From this perspective, to the extent to which a being experiences freedom could simply be considered the extent to which that being is ignorant of the actual causation of their experiences of freedom.

[4:7] On the other hand, if primary and secondary qualities only explain the deterministic categories of cause and effect, then there either needs to be one or more other "types" of qualities to explain the "free will" category of cause and effect, or there needs to be a better explanation using the existing primary and secondary qualities distinction in order to not only explain the experience of free choice, but to also explain and justify the concept of free choice in the selection of moral purposes and ends.

[4:8] However, free choice has several conceptual problems some of which are as follows:

1. Compatibilism or soft determinism

[4:9] If free choice is a cause and effect relationship then how could the "caused effect" be defined as free and not determined? One perspective, called compatibilism or soft determinism, is the claim that although all effects are caused, i.e. determined, some causes can be defined as "free." The compatibilist may make a distinction between determined acts that are free and determined acts that are unfree by defining a free act as, "any act that involves no compulsion or coercion by another person," or "any act that is derivable from pure rational reason" or "an act that would not have been chosen if the agent had had different desires."

[4:10] However, since by definition all causes "cause" or "determine effects," it follows that the distinction between free causes, which may for example involve causes that have no coercion or causes that are based on pure rational reasoning are still causes that determine particular effects. As a result the incompatibilist argues that determinism and free will are totally incompatible concepts and either the universe is purely deterministic—hard determinism, or the universe is not deterministic—libertarian. (Not to be confused with libertarian as a political concept.)

2. Uncaused effects

[4:11] If free will is not a cause effect relationship then free will becomes an uncaused effect. However, what exactly would it mean to have an uncaused free choice effect caused by a free choice cause that does not exist? Free will construed as an uncaused effect becomes a logical contradiction.

[4:12] The concept of free will is generally not thought of or experienced as an uncaused effect, rather free will is generally conceived of and experienced as being a type of "cause," i.e., a free will cause. An uncaused effect is not only a logical contradiction it also does not correspond to what people actually experience as free will.

3. Indeterminable effects

[4:13] Another perspective is the indeterminable effects, where one cause can result in more than one possible free will effects.

However, this explanation of free will is also lacking in that the causal explanation of why a particular cause resulted in one or more particular effects rather than one or more different particular effects would still have to be address. In other words, the cause effect relationship still ends up being deterministic even if it is not possible to determine what the specific effect is going to be between the effect options. This also is not what most people mean or experience when they talk about a free will causing the determination of a particular effect.

4. Indeterminable causation

[4:14] Indeterminable causation is similar to indeterminable effects except that instead of a choice that may cause one or more particular free will effects, with indeterminable causation it is not possible to define what the causation options even are of the free will effect. If free will is indeterminable in terms of causation then it would follow that free will effects would not be susceptible to empirical proof, as the cause and effect relationship would be indefinable. The establishment of empirical claims is a necessary condition for scientific empirical verification. In other words, if a scientific claim is incapable of being established by empirical evidence with determined cause effect relationships, then it cannot be a scientific empirical claim as all empirical claims must have measurable attributes and determined cause and effect relationships.

[4:15] All categories of the empirical sciences are based on evidence and verification as that is how science makes its claims and becomes self-correcting. If free choice cannot be empirically established then it also follows that free choice is not an empirical scientific claim.

C. Freedom As An Axiom or Postulate

[4:16] Two possible solutions to the above intractable problems regarding free will or free choice are to:

Option 1: [4:17] Claim that free choice does not exist and that freedom is an illusion caused by the ignorance of causation, or

Option 2: [4:18] Claim that the existence of free choice is an axiom or postulate within the context of subjective experiences.

1. Cognitive freedom is intuitively agreeable and practical

Option 1: [4:19] The claim that free choice does not exist is counterintuitive and is also not helpful in accomplishing the moral end of pluralistic decision-making.

Option 2: [4:20] The claim that free choice is an axiom or postulate is both intuitively agreeable and is also helpful in accomplishing the moral end of pluralistic decision-making. Freedom, of course, is not just some random axiom or postulate any more than the axioms and postulates of mathematics are random.

2. Cognitive freedom as a first principle is unprovable

[4:21] All first principles are by definition epistemologically unprovable. However, hardly anyone questions the logic of mathematics based on the fact that it is a cognitive system that by necessity begins with axioms and postulates.

[4:22] So also with the intersubjective cognitive system of moral principles, morality must by necessity begin with a first principle. Like mathematics, most people do not find that as being particularly problematic as all knowledge or systems of thought must start out with an unprovable first principle, and for moral decision-making that first principle or postulate is freedom.

3. Rejection of hard determinism for cognitive experiences is reasonable

[4:23] If there is no free-will and all actions are determined then all events are necessitated by earlier events and therefore all present and future events would be as fixed and unalterable as the past is fixed and unalterable.

[4:24] It has been argued that if hard determinism is true, then there would be no justification for holding others morally accountable for their actions.

[4:25] The only possible justification for holding others morally accountable would be for behavior modification, but even the "choice" of using stimulus response would also have to be considered determined and the concept of justice would also have to be reconsidered. However, this position is so counter intuitive to all that is known about morality and how moral agents experience their subjective life, that even if hard determinism is a logical possibility, it fails dramatically in explaining how beings actually and practically live and experience their lives.

[4:26] Therefore, for subjective cognitive experiences the rejection of the deterministic point of view, for the acceptance of the assumption of cognitive freedom, is a reasonable and practical position even though determinism is the case for the phenomenal world.

D. Consistency With Hume, Kant, Mill, Moore, and Dawkins

[4:27] The primary and secondary qualities distinction with the assumption of freedom is now successful in avoiding David Hume's "is-ought" problem and also G.E. Moore's naturalistic problem as presented in the beginning of this section. Since secondary qualities and freedom—"mind dependent qualities," are kept distinct from the primary qualities—"mind independent qualities," it follows that prescriptive morality—"ought," is not being formulated by an appeal to primary qualities—"is," and so the naturalistic fallacy in which mind dependent secondary qualities are incorrectly used to describe mind independent primary qualities is avoided.

[4:28] The deterministic primary and secondary quality distinction along with the assumption of cognitive freedom is also consonant with Immanuel Kant's distinction between the phenomenal realm that is completely deterministic and the noumenal realm that is completely rational and based on the axiom or postulate of freedom. The primary qualities can be thought of as the description of the deterministic phenomenal realm and the secondary qualities in combination with the axiom or postulate of freedom, can be thought of as the experience of the noumenal realm.

[4:29] The deterministic primary and secondary distinction along with the assumption of cognitive freedom is also in agreement with John Stuart Mill's recognition that there can only be empirical proofs of "means to ends" but that there can be no empirical proof of an "ultimate end" as ends for Mill are based on the axiom or postulate of happiness. The "means to ends" refers to the deterministic primary and/or secondary qualities and their cause and effect relations, and the "ultimate end" is determined by the subjective cognitive experience of choice and/or axioms/postulates.

[4:30] Lastly, the deterministic primary and secondary distinction with the assumption of cognitive freedom is also in agreement with Richard Dawkins, an evolutionary biologist, who in addition to physical genes appeals to the natural selection of nonphysical cognitive memes. Freedom and the subjective cognitive faculties would be such nonphysical cognitive memes that would be susceptible to memetic natural selection as the cultural memetic attributes create environments that promote the reproduction and survival of the species.

[4:31] The distinction between deterministic primary and secondary qualities, along with the axiom or postulate of cognitive freedom, avoids many of the problems presented so far that are associated with morality.

Summary: Determinism & Freedom

[4:32] Both primary qualities and secondary qualities only address deterministic concepts. Mind-dependent secondary qualities are just as empirically determined as the mind-independent primary qualities, as determinism is not a matter of degree. Physical experiments indicate that all physical effects have physical causes and cognitive experiences also indicate that all cognitive effects have physical/cognitive causes. Since both physically and cognitively all effects have causes both primary qualities and secondary qualities appear to be all determined.

[4:33] The philosophical issue, if determinism is the case, is how to explain the empirical fact that beings cognitively experience freedom.

1. Compatibilism or soft determinism

[4:34] This point of view agrees that all effects have causes or are determined, but disagrees that determinism is antithetical with freedom. Freedom from this point of view is defined as: (a) determined causes that involve no external compulsion or coercion, (b) determined causes that are derivable from pure rational reason, (c) determined causes that would have resulted in a different action if the agent had had different desires, (d) determined causes that are impossible to establish as the causation of a particular effect, or (e) a determinate cause that can establish a causation of equal probability of one or more effects.

2. Incompatibilism

[4:35] The incompatibilism position argues that determinism and freedom are in fact antithetical with each other and is represented by hard determinists, libertarians, dualists, and holistic dualists.

a. [4:36] The hard determinist position is that if determinism is true then it is true of all aspects of the universe and there is no freedom regardless of the experiences of cognitive beings. Cognitive freedom from this point of view is an illusion.

b. [4:37] The libertarian position is that: (1) determinism is not true, and (2) the universe is not determined by cause and effect relations. Determinism from this point of view is a misconception as empiricism can only observe that an effect temporally comes after a cause, not that it was necessarily determined.

[4:38] (One critique of the notion that effects are not caused is that it is not just a logical contradiction of an analytic statement, like "I am a married bachelor," but it also results in synthetic statement conclusions that could claim that it is just as reasonable to conclude that the sun will not rise in the morning as to say that it will. (Hume footnote) This position would question the very possibility of attaining any cause effect knowledge and would explain the notion of cause and effect, for example, as an emotive experience.)

c. [4:39] Dualism is both an incompatibilist position and a compatibilist position that asserts that for primary qualities hard determinism is true, and at the same time asserts that for secondary qualities compatibilism is true. This is accomplished by having two metaphysical realities that exist simultaneously yet independently of each other. The physical reality is the reality of the empirical cause and effect relationships in which determinism exists. The immaterial reality is the reality of the cognitive in which some experiences are determined, such as the experience of the color green, and some experiences are free, a result of real choices or self-direction that results in the experience of freedom, i.e. compatibilism.

3. Holistic dualism

[4:40] Holistic dualism is the position that not only recognizes the helpfulness in making the dualistic distinction for discussion and evaluation, but also recognizes that in the end the distinction between the two realms must give way to a holistic worldview. This position allows for the recognition of determinism in both the physical and immaterial reality yet at the same time also allows for axiomatic freedoms, or postulates of freedom as part of certain types of cognitive activities. The justifications of these axioms and postulates are very similar to the justifications of the axioms and postulates of mathematics. This holistic view is not only a synthesis of compatibilism and incompatibilism but it also emphasizes the symbiotic relationship between the material and immaterial realities. Without the mind, the body does not function, without the body the mind does not function. The mind and body are not only dependent on each other they are actually in the end, one and the same entity or reality resulting in the experience of what is in fact self-identity.

[4:41] Holistic dualism successfully avoids Hume's "is-ought" problem by allowing for the development of rational moral statements of ought that are independent of and without appeal to empirical evidence.

[4:42] Holistic dualism also successfully avoids Moore's naturalistic fallacy as it is able to keep clear the distinction between that which the mind experiences from the stimulation or causation of such experiences.

[4:43] Holistic dualism is consonant with Kant's deterministic phenomenal realm and his noumenal realm that includes freedom. Kant also was holistic in that although he made a clear distinction between the phenomenal and noumenal realm, he also thought that they were in the end only "concepts of the mind" that made it possible to understand what was really a single holistic reality.

[4:44] Holistic dualism is in agreement with Mill in his recognition of determined cause and effect relationships of means to ends, yet at the same time recognizing that ends must be freely chosen, and since an ultimate end is not a means to anything else they are empirically unprovable.

[4:45] Lastly, holistic dualism is consistent with evolution and in particular with Dawkin's memetic natural selection. There are the primary qualities which are independent of the mind and are wholly determined by evolution, and there are the secondary qualities of the mind which are compatible with both memetic natural selection, and freedom qualities of self-directedness.

V. Language

A. Language as Sense Data

[5:1] It is now necessary to investigate how it is even possible that this epistemological and metaphysical discussion using language is occurring and what the implications of the uses of language are for morality. Using language to discuss morality raises some interesting issues regarding the nature and limits of language in the transference or representation of knowledge, and whether or not language is the nature of reality for some types of thoughts.

[5:2] One perspective is that language is being used to communicate ideas, but that the ideas themselves are not being directly communicated to the recipient, rather the recipient can only cognitively perceive that which the language presents, much like sense data causing cognitive experiences.

[5:3] First the perceiver is stimulated by language, then the perceiver forms ideas that the language was attempting to communicate. However the language itself has little if any resemblance at all to the idea that is being communicated much like the experience of the cognitive quality of "green" in contrast with the "5,300 angstroms" of light that is the causation of the experience. Therefore, with this perspective, language is only a type of sense data that stimulates ideas, but are not the actual ideas themselves.

[5:4] If language, as so described, is a type of sense data, then the following issues would have to be addressed:

[5:5] What is the relationship between language and its ability to stimulate thoughts and experience? Is it a determined relationship of cause and effect or is it both a determined relationship of cause and effect and a freely influenced mental relationship of the mind as well? If it's a determined relationship of cause and effect then language would be independent of the activities of the perceiver's mind. If the mind also contributes to the cause and effect relationship and if the mind's participation includes the assumption or postulate of freedom, then language would be something different than a deterministic cause effect relationship with the mind.

[5:6] If language is an abstract representation of an idea, and if the language representation therefore has little if any resemblance at all to the idea it represents, and if the subjective cognitive experiences of the perceiver of the language also has little if any resemblance at all to the language, then it follows that the subjective cognitive experiences of the perceiver caused by language could also have little if any resemblance at all to the ideas which: a) the language claims to be communicating, and b) the perceiver usually assumes as being communicated.

[5:7] If all the subjective cognitive experiences caused by both the sense data of language, and all of the other perceptions, are all that a being can epistemologically know about the world, then the scope of the determination of the metaphysical nature of reality has been greatly reduced to that of how a being's cognitive faculties are able to perceive, interpret and integrate their own subjective experiences. In other words, the reality of the world would then be the activity of the perceiver's own mind, resulting in a solipsistic point of view in which the self's cognition is really all that can be known.

[5:8] After all to claim to have knowledge outside of a being's own subjective cognitive experiences is absurd, as all knowledge known to a being can only be a subjective cognitive experience.

B. Language as Thought

[5:9] Another perspective on language is that thoughts are inseparable from language. In other words, thoughts are language, and languages are thoughts, i.e., without language there would be no thoughts and without thoughts there would be no language.

[5:10] From this perspective, thoughts are formed within the framework of language, and when the language is communicated or transferred to others, the perceiving mind acquires the transferred language and then acquires the language of thought itself.

[5:11] A benefit of such a description is that communication then becomes the direct transferring of a subjective language experience—a thought, to that of another being's subjective language experience—the same thought, with no intermediary transformations as with sense data.

[5:12] If language as so described is identical with thought, then the following issues would have to be addressed:

[5:13] If language is thought and thought is language, then the types of thoughts that are possible are directly related to the language framework that is being used. Simple language frameworks would presumably result in simpler thoughts and more complex language frameworks would have the potential of more complex thoughts.

[5:14] In other words, the potential to have complex thoughts with a simple language framework is lower than with a sophisticated language framework.

[5:15] Using the language of mathematics, for example, the degree to which an individual has the proficiency of various mathematical languages, e.g., trigonometry, geometry, calculus, differential equations, topology, etc., is directly proportional to the individual's potential to form complex understandings using those concepts.

[5:16] Likewise, the degree to which an individual has the proficiency of various linguistic tools and concepts is also directly proportional to the individual's potential to form complex understandings using those concepts.

[5:17] Suppose a person believed that reality was a purely experiential linguistic construct.

[5:18] If that were the case then the "linguistic construct" would be empirically unverifiable because the "linguistic construct" is all that reality is. In other words, reality could never be in a position to be independently established or proven to be the case since the linguistic construct is all there is for the verification of itself. Reality from this point of view would be incomprehensible or meaningless outside of language even if such an outside reality did in fact exist.

[5:19] If thoughts can only occur within language then beings that have no language would have no thoughts. Therefore, if moral considerability were to be attached, for example, to the ability to experience the thoughts of one or more of the principles of autonomy (self-rule), beneficence (do good), nonmaleficence (do no harm), and justice (be fair), and if humans were to conclude that they were the only beings that use language, then it would follow that humans would be the only beings to which moral considerability would be applicable. The ancient Greeks thought that the Greek language was the only true language and anyone who did not speak Greek was defined as a barbarian.

[5:20] One way out of this is to expand rather than contract the definition of language. However, another interesting and problematic question is how far the definition of language can be expanded. Does a language have to be vocal or written? What about body movements? Are emotions a type of language? What about pleasures and pains? Perhaps all sentient experiences are types of languages either to the experiencer, others, or both.

[5:21] If the notion of language is expanded to include all knowledge that all sentient or perceivable beings experience, then a full circle has been made with regard to language as the language framework has been broken down and is now being defined simply as any subjective cognitive experience. To define a language framework simply as any subjective cognitive experience would make the definition of language either meaningless or at least tautological as all that can be known by definition is already a cognitive experience and language would therefore not provide any type of synthetic additive knowledge or specific communicative activity to the subjective experiencer.

[5:22] If language, whether mathematical, linguistic, diagrammatic, emotional, experiential, musical, etc. is in the same category as the other sense perceptions, then language is likewise a purely subjective cognitive experience and is no longer able to explain how one subjective cognitive experiencer is able to communicate to another subjective cognitive experiencer.

C. Language as Pluralistic

[5:23] All of the above positions and arguments of the nature, and function of language have credibility under certain conditions. In other words, language is pluralistic in its form and function. For example, the language of mathematics is particularly useful in the analysis of sense data but is not useful in the communication of emotions or historical events. In contrast body language seems to be particularly effective in communicating the emotions of love, compassion, and physical feelings of pain, pleasure, and enjoyment. Verbal and written language is particularly useful in the communication of history, plans and goals, and is sometimes inextricably part of cognitive thoughts. So although it is the case that many types of thinking can be independent of verbal or written language, it is also recognized that many thoughts are formed within a language framework. The experiences of the mind are wide and varied and some thoughts and experiences are clearly dependent on a particular language framework, some thoughts and experiences use differing language frameworks, and other thoughts and experiences are totally independent of any type of language framework. Obviously, those types of experiences that are independent of language are going to be more difficult if not impossible to communicate effectively through the use of language. Those types of experiences that are dependent on language are going to be more effectively communicated to others through the use of language especially if the language of the thought or experience is the same as the language that is being used to communicate the thought or experience. Certainly there can be representative problems when one type of language framework, say verbal language, is trying to be communicated by another type of language framework, say body language, as is exemplified in the game of charades where participants try to act out a word or phrase and the teammates try and guess what the word or phrase is.

[5:24] Morality is certainly a communicative activity that is dependent on a pluralistic variety of language frameworks some being verbal, written, body language, etc.

[5:25] Going back to the question as to whether or not a person can know any of the attributes of primary qualities other than that they are mind independent can now be better addressed. For example, electrons, protons, and neutrons, are mental concepts described by the language of mathematics and physics yet they are also asserted as existing independently of such conceptions.

[5:26] An electron does not literally mean the linguistic word, or mathematical statement, as some have claimed, however it certainly may be the case that the linguistic word or mathematical statement is all that a person can and do know of such entities. However, what a person does know is also a "type of reality" that helps them to understand the origins, processes, and future predictions of such subjective entities.

[5:27] For example, the practical production of atomic bombs and nuclear reactors are possible because linguistic atomic knowledge is epistemological knowledge of at least a type of metaphysical reality.

[5:28] If other theories of linguistic knowledge do not account for the fact that atomic bombs and nuclear reactors are about "reality" independent of language then so much the worse for those theories, as practically, those positions have been proven to be wrong.

[5:29] In other words, although it is logically impossible to experience primary qualities, if by definition all experiences are in fact subjective, it is still the case that science is able to use the concepts and applications of primary qualities for among other things, technological advances, and reproductive success.

[5:30] If all that people can know are in fact subjective cognitive experiences, then it follows that the perceiver is in an extreme form of solipsism in which the self's experiences are all that the perceiver can ever know. However, people also know that practically, and by natural selection, that perceivers do in fact conduct themselves socially, and perceivers do in fact interact with the environment around them, therefore the solipsism must not be total but only partial.

[5:31] A helpful analogy might be the hermeneutical circle that states: in order to understand the whole a person needs to understand the parts, but to understand the parts the person needs to understand the whole—i.e., if it's a vicious circle then it would be impossible to understand or learn. However, practically it is known that when people read an article they can actually come to understand or learn what the article is communicating. Therefore, the hermeneutical circle cannot be a completely vicious circle.

[5:32] Likewise, people know that perceivers are not totally solipsistic, in which the self's experiences are all that the perceiver can ever know, and they are able to practically extend themselves beyond their own experiences and interact with others and the environment. This is known because if this were not the case, then there would have been no reproduction, and without reproduction, the genetic line would have gone extinct, i.e., natural selection. It may be the case that morality is in fact a subjective determination of values, yet practically moral agents do have intersubjective agreements with others. Memes such as moral principles are transmitted by the process of natural selection from one generation to another and people within society are able to come to practical and pluralistic moral decision-making agreements because of these intersubjective moral agreements.

[5:33] If this were not the case, then natural selection would have already selected these individuals out, before the solipsistic characteristics had time to develop.

D. Language As A Cross Over To The Incommunicable

[5:34] Language helps those who communicate cross over the linguistic descriptions into the realm of abstract understanding, which is the incommunicable. The experience of the color "green" is again a good example of an incommunicable experience. (Green, not in terms of wavelength, but in terms of the experiential or subjective quality of greenness.) Greenness is not a word, and it is not an attribute of an atom (atoms are smaller than a wavelength of light and therefore they cannot individually reflect light which makes them colorless).

[5:35] The experience of greenness is nothing other than a subjective incommunicable experience. However, this does not mean that subjective experiences are relative, rather through the process of intersubjective agreements it can be determined that most people actually share quite similar subjective experiences of color.

[5:36] Ophthalmologists, for example, are able to systematically test for color blindness, verifying the similarity of subjective experiences. Red, green, blue, (RGB) televisions, and cameras are able to "mix" the pixels with consistent results, which would never be possible if color experiences were to be relative for each subjective perceiver. Certainly there can be defects in a person's ability to have shared sense data experiences, but that is the exception rather than the rule.

[5:37] Colorblind testing charts, called Ishihara plates, are often used to check for color deficiencies for trichromatic humans. This empirical test only works because trichromatic individuals see colors more similarly than dissimilarly.

[5:38] If color experiences were random or relative, then such empirical color sensitivity tests would not work. The fact of the matter, is that such sensitivity tests do work, which establishes that subjective cognitive experiences of color are more determined and consistent with others than nondetermined and dissimilar.

[5:39] Intersubjective agreements are sufficient evidence that there are shared subjective incommunicable experiences. In other words, just because an experience is subjective and incommunicable, it does not follow that the experiences are necessarily relative. An example of such shared intersubjective moral agreements are the broad and general moral principles of: autonomy (self-rule), beneficence (do good), nonmaleficence (do no harm), and justice (be fair).

[5:40] These principles have broad and general intersubjective agreements as to their value, and are not in conflict with many, if not most, worldviews.

[5:41] Therefore, although people may interpret or understand language differently, through the use of proper hermeneutical approaches, there is more intersubjective agreement with regard to language than disagreement. If language were to be completely relative with regard to the communication of shared incommunicable experiences, then language would have had no reproductive function and therefore would have never been naturally selected. Language exists precisely because it is effective in communicating ideas and is therefore effective in communicating the concepts relating to moral principles.

Summary: Language

[5:42] A necessary topic in any discussion of epistemology and metaphysics is language. Knowledge and reality are communicated and some claim even constructed by language. This section discussed language as sense data, thought, pluralistic, and as a cross over to the incommunicable.

A. Language as sense data.

[5:43] This description equates language to be much like the primary and secondary quality discussion. There is a thought or idea, and the communicator then uses language to describe the thought or idea to another being, who then translates the perceived language into their own thought or idea.

[5:44] 1. Language seems to be able to causally determine particular thoughts and ideas. However, it also seems to be the case that the mind has the ability to freely influence the conception of the thought or idea. Therefore, it appears that there is a synthesis between determinism and freedom with regard to the conception, communication, and understanding of thoughts and ideas.

[5:45] 2. If language has little if any resemblance at all to thoughts and ideas, and if what the perceiver perceives is the language and not the actual thoughts and ideas, it follows that it is possible that thoughts and ideas as perceived by the perceiver could also have little if any resemblance to the original thought or idea. Therefore language as abstract representations of ideas results in questionable communication.

[5:46] 3. If subjective cognitive experiences are all that can be epistemologically known, then what can be metaphysically determined to exist has been greatly reduced to that of the mind.

B. Language as Thought.

[5:47] Another perspective is that language is thought and thought also only exists as language. As so described then language is a direct transferring of the subjective language experience to another being's subjective language experience without any intermediary transformations. If true, then: (1) simple languages would have a tendency to have more simple thoughts and simple thoughts would also result in simple languages, (2) reality would be a purely experiential linguistic construct and reality therefore would not be comprehensible independent of the language construct, and (3) beings that have no language would therefore be beings that have no thoughts.

C. Language as Pluralistic.

[5:48] Language is manifested in many different ways, verbal, written, body movements, music, mathematics, computer programming, art, etc. Language could be expanded to include any subjective cognitive experience but then language becomes synonymous to cognitive experience and it looses its distinctive meaning.

[5:49] The synthetic approach is to recognize the truth of a variety of language frameworks depending on the circumstances. The language framework of mathematics is particularly successful at analyzing data but not very successful at communicating emotions, or historical events. The language framework of the body is good at communicating emotions. The language framework of the verbal is good at communicating events, plans, goals and cognitive thoughts, etc.

D. Language as a crossover to the incommunicable.

[5:50] Some thoughts are totally independent of any particular language framework, and other thoughts are totally dependent on a particular language framework. Experiences that are independent of, or part of, a different language framework that is being used to communicate it can compromise or even eliminate the ability to communicate such experiences as exemplified in the game of charades.

[5:51] Although all that can be communicated is that which can be experienced, and although experiences can be quite different from the mind independent reality, it is still the case that language has, through natural selection, proven itself to be practical enough for persons to be able to interact in the world and to reproduce. The hermeneutical circle is an example of how vicious circles are often times not all that vicious, and likewise, a being's solipsistic knowledge does not necessarily isolate the being from others and the world around them.

[5:52] Language is able to cross over to the incommunicable. The experience of green, or an emotion is certainly not a concept that is part of a language framework, but language is able to "point to" or "refer to" such shared experiences, or intersubjective agreements. Color blind testing charts are an example of such shared intersubjective agreements, indicating that just because an experience is subjective it does not necessarily mean that the experience is relative. In fact, the opposite seems to be the case in that there seems to be more universal intersubjective agreements than disagreements.

[5:53] This is especially true with ethics, or moral principlism. There are many universal moral values that all persons share even though there may be great differences as to the personal or social beliefs as to how to act on such values. For example, humanity has the universal family values of reproduction, protection of children, and education even though there are great personal and social differences as to the beliefs as to how to best implement those values. These universal values have arisen by natural selection because those who did not have those family values had a greater tendency for extinction, and those who did have those family values had a greater tendency for reproductive success.

[5:54] Autonomy, (self-rule), beneficence (do good), nonmaleficence (do no harm), and justice (be fair), are also such universal intersubjective values that have arisen by natural selection. However, what are not held as universal intersubjective agreements are the personal and social beliefs as to how to specify, weigh, and balance those principles.

[5:55] Holistic dualism successfully explains how a nonpurposive deterministic world has evolved to the point of allowing for the subjective cognitive creation of purpose and freedom. Purpose and freedom are the necessary conditions for moral accountability, as exemplified by Principlism. Holistic dualism is not just a symbiotic relationship between two distinct metaphysical realities, rather the ultimate understanding is the realization that metaphysical dualism is a helpful reductive epistemological approach that is effective in communicating and explaining various aspects of reality that in the end is metaphysically monistic. This is the monistic synthesis of what has historically been distinctly dualistic, and language is the means, and perhaps even the content, of this description of holistic dualism.

Overview & Conclusion

[6:1] Morality is an academic discipline both in terms of epistemology and metaphysics. This approach limits the study to empirical and rational deliberations of the epistemic origins, nature, limits, and justification of the knowledge of morality along with the metaphysical establishment of the nature, properties, and attributes of moral principles.

[6:2] One major difficulty that all ethicists must address is what is the origin and nature of freedom. Either determinism is the case or it is not the case, either freedom exists or it doesn't exist. The universal academic acceptance of evolution and natural selection points to determinism as the answer. Even the distinctions between primary and secondary qualities results in deterministic evaluations. However, freedom can be justified as an acceptable axiom or postulate, and even though freedom may not be empirically provable, freedom is intuitively agreeable and practical. Mathematics starts off with many unprovable axioms and postulates with no weakening effect to its analytic structure. Combining the primary and secondary qualities distinction, along with the axiom or postulate of freedom, addresses or avoids David Hume's "is-ought problem, along with G.E. Moore's naturalistic fallacy, is consonant with Immanuel Kant's deterministic phenomenal realm and his assumption of freedom in the noumenal realm, and agrees with John Stuart Mill's deterministic proofs of "means to an end" and his freely chosen unprovable "ultimate ends." Such varied logical consistency is evidence that the approach presented for the justification of freedom along with evolutionary determinism is valid and sound.

[6:3] Another major issue that all ethicists must address is what is language and is it able to communicate the ideas and concepts of morality. Several perspectives were presented such as language being similar to sense data, identical to thought, pluralistic, and a tool for crossing over to experience the incommunicable. In the end it is shown that a wide variety of language communications are appropriate for differing types of communications. Mathematics can effectively evaluate sense data but not emotions or history. Body language can effectively communicate emotions, pain and pleasure but not sense data. Verbal and written language can effectively communicate history, purposes and ends and at times may even be identical with thought itself. Lastly there are some thoughts and experiences that transcend any type of communicative frameworks making them incommunicable. Communication is not something that can be reduced to a single type of activity, rather communication is wide and varied just as experiences are. However, as effective as communication can be, it needs to be recognized that communication certainly cannot directly communicate the incommunicable, and there are always epistemological issues of just how effective or accurate communication can be of any type of subjective cognitive experience. Yet if the incommunicable subjective ideas are shared by intersubjective agreements, then language can have the ability of "pointing" towards the shared experiences, and the incommunicable can, for all practical purposes, become communicable.

[6:4] This is a work that will linguistically describe how a non-purposive deterministic reality has evolved through the process of natural selection into the cognitive reality that now includes the ability to experience moral freedom.

***

II. MID-LEVEL PRINCIPLES

Overview

[i:1]

Philosophers in the field of moral decision-making have traditionally used either the theory model or the intuition model for describing how moral decisions are, or should, be made. However, when these models are used independently of each other, they each have serious limitations and inconsistencies and certainly are not very practical in pluralistic environments.

[i:2] Five major problems and considerations that need to be taken into account with the pure theory model are: gray areas, intuitions are used, metaphysical disagreements do occur, infinite regress, and criteria. Three major problems and considerations that need to be taken into account with the pure intuition model are: theories are used, theories would not be needed, and moral disagreements would not be resolvable.

[i:3] After the major problems and considerations of both the theory and intuition models of moral decision-making are investigated the basic moral framework will then be tested to show how the process of moral decision-making using mid-level principles could actually work in a decision-making process.

[i:3] Chapter 3: Informed Consent, will focus on information disclosure for an ideal society, and chapter 4: Principlism, will then provide the substantive content of mid-level principles completing the development of the moral framework called Principlism.

I. The Theory Model

A. Definition

1. Top to bottom

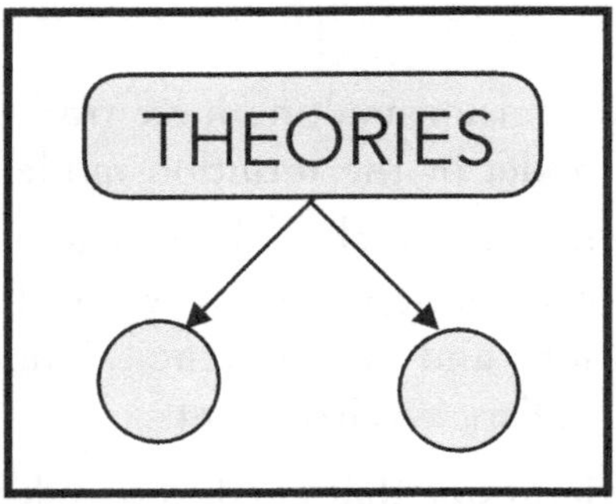

[1:1] The theory model is the moral position, which justifies what is right or wrong by reasoning "down" from a theory. The agent starts with a moral theory and deduces from that theory what action is logically consistent with the moral theory. The theory model emphasizes general norms and ethical theory(ies) as the starting point for decision-making.

[1:2] If a deductive argument is valid reasoning involving inferences from the general to the specific, or from the "top-down," then this model could have been called the deductive model. However, it seems that not all deductive arguments go from the general to the specific. Here is a counter example of a valid deductive argument that goes from the specific to the general:

COUNTER EXAMPLE **Deductive argument going from specific to general:**
Bob is moral (Specific)
:. **Therefore** Anyone who knows Bob knows someone who is moral. (General)

[1:3] As a result, it is more appropriate to call this the *theory model* instead of the deductive model.

[1:4] Mill's utilitarianism, or the greatest-happiness theory, and Kant's deontological, or duty theory, are often times used as examples of this top-down theoretical approach.

2. General to particulars

[1:5] The theory model is a covering-precept model in which justification is from the "top-down" perspective, i.e., it usually goes from the general to the particulars. The theory model also emphasizes the fact that when there is an established body of general guidelines, it is appropriate to make decisions by reasoning from those guidelines or theories. The theory model, as a result, presents a system that has a tendency to resist individual and social change as it only uses the traditionally established guidelines and/or theories.

B. Problems With The *Pure* Theory Model

1. Gray areas

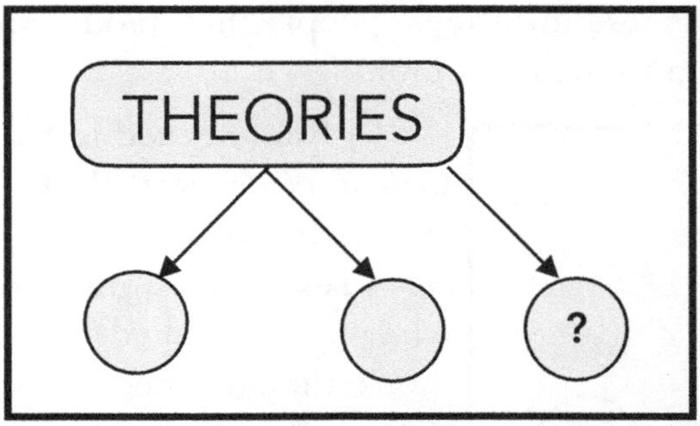

[1:6] Many times when trying to apply a particular theory, the theory does not directly address the issue(s) at hand. This is not necessarily a fault with the theory; rather, it is just a natural limitation of theories. For example, the Bible, if conceived of as a moral theory,[1] may give guidance on how persons ought to conduct their lives in general, yet may be unclear about specific contemporary issues such as corporate buyouts, or freedom of speech on the Internet.

[1:7] Theory(ies) may be applicable in these situations; yet in terms of direct guidance, it becomes gray or unclear as to how the application of those theory(ies) should be made. Therefore, the theory model by itself is not a sufficient or comprehensive enough model for moral decision-making.

2. Intuitions are used

[1:8] It is clear to most philosophers that in addition to making decisions through the use of, or the application of theories, i.e.,

[1] It may be inappropriate to categorize the Bible as a moral theory as it is dependent on revealed religion. However, the example of the Bible as a moral theory is used here for two reasons: 1. the Bible is one of societies most common perspectives appealed to, and 2. the development of more sophisticated moral theories such as utilitarianism and deontological theories have not yet been developed in this text.

"top-down," there are also times in which decisions are made intuitively from the "bottom-up." In other words, sometimes agents modify or develop their theory(ies) from particular judgments that they "know" or "intuit" are morally right.

[1:9] The argument is that the theory model alone is not enough. Moral agents also need to, and do in fact at times approach decision-making intuitively. For example, some people "saw" or "intuited" the injustice that was being done toward women and enslaved people, not through the application of any particular theory, but by intuition. From these intuitions, people then modified their theory(ies) to conform to their intuitions.

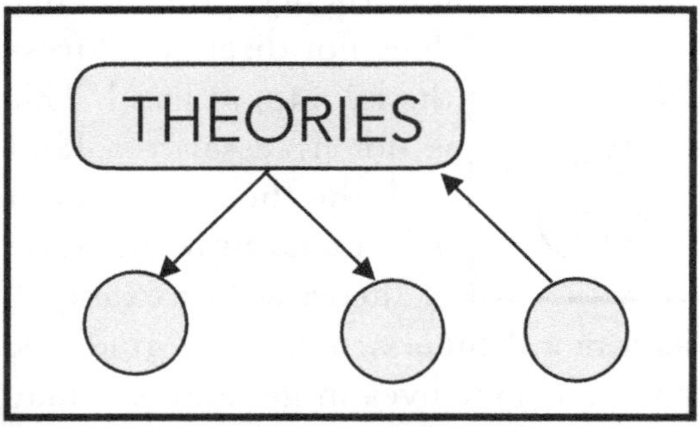

[1:10] Kant argued in his *Critique of Practical Reason* for the use of three *a priori* presuppositions or what is also called intuitions thought necessary for the establishment of the *summum bonum,* or the greatest good. Kant's presupposed moral trinity is freedom, immortality, and God.

> [1:11] "In order to extend a pure cognition *practically,* there must be an *a priori purpose* given, that is, an end as object (of the will), which independently of all theological principles is presented as practically necessary by an imperative which determines the will directly (a categorical imperative), and in this case that is the *summum bonum.* This, however, is not possible without presupposing three theoretical conceptions (for which, because they are mere conceptions of pure reason, no corresponding intuition can be found, nor consequently by the path of theory any objective reality), namely, freedom, immortality, and God. ... [B]ecause practical reason indispensably requires their existence for the possibility of its object, the *summum bonum,* which practically is absolutely necessary, and this justifies theoretical reason in assuming them. But this exten-

> sion of theoretical reason is no extension of the speculative."[2]

[1:12] However, Kant's presuppositions are not intuitions because his definition of intuition was that of *a posteriori* knowledge, or that which comes from the sensible.[3] However, if intuitions were to be conceived of as presuppositions that are not provable by any type of sensible perceptions, then it would seem that Kant also held to the position that intuitions are needed and that the theoretical approach is not a sufficient or comprehensive enough model for moral decision-making.

[1:13] Mill in his utilitarian, or greatest-happiness theory also argued that all questions about ultimate ends, which are what theories propose to elaborate, couldn't be proven.

> [1:14] "Questions of ultimate ends are not amenable to direct proof. Whatever can be proved to be good must be so by being shown to be a means to something admitted to be good without proof. The medical art is proved to be good by its conducing to health; but how is it possible to prove that health is good? The art of music is good, for the reason, among others, that it produces pleasure; but what proof is it possible to give that pleasure is good? ... We are not, however, to infer that its acceptance or rejection must depend on blind impulse or arbitrary choice. ... The subject is within the cognizance of the rational faculty."[4]

[1:15] Since, all consequential theories must be based on an end, it is clear that Mill did not think that a pure theory model of moral decision-making was a comprehensive enough model i.e., independent of any empirical evidence.

> [1:16] "The only proof capable of being given that an object is visible is that people actually see it. The only proof that a sound is audible is that people actually hear it. ... In like manner, I apprehend, the sole evidence it is possible to produce anything is desirable is that people do actually desire it. If the end which the utilitarian doctrine proposes

---

[2] Kant, *Critique of Practical Reason*, p. 161-162.

[3] A fuller discussion on Kant's concept of intuition is presented in the next section: II The Intuition Model. [2:1]

[4] Mill, *Utilitarianism*, Chapter 8, [I:35-43].

> to itself were not, in theory and in practice, acknowledged to be an end, nothing could ever convince any person that it was so. ... Happiness has made out its title as one of the ends of conduct and, consequently, one of the criteria of morality."[5]

[1:17] Both Kant and Mill, who have traditionally been labeled as deontological and consequentialistic theories respectively, are clearly not *pure* theories, i.e., both recognized the need to have certain presuppositions, or intuitions, for the establishment of freedom, or of their *summum bonum*.[6] The following is a quote from Kant that descriptively states that we reciprocally presuppose freedom in order to think of ourselves as being able to choose to follow moral principles, and at the same time we find ourselves obliged to obey moral principles because we are free.

> [1:18] "...One must frankly admit that there is here a sort of circle from which, so it seems, there is no way to escape. In the order of efficient causes we **assume** that we are free so that we may think of ourselves as subject to moral laws in the order of ends. And we then think of ourselves as subject to these laws because we have attributed to ourselves freedom of the will. Freedom and self-legislation of the will are both autonomy and are hence reciprocal concepts."[7]

[1:19] Both Kant and Mill clearly believed that all moral agents use much more than just a theory model as the theory model by itself is not a sufficient or comprehensive enough model for moral decision-making.

---

5 Mill, *Utilitarianism*, Chapter 8, [IV:9-15].

6 See endnotes 26 and 27. Mill, *Utilitarianism*, Chapter 8, [I:33-43], [IV:1-15].

7 Immanuel Kant, *The Groundwork for the Metaphysics of Morals*, (1785), Translated by James W. Ellington, (Indianapolis: Hackett Publishing Company, 1981). pp. 50-52, [447-450].

Freedom Must Be Presupposed as a Property of the Will of All Rational Beings.

3. Metaphysical disagreements

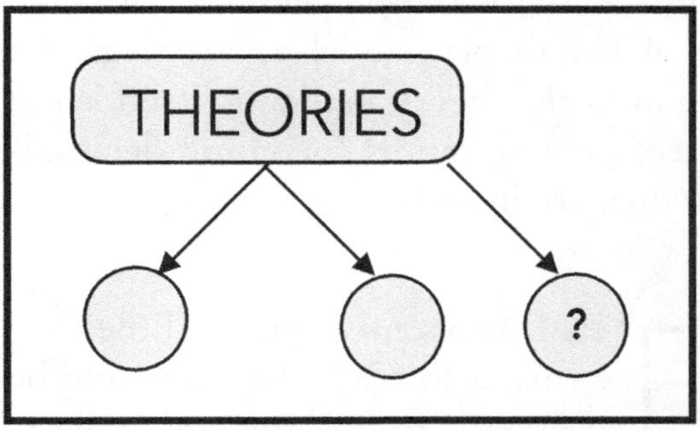

[1:20] Even when individuals approach a decision using the very same theory(ies), often times there still can be no agreement because they disagree on metaphysical, scientific, or religious interpretations.

[1:21] For example, two people may argue from the very same theory(ies) about whether abortion is permissible or not and still not come to an agreement because of differing views or intuitions on whether a fetus is a person or not. This fact does not discredit the theory model, it just shows that decision-making in many circumstances needs a much more comprehensive moral model.

4. Infinite regress

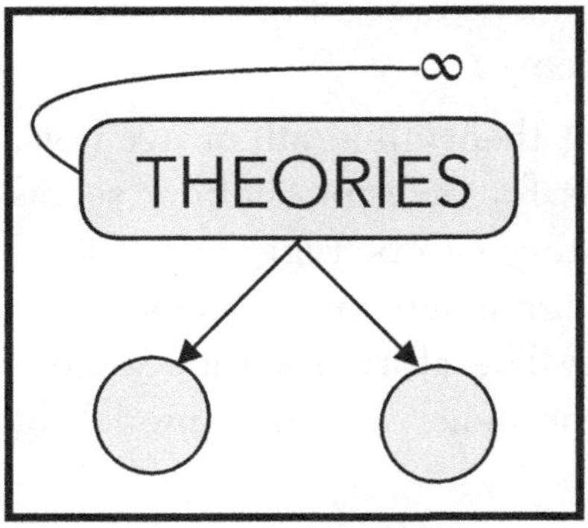

[1:22] Another problem with trying to develop a pure theory model for moral decision-making is the problem of how to "justify" our "first principle" or primary theory. There is really only two "types" of justifications—external justification and internal justification. An external justification is a justification that does not appeal to what is being justified. In contrast, an internal justification is a justification that appeals to what is being justified and has often times been classified as "begging the question" or as a "circular argument."

[1:23] If an external justification of the theory is given, then it would be reasonable to expect a justification of the justification, and then to justify the justification of the justification, *ad infinitum*, i.e., there is the development of an infinite regress of justification, e.g., "turtles all the way down." The only way out of this infinite regress is to realize that the first principle or theory has to be accepted axiomatically, i.e., inductively. Therefore, it is not even possible to conceive of the theory model as existing as a pure decision-making method as the theory model by itself is not a sufficient or comprehensive enough model for moral decision-making as axioms, or intuitions, are inductively necessary.[8]

5. Criteria

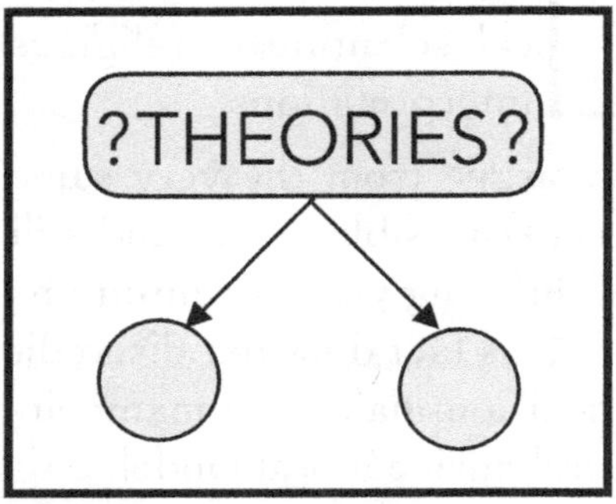

[1:24] Currently, there is little consensus as to what criteria would be necessary for a general theory. Therefore, if there can be no consensus as to the criteria, then there can be no consensus as to which theory(ies) "qualify" or are "best" for the making of moral decisions.

[1:25] For example, should utility, logical consistency, greatest happiness, virtue, duty, pragmatism, divine command, or benefits v. burdens be used in the determination of the "best" decision-making theory?

[1:26] The idea that there can be one theory that all, or even one person, will use in all circumstances for decision-making seems to be idealistic, and it appears, if history can be regarded as a reliable guide, that there will be no agreement or consensus any time in the near or immediate future. Therefore, the theory model by itself is not a sufficient or comprehensive enough model for moral decision-making.

8 Similar to the theorems, proven by Kurt Godel in 1931. The first incompleteness theorem states that no consistent system of axioms whose theorems can be listed by an "effective procedure" is capable of proving all facts about natural numbers. There will always be statements about the natural numbers that are presupposed to be true, i.e., axiomatic, but that are unprovable within the system. The second incompleteness theorem shows that if such a system of presuppositions, or axioms, are capable of proving certain basic facts about the natural numbers, then the system itself cannot prove its own consistency.

II. The Intuition Model

A. Definition

1. Bottom Up

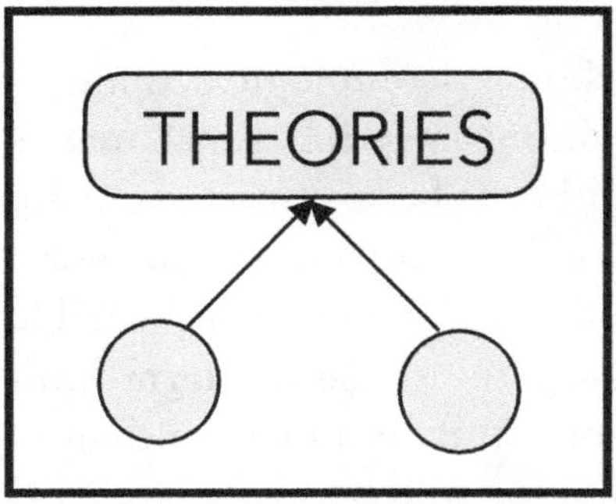

[2:1] The intuition model is an individual-case model in which justification is from a bottom-up perspective, i.e., analysis goes from particulars to the general. The intuition model, as a result, presents a system that is very conducive to change as it is not based on a generally accepted moral theory or doctrine.

[2:2] If the definition of an inductive argument is the use of correct inferences going from the specific to the general, or from the "bottom-up," then this model could have been called the inductive model. However, it seems that not all inductive arguments go from the specific to the general, e.g., here is an example of an inductive argument that seems to go from the general to the specific:

[2:3]

COUNTER EXAMPLE **Inductive argument going from general to specific:**
All NBA basketball players made a lot of money this year. (General)
:. **Therefore** (Some specific NBA player) will make a lot of money next year. (Specific)

[2:4] As a result, instead of calling this the inductive model, it will be called the intuition model.

2. Particulars to general

[2:5] The intuition model is the position in which the justification of what is right or wrong is based on the use of intuition or conscience.

[2:6] Starting with what is intuitively known to be right or wrong there is the development of moral theory(ies) that reflects the intuitive "knowledge." Intuition emphasizes existing social agreements and practices as the starting point from which to develop general norms and theories that are derivative in nature.

3. Kant's deontological theory

[2:7] Some people have classified Kant's deontological philosophy of morality as intuitionism. Intuitionism in this sense means *a priori* knowledge, or knowledge without the use of sense data. However, Kant used the term intuition in a much different sense. Kant used the term intuition to indicate *a posteriori* or sensible knowledge, whereas, the common usage is to use the term intuition as representing the immediate or intuitive understanding of something without conscious reasoning or study.

[2:8] If the term "intuition" is used as *a posteriori* knowledge then rendering Kant's moral philosophy as a type of intuitionism could not be any further from the truth and would indicate a misunderstanding of Kant's moral philosophy. Calling Kant's moral philosophy intuitionism would be to confuse Kant's phenomenal philosophy—*a posteriori* knowledge—with his noumenal philosophy—*a priori* knowledge. Kant rejects the idea of intuition—*a posteriori* knowledge—as having any part of his moral philosophy.[9, 10, 11, 12]

[2:9] Kant maintains that *a posteriori* intuition is definitely not part of his deontological theory. However, Kant's position does presuppose three theoretical conceptions of pure reason: free-

---

[9] Kant, *Critique of Practical Reason*, p. 89.

The physical law being a law to which the object of sensible intuition, as such, are subject, must have a schema corresponding to it—that is, a general procedure of the imagination. ... However, the law of freedom (that is, of a causality not subject to sensible conditions), and consequently the concept of the unconditionally good, cannot have any intuition, nor consequently any schema supplied to it for the purpose of its application *in concreto*. Consequently, the moral law has no faculty but the understanding to aid its application to physical objects.

[10] Ibid., p. 111.

The Analytic of pure theoretic reason had to do with the knowledge of such objects as may have been given to the understanding, and was obliged therefore to begin from intuition, and consequently (as this is always sensible) from sensibility; and only after that could advance to concepts (of the objects of this intuition), and could only end with principles after both these had preceded. On the contrary, since practical reason has not to do with objects so as to *know* them, but with its own faculty of realizing them (in accordance with the knowledge of them), that is, with a will which is causality, inasmuch as reason contains its determining principle; since consequently it has not to furnish an object of intuition, but as practical reason has to furnish only a law (because the notion of causality always implies the reference to a law which determines the existence of the many in relation to one another); hence a critical examination of the Analytic of reason, if this is to be practical reason (and this is properly the problem), must begin with the *possibility of practical principles a priori.*

[11] Ibid., pp. 126-127.

Freedom, a *concept of the reason*, being a transcendent concept, cannot have any intuition corresponding to it, yet the *concept of the understanding*—for the synthesis of which *the former* demands the unconditioned—(namely, the concept of causality) must have a sensible intuition given, by which first its objective reality is assured.

[12] Ibid., pp. 163-164.

... [C]ategories have their seat and origin in the pure understanding, simply as the faculty of thought, before and independently of any intuition ...

dom, immortality, and God.[13] The point being that when Kant says his moral theory does not use any intuitions the reader must be aware that Kant is not using the term in its current popular sense. Therefore, if intuition is used with the understanding of being *a priori*—independent of sense data, and if Kant's deontological moral framework is based on *a priori* presuppositions, then Kant's framework can be considered to be a type of intuitionism.

[2:10] However, the reason Kant's *a priori* presuppositions works for Kant is because he believed that the mind has natural predispositions or moral endowments. No one has a duty to acquire such natural dispositions because the natural dispositions are the very basis of the moral agent's receptiveness to duty. The natural predispositions of the mind is that which makes it possible for a being to be able to experience duty and therefore it would be impossible to have a duty to acquire such a predispositions. If those natural predispositions are not present, then it would be impossible for the mind to experience any kind or type of duties. However, Kant believed that every human being has those natural cognitive predispositions or moral endowments and therefore,

---

[13] Kant, *Critique of Practical Reason*, p. 161-162.

In order to extend a pure cognition *practically*, there must be an *a priori purpose* given, that is, an end as object (of the will), which independently on all theological principles is presented as practically necessary by an imperative which determines the will directly (a categorical imperative), and in this case that is the *summum bonum*. This, however, is not possible without presupposing three theoretical conceptions (for which, because they are mere conceptions of pure reason, no corresponding intuition can be found, nor consequently by the path of theory any objective reality), namely, freedom, immortality, and God. ... [B]ecause practical reason indispensably requires their existence for the possibility of its object, the *summum bonum*, which practically is absolutely necessary, and this justifies theoretical reason in assuming them. But this extension of theoretical reason is no extension of the speculative.

because of those predispositions, every human being has moral obligations.[14]

[2:11] The natural predispositions or moral endowments are: moral feeling, conscience, love of one's neighbor, and respect for oneself.[15] Once again, it is by virtue of these moral endowments

---

[14] Kant, *The Metaphysics of Moral; The Doctrine of Virtue,* p. 159, [6:399].

There are certain moral endowments such that anyone lacking them could have no duty to acquire them. –They are *moral feeling, conscience, love* of one's neighbor, and *respect* for oneself. There is no obligation to have these because they lie at the basis of morality, as *subjective* conditions of receptiveness to the concept of duty, not as objective conditions of morality. All of them are natural predispositions of the mind for being affected by concepts of duty, antecedent predispositions on the side of *feeling*. To have these predispositions cannot be considered a duty; rather, every human being has them, and it is by virtue of them that he can be put under obligation. –Consciousness of them is not of empirical origin; it can, instead, only follow from consciousness of a moral law, as the effect this has on the mind.

[15] Kant, *The Metaphysics of Morals; The Doctrine of Virtue, pp. 160-162, [6:400-403].*

Moral Feeling: This is the susceptibility to feel pleasure or displeasure merely from being aware that our actions are consistent with or contrary to the law of duty.

Conscience: For Kant it is a kind of "second-order" reflection on how well we are making or have made our choices. We do not have a duty simply to *have* a conscience. We have a conscience whether we want one or not. However, since we can never be sure about the purity of our intentions, judgments of conscience apparently are limited to questions about the moral *legality* of our behavior and about whether we have tried or are trying as hard as possible to act dutifully. So holy are the judgments of our conscience that we cannot avoid thinking of them as if they were divine verdicts. It is also not possible to have an erring conscience as you cannot be mistaken in your subjective judgment as to whether you have submitted something to your practical reason. To act in accordance with conscience cannot itself be a duty; for if it were, there would have to be yet a second conscience in order for one to become aware of the act of the first. The duty here is only to cultivate one's conscience.

Love of Human Beings: *Duty to love* is an absurdity. But *benevolence,* as conduct, can be subject to a law of duty. "You ought to *love* your neighbor as yourself" does not mean that you ought immediately (first) to love him and (afterwards) by mean of this love do good to him. It means, rather, *do good* to your fellow human beings, and your beneficence will produce love of them in you.

Respect: It is not correct to say that a human being has a *duty of self-esteem*; it must rather be said that the law within him unavoidably forces from him *respect* for his own being and this feeling is the basis of certain duties, that is, of certain actions that are consistent with his duty to himself.

that puts the individual under moral obligation and therefore having such traits cannot be an obligation to acquire.

[2:12] Moral feeling: the natural predisposition of the mind that gives it the ability to experience pleasure or displeasure from the awareness that their actions are consistent or not consistent with *a priori* duty.

[2:13] Conscience: the natural predisposition of the mind that gives it the ability to experience second-order reflections, or judgments, on how pure the mind's intentions are when fulfilling a duty. However, because of the current state of imperfection it is impossible to have perfectly pure intentions of fulfilling one's duty simply because of duties sake.

[2:14] Love: the natural predisposition of the mind that gives it the ability to have benevolent interests towards others in helping them attain that which they believe, and/or will, make others happy.

[2:15] Self-Respect: is the natural predisposition of the mind that gives it the ability to experience self-esteem because of its recognition that the mind itself is the very source of moral duty. Moral duty is self-generating and the recognition of such results in awe of oneself, i.e., self-respect.

[2:16] To the extent that Kant's deontological theory uses *a priori* presuppositions and cognitive dispositions—moral endowments, and to the extent that they can be considered to be types of intuitions, is the extent towards which Kant's moral position is pluralistic in nature, i.e., theoretical and intuitional.

4. Mill's utilitarian theory

[2:17] Mill's utilitarian theory also uses the intuition model with his notion of the feeling of justice—a powerful sentiment and clear perception of certainty resembling an instinct, an inherent quality in things of something absolute, distinct from the consequences, and in concept even opposed to consequences, though in the long run never disjoined from the consequences.

> [2:18] "… justice. The powerful sentiment … [having] certainty resembling an instinct … the just must have an exis-

tence in nature as something absolute, generally distinct from every variety of the expedient and, in idea, opposed to it, though never, in the long run, disjoined from it in fact."[16]

[2:19] Mill points out that the instinct of justice may have been bestowed on moral agents by nature as a peculiar type of instinct, similar perhaps to Kant's natural predispositions or moral endowments.

[2:20] However, just like how other animal instincts that prompt the individual to act in particular ways need to be controlled and enlightened by higher reason, so also, Mill argues, that the instinct of justice that prompt the individual to judge in a particular way also needs to be controlled and enlightened by higher reason.

> [2:21] "If we have intellectual instincts leading us to judge in a particular way, as well as animal instincts that prompt us to act in a particular way, there is no necessity that the former should be more infallible in their sphere than the latter in theirs."[17]

---

[16] Mill, *Utilitarianism*, Chapter 8, [5:1-2].

... justice. The powerful sentiment and apparently clear perception which that word recalls with a rapidity and certainty resembling an instinct have seemed to the majority of thinkers to point to an inherent quality in things; to show that the just must have an existence in nature as something absolute, generically distinct from every variety of the expedient and, in idea, opposed to it, though (as is commonly acknowledged) never, in the long run, disjoined from it in fact.

[17] Mill, *Utilitarianism*, Chapter 8, [5:5].

The feeling of justice might be a peculiar instinct, and might yet require, like our other instincts, to be controlled and enlightened by a higher reason. If we have intellectual instincts leading us to judge in a particular way, as well as animal instincts that prompt us to act in a particular way, there is no necessity that the former should be more infallible in their sphere than the latter in theirs; it may as well happen that wrong judgments are occasionally suggested by those, as wrong actions by these.

[2:22] Mill explains how the natural sentiments or instincts of: self-defense, and the feeling of sympathy towards others,[18] results in the mental experience of justice as a secondary quality like our subjective experience of color.[19] It may be the case that justice is a derivative feeling of self-defense and sympathy but the mental conception of justice in the end becomes like the experience of color, i.e., a determined subjective cognitive experience. As a result, justice is the name given to social utilities which are so important, that they are more absolute and imperative as a class of utilities, and as a result, our sentiments or feelings guards justice not only as a difference in degree of social utility, but actually regards justice as being different kind, i.e., independent of consequences, or in other words, absolute.[20] In other words, the theory model by itself is not sufficient or comprehensive enough model for describing how moral agents do in fact make moral decisions.

---

[18] Mill, *Utilitarianism*, Chapter 8, [5:109].

Now it appears to me that the desire to punish a person who has done harm to some individual is a spontaneous outgrowth from two sentiments, both in the highest degree natural and which either are or resemble instincts: the impulse of self-defense and the feeling of sympathy.

[19] Mill, *Utilitarianism*, Chapter 8, [5:10].

For the purpose of this inquiry it is practically important to consider whether the feeling itself, of justice and injustice, is, *sui generis* like our sensations of color and taste or a derivative feeling formed by a combination of others.

[20] Mill, *Utilitarianism*, Chapter 8, [5:246].

Justice remains the appropriate name for certain social utilities which are vastly more important, and therefore more absolute and imperative, than any others are as a class; and which, therefore, ought to be, as well as naturally are, guarded by a sentiment, not only different in degree, but also in kind.

B. Problems With The Pure Intuition Model

1. Theories are necessary

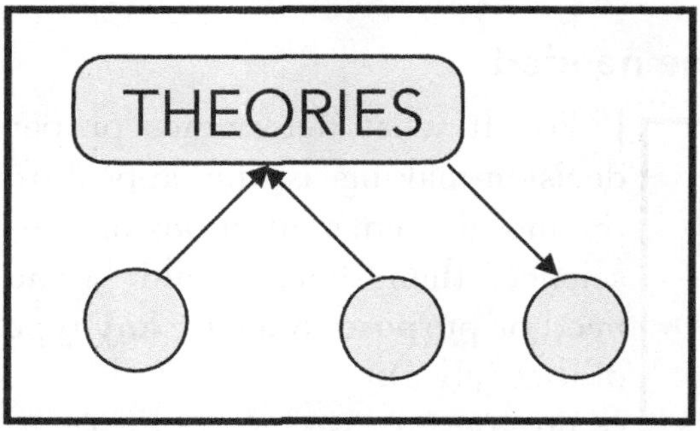

[2:24] It is clear to most philosophers that in addition to making decisions through the use of intuitions, i.e., "bottom-up," that there are also times in which decisions are made by the theory model—from the "top-down." In other words, sometimes moral agents do in fact "apply" or "reason" from an accepted theory(ies) in order to determine what would be the "best" or "right" decision. Therefore, the argument is that the intuition model, like the theory model, is not sufficient or comprehensive enough model for moral decision-making.

[2:25] In addition to making decisions intuitively, there is also the need to approach decision-making through the use of theories. For example, some people just did not "see" or "intuit" the injustice that was being done toward women and enslaved people. However, through the application of the Constitution of the United States, or the application of any number of moral theories, people were then able to reason down to the conclusion that Women and enslaved people were in fact being treated unjustly and that their autonomy was being violated. Reasoning from theories, people were then compelled to modify their intuitions to conform to their theory(ies).

[2:26] Mill argued that intuitionism that does not acknowledge a first principle, i.e., in this context a theoretical approach, will end up being an approach that only justifies each person's feelings, desires, and/or prejudices.[21]

---

[21] Mill, *Utilitarianism*, Chapter 8, [1:26].

The nonexistence of an acknowledge first principle [theory] has made ethics not so much a guide as a consecration of men's actual sentiments.

[2:27] It appears that both the theory model and the intuition model are both needed and used for the making of moral decisions.

2. Theories would not be needed

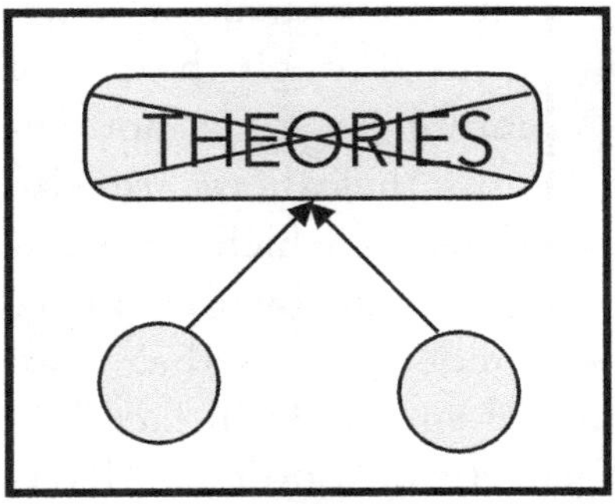

[2:28] If what determines proper decision-making is the appeal to the moral agent's intuitions or conscience, then there would be no need or purpose to devise any type of theory(ies).

[2:29] It makes no sense to develop theory(ies) if they can never be used to override one's intuitions or conscience. General theories would not be needed; only intuitions and conscience would be needed.

[2:30] However, it is known through experience that intuitions are at times conformed to particular theories. For example, many people had pejorative intuitions of women and enslaved people that could not, and did not change until these two groups were recognized as participants under the theory of "human rights." It is interesting how historically there have been individuals with considerable mental endowments and who held to very high moral standards but were still very prejudicial without even the slightest indication that they were aware of this defect.[22]

Kant and Hume, two of the most important and well thought out moral philosophers of all time were not immune from the intu-

[22] Mill, *Utilitarianism*, Chapter 8, [2:151].

... [P]ersons, even of considerable mental endowment, often give themselves so little trouble to understand the bearings of any opinion against which they entertain a prejudice, and men are in general so little conscious of this voluntary ignorance as a defect that the vulgarest misunderstandings of ethical doctrines are continually met with in the deliberate writings of persons of the greatest pretensions both to high principle and to philosophy.

itive prejudices of their eighteenth century environment.[23, 24, 25,]

---

[23] Immanuel Kant, *Observations On The Feeling Of The Beautiful And Sublime,* (1763), Translated by John T. Goldthwait, (Berkeley: University Of California Press, 1960), Translator's Introduction, p. 81.

The virtue of a women is a *beautiful virtue*. That of the male sex should be a *noble virtue*. Women will avoid the wicked not because it is unright, but because it is ugly; and virtuous actions mean to them such as are morally beautiful. Nothing of duty, nothing of compulsion, nothing of obligation! Woman is intolerant of all commands and all morose constraint. They do something only because it pleases them, and the art consists in making only that pleases them which is good. I hardly believe that the fair sex is capable of principles, and I hope by that not to offend, for these are also extremely rare in the male.

[24] Ibid., pp. 93-94.

A woman is embarrassed little that she does not possess certain high insights, that she is timid, and not fit for serious employments, and so forth; she is beautiful and captivates, and that is enough. On the other hand, she demands all these qualities in a man, and the sublimity of her soul shows itself only in that she knows to treasure these noble qualities so far as they are found in him. How else indeed would it be possible that so many grotesque males faces, whatever merits they may possess, could gain such well bred and fine wives! Man on the other hand is much more delicate in respect to the beautiful charms of woman. By their fine figure, merry naïveté, and charming friendliness he is sufficiently repaid for the lack of book learning and for other deficiencies that he must supply by his own talents.

[25] In a note to his essay "Of National Characters", Hume says: "I am apt to suspect the Negroes to be naturally inferior to the Whites. There scarcely ever was a civilized nation of that complexion, nor even any individual, eminent either in action or speculation. No ingenious manufactures amongst them, no arts, no sciences. On the other hand, the most rude and barbarous of the Whites, such as the ancient Germans, the present Tartars, have still something eminent about them, in their valor, form of government, or some other particular. Such a uniform and constant difference could not happen, in so many countries and ages, if nature had not made an original distinction between these breeds of men. Not to mention our colonies, there are Negro slaves dispersed all over Europe, of whom none ever discovered any symptoms of ingenuity; though low people, without education, will start up amongst us, and distinguish themselves in every profession. In Jamaica, indeed, they talk of one Negro as a man of parts and learning; but it is likely he is admired for slender accomplishments, like a parrot who speaks a few words plainly." David Hume, *Essays and Treatises on Several Subjects,* 2 vols. (Edinburgh, 1825), I, 521-522 "Of National Characters" was first published in 1748.

Ibid., (Translator's Notes), p. 123.

26

[2:31] Mill describes how historically accepted social prejudices move from being considered "socially expedient" to that of being universally stigmatized and condemned as being morally wrong. Mill believed that all social inequalities would sooner or later meet this fate, as the entire history of social improvements has followed such a progression.[27]

[2:32] Intuitions by themselves may certainly, as shown above, result in some outrageously immoral beliefs and decisions. It is at these times especially that the need for theories becomes evident. Moral theories are able to override or help in the conforming of

---

[26] Ibid., pp. 110-111.

The Negroes of Africa have by nature no feeling that rises above the trifling. Mr. Hume challenges anyone to cite a single example in which a Negro has shown talents, and asserts that among the hundreds of thousands of blacks who are transported elsewhere from their countries, although many of them have even been set free, still not a single one was ever found who presented anything great in art or science or any other praiseworthy quality, even though among the whites some continually rise aloft from the lowest rabble and through superior gifts earn respect in the world. So fundamental is the difference between these two races of man, and it appears to be as great in regard to mental capacities as in color. The religion of fetishes so widespread among them is perhaps a sort of idolatry that sinks as deeply into the trifling as appears to be possible to human nature. A bird feather, a cow's horn a conch shell, or any other common object, as soon as it becomes consecrated by a few words, is an object of veneration and of invocation in swearing oaths. The blacks are very vain but in the Negro's way, and so talkative that they must be driven apart from each other with thrashings.

[27] Mill, *Utilitarianism*, Chapter 8, [5:235-238].

All persons are deemed to have a *right* to equality of treatment, except when some recognized social expediency requires the reverse. And hence all social inequalities which have ceased to be considered expedient assume the character, not of simple inexpediency, but of injustice, and appear so tyrannical that people are apt to wonder how they ever could have been tolerated—forgetful that they themselves, perhaps, tolerate other inequalities under an equally mistaken notion of expediency, the correction of which would make that which they approve seem quite as monstrous as what they have at last learned to condemn. The entire history of social improvement has been a series of transitions by which one custom or institution after another, from being a supposed primary necessity of social existence, has passed into the rank of a universally stigmatized injustice and tyranny. So it has been with the distinctions of slaves and freemen, nobles and serfs, patricians and plebeians; and so it will be, and in part already is, with the aristocracies of color, race, and sex.

intuitions to the accepted theories aiding in the development of moral progress.

3. Disagreements would be unresolvable

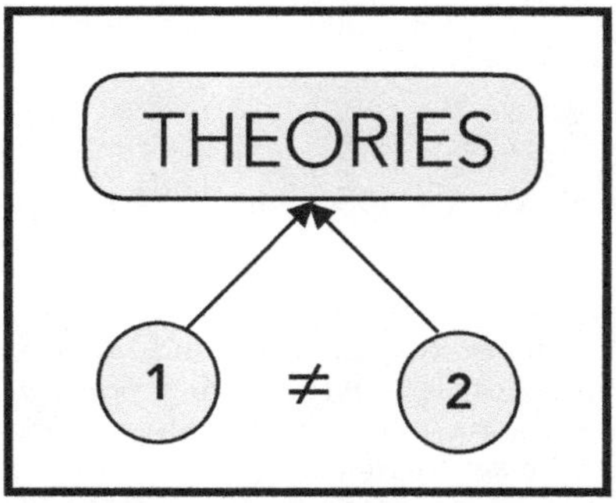

[2:33] Use of a pure intuition model for moral decision-making will give little help in the adjudication of disputes. For example, within the intuition model, how would two equally informed and dispassionate individuals come to an agreement when their intuitions and/or consciences disagree? Intuitionism provides no means of conflict resolution.

[2:34] For example, suppose two parents have a child who is sick. One parent intuits that morally the child should get medical treatment and the other parent intuits that morally the child should not get medical treatment. Although the child either will or will not in fact get medical treatment, the intuition model gives no guidance as to how to resolve or adjudicate these conflicting intuitions and in the end the result will be "might makes right."[28]

[2:35] As a result, the intuition model, as important as it is, is not a sufficient or comprehensive enough model for describing how

---

[28] Kant, *Metaphysics of Morals,* Introduction by Roger J. Sullivan, p. xi.

Reason can point out that, regardless of how people in fact tend to treat each other, the state of nature necessarily lacks *public* justice. In cases of dispute each person's thinking is limited to his or her own estimate of what is right and good, for there is no impersonal mediator. Consequently, persistent differences can be settled in the end only by force. In a state of nature might truly does make right. However, within a civil arrangement there can be a "rightful condition" between individuals, in which the principle of right is publicly recognized and disputes are conclusively arbitrated by a competent and objective legal tribunal, enabling everyone to enjoy their rights.

moral agents make moral decisions.[29],

---

[29] Kant, in his Preface to his Metaphysics of Morals; Doctrine of Virtue, p. 141 [6:375-376], says the following:

"A *philosophy* of any subject is a system of rational knowledge from concepts) requires a system of *pure rational* concepts independent of any conditions of intuition, that is, a *metaphysics*. –The only question is whether every *practical* philosophy, as a doctrine of duties, and so too the *doctrine of virtue* (ethics), also needs *metaphysical first principles,* so that it can be set forth as a genuine science (systematically) and not merely as an aggregate of precepts sought out one by one (fragmentarily). –No one will doubt that the pure doctrine of right needs metaphysical first principles; for it has to do only with the *formal condition* of choice that is to be limited in external relations in accordance with laws of freedom, without regard for any *end* (the matter of choice). Here the doctrine of duties is, accordingly, a mere *scientific doctrine. (footnote:…* A practical philosopher is one who makes the *final end of reason* the principle *of his actions* and joins with this such knowledge as is necessary for it. Since this knowledge aims at action it need not be spun out into the finest threads of metaphysics, unless it has to do with a duty of right. In that case *what is mine* and *what is yours* must be determined on the scales of justice exactly, in accordance with the principle that action and reaction are equal, and so with a precision analogous to that of mathematics; but this is not necessary when it has to do with a mere duty of virtue. For what counts in the latter case is not merely knowing *what* it is one's duty to do (because of the ends all men have by their nature this is easily stated); it is primarily the inner principle of the will, namely that consciousness of this duty be also the incentive of actions.)

But in this philosophy (the doctrine of virtue) it seems directly contrary to the idea of it to go all the way back to *metaphysical first principles,* so as to make the concept of duty, though purified of anything empirical (any feeling), the incentive. For what sort of concept can be made of the force and Herculean strength needed to subdue the vice-breeding inclination if virtue is to borrow its weapons from the arsenal of metaphysics, a speculative subject that few know how to handle? Hence all doctrine of virtue, in lecture halls, from pulpits, or in popular books, also becomes ridiculous if it is decked out in scraps of metaphysics. –But it is not useless, much less ridiculous, to investigate in metaphysics the first grounds of the doctrine of virtue; for someone, as a philosopher, has to go to the first grounds of this concept of duty, since otherwise neither certitude nor purity can be expected anywhere in the doctrine of virtue. …

But in fact no moral principle is based, as people sometime suppose, on any *feeling* whatsoever. Any such principle is really an obscurely thought *metaphysics* that is inherent in every human being because of his rational predisposition, as a teacher will readily grant if he experiments in questioning his pupil *socratically* about the imperative of duty and its application to moral appraisal of his actions. …

30

4. Intuitions can lead to heuristic errors

[2:36] Heuristics is another name given to the use of the intuitive approach to decision-making in which the decision-maker goes from particular instances to the making of general statements—bottom up, shortcutting rational analysis—top down. The intuition model generally works well but can also lead to systematic heuristic errors.

[2:37] One of the many types of inductive errors is based on availability of examples. Tversky and Kahneman determined that "When the size of a class is judged by the availability of its instances, a class whose instances are easily retrieved will appear more numerous than a class of equal frequency whose instances are less retrievable."[31]

[2:38] For example when people were asked if there were more words on a page that ended in "ing" or more words on a page that ended with the letter "n" being the second to last letter of a word, more people erroneously answer that there were more words ending in "ing" than with "n" being the second to the last letter of a word. Of course that would be impossible as "n" is the second to last letter in words ending in "ing." These erroneous conclusions happen because people psychologically are using the "availability heuristic," to answer difficult questions. Words ending in "ing" are much easier to come up with so even if there are an equal number of instances of words ending in "ing" and words having the letter "n" being the second to last letter of a word, people will still conclude that there are more instances of words

---

[30] Kant, in his Preface to his Metaphysics of Morals; Doctrine of Virtue, p. 141 [6:375-376], a continuation of previous citation:

If one departs from this principle and begins with pathological or pure aesthetic or even moral *feeling* (with what is subjectively rather than objectively practical); if that is, one begins with the matter of the will, the *end*, instead of with the form of the will, the *law*, in order to determine duties on this basis, then there will indeed be no *metaphysical first principles* of the doctrine of virtue, since feeling, whatever may arouse it, always belongs to the *order of nature*."

[31] Tversky and Kahneman, Science, New Series, Vol. 185, No.1457. (Sep. 27,1974), p. 1127.

ending in "ing." As a result, using the "availability heuristic" can lead to serious errors of fact that can result in excessive fears of low risks events, such as a terrorist attack, and the neglect of high risks events, such as getting in a car accident.[32]

Perhaps a better example is that in the United States it has been statistically determined that there is a greater risk of dying from a T.V. set falling on top of them then dying as a result of a terrorist attack. However, most people, and public policy decision-making, are erroneously much more afraid of terrorists than their T.V. sets. One major reason for this is that there are numerous terrorists accounts to recall and next to no recollection of any T.V. accidents accounts, i.e., the availability heuristic error.

[2:39] A couple of other examples or types of heuristic errors are that of representativeness heuristic error, and adjustment anchoring heuristic error. The representativeness heuristic is the psychological propensity to evaluate probabilities in such a way that to the degree to which "A" represents "B" is the degree towards which "A" comes from "B." An example of a representativeness heuristic error might be the conclusion that an emotional event implies an emotional cause. The heuristic error is that the cause could be something other than emotional. Adjustment anchoring heuristic is when differing starting points psychologically influences individuals to be biased toward the initial starting point. For example, in complex systems there may be multiple components that have a low probability of failure, but when put together it results in a very high rate of failure. The heuristic error is that people will have a tendency to underestimate the probabilities of failure of complex systems that are composed of multiple low risk components.[33]

[2:40] In other words, the use of intuitions—bottom up, independent of other rational approaches, such as theories, can lead to systemic intuitive errors. Therefore a more pluralistic ap-

---

32 Sunstein, Moral Heuristics, Chicago, 2003, p. 3.

33 Tversky and Kahneman, Science, New Series, Vol. 185, No.1457. (Sep. 27,1974), p. 1124-1131.

proach that implements checks and balances is needed as the intuition model, as important as it is, is not a sufficient or comprehensive enough model for describing how moral agents do or should make moral decisions.

III. The Synergistic Model

A. Definition

1. Back and forth

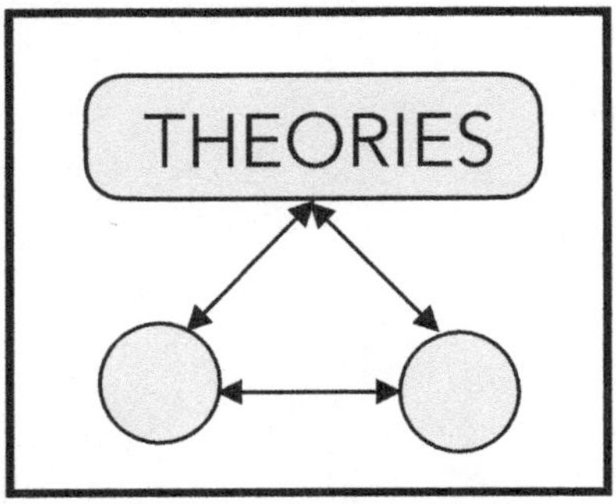

[3:1] The synergistic model is the position in which the justification of what is right or wrong is done not by using either a pure theory model, or a pure intuition model. The synergistic model is a back-and-forth process—starting with particulars and going to the general and back to the particulars and so on and so forth. This is a constant process that never really comes to closure as new decisions in different contexts are constantly having to be made.[34]

2. Synergistic

[3:2] The synergistic model combines the theory model and the intuition model using the process of reflective-equilibrium. It combines the covering-precept model in which justification is from the "top-down," and the individual-case model in which justification is from the "bottom-up," using a process of reflective-equilibrium in which individuals take their accepted intuitions, norms, and theories, mirror them back and forth, making appropriate changes, until an equilibrium or balance is achieved.

---

[34] Kant, *Metaphysics of Morals,* p. 167, [6:409].

Virtue is always *in progress* and yet always starts *from the beginning*. –It is always in progress because, considered *objectively,* it is an ideal and unattainable, while yet constant approximation to it is a duty. That it always starts from the beginning has a *subjective* basis in human nature, which is affected by inclinations because of which virtue can never settle down in peace and quiet with its maxims adopted once and for all but, if it is not rising, is unavoidably sinking. For, moral maxims, unlike technical ones cannot be based on habit (since this belongs to the natural constitution of the will's determination); on the contrary, if the practice of virtue were to become a habit the subject would suffer loss to that *freedom* in adopting his maxims which distinguishes an action done from duty.

B. Strengths

[3:3] The synergistic effect is that the whole is greater than the sum of its parts.

[3:4] In-other-words, the synergistic combination of the theory model, the intuition model, and the process of reflective-equilibrium is one that creates a decision-making model that is far superior than what would be expected from the simple addition of the two models. This combination results in a reciprocal relationship that is not only mutually constraining, but also one in which the moral conclusions do not have the limitations that each of the processes have when used alone.

C. Weaknesses

1. Jack-of-all-trades and master of none

[3:5] Kant argued, in the Critique of Practical Reason, that in our syncretistic age[35] we have:

[3:6]

SYNCRETISTIC AGE
* 1. Taken contradictory principles of morality
* 2. Combined them together.
.: **Therefore** 3. Developed shallow and dishonest systems of morality.

[3:7] This syncretistic process is done for the purpose of pleasing everyone in a pluralistic society that is content to know something of everything and nothing thoroughly, i.e., to be a jack-of-all-trades and master of none.[36]

---

[35] Even though this argument was published in 1787 it is clear that it still holds for our current contemporary era.

[36] Kant, *Critique of Practical Reason*, p. 38.

Consistency is the highest obligation of a philosopher, and yet the most rarely found. The ancient Greek schools give us more examples of it than we find in our syncretistic age, in which a certain shallow and dishonest systems of compromise of contradictory principles is devised, because it commends itself better to a public which is content to know something of everything and nothing thoroughly, so as to please every party. [Literally, "to have a firm seat in any saddle." —Kant's father was a saddler.]

2. A new true philosophy

[3:8] John Stuart Mill in the opening paragraph of his book, Utilitarianism, published in 1861, argued that little progress has been made with respect to the determination of the criterion of right and wrong. The foundations of morality has always been the main problem in philosophy and it has been this issue that has occupied the most gifted intellects and divided them into various schools of thought. After two thousands years the discussions still continue with no agreement in sight.[37]

[3:9] Today is no closer to coming to a unified agreement on the summum bonum (ultimate good) than when Mill wrote this in 1861. If anything, there is probably more disagreement over the foundation of morality in the contemporary world than at any other time in history. However, people have been making moral decisions for thousands of years and will continue to do so.

[3:10] Kant argued that if a contemporary philosopher were to discover "the true moral philosophy" then that would in effect say that before people renounced their previous untrue moral philosophy, they would be using a false moral philosophy. Not only that, but it would also follow that all people previous to the time of the discovery of "the true moral philosophy," that they would have all been using a false moral philosophy and therefore they would have all been either immoral agents, or at the very

---

[37] Mill, *Utilitarianism*, Chapter 8, [1:1-3].

There are few circumstances among those which make up the present condition of human knowledge more unlike what might have been expected, or more significant of the backward state in which speculation on the most important subjects still lingers, than the little progress which has been made in the decision of the controversy respecting the criterion of right and wrong. From the dawn of philosophy, the question concerning the *summum bonum*, or, what is the same thing, concerning the foundation of morality, has been accounted the main problem in speculative thought, has occupied the most gifted intellects and divided them into sects and schools carrying on a vigorous warfare against one another. And after more than two thousand years the same discussions continue, philosophers are still ranged under the same contending banners, and neither thinkers nor mankind at large seem nearer to being unanimous on the subject than when the youth Socrates listened to the old Protagoras.

least amoral agents. This perspective, of course, would be arrogant, conceited, and belittling.[38]

[3:11] If it is true that there can be only one true philosophy and if it is true that the synergistic model is a new true philosophy then it is a valid deductive argument to conclude that it is true that all previous philosophies were in fact false.[39] The deductive argument is as follows:

[3:12]

---

[38] Immanuel Kant, *The Metaphysics of Morals; Preface to Doctrine of Right*, (1785), Translated by Mary Gregor, (New York: Cambridge University Press, 1996), pp. 4-5, [6:207].

It sounds arrogant, conceited, the belittling of those who have not yet renounced their old system to assert that before the coming of the critical philosophy there was as yet no philosophy at all. ... — So anyone who announces a system of philosophy as his own work says in effect that before this philosophy there was none at all. For if he were willing to admit that there had been another (and a true) one, there would then be two different and true philosophies on the same subject, which is self-contradictory.

[39] Kant, *The Metaphysics of Morals; Preface to Doctrine of Right*, pp. 4-5, [6:207].

It sounds arrogant, conceited, the belittling of those who have not yet renounced their old system to assert that before the coming of the critical philosophy there was as yet no philosophy at all. — In order to decide about this apparent presumption, it need but be asked *whether there could really be more than one philosophy*. Not only have there been different ways of philosophizing and of going back to the first principles of reason in order to base a system, more or less successfully, upon them, but there had to be many experiments of this kind, each of which made its contribution to present-day philosophy. Yet since, considered objectively, there can be only one human reason, there cannot be many philosophies; in other words, there can be only one true system of philosophy from principles, in however many different and even conflicting ways one has philosophized about one and the same proposition. So the *moralist* rightly says that there is only one virtue and one doctrine of virtue, that is, a single system that connects all duties of virtue by one principle, the *chemist,* that there is only one chemistry (Lavoisier's); the *teacher of medicine,* that there is only one principle for systematically classifying diseases (Brown's). Although the new system excludes all the others, it does not detract from the merits of earlier moralists, chemists, and teachers of medicine, since without their discoveries and even their unsuccessful attempts we should not have attained that unity of the true principle which unifies the whole of philosophy into one system. — So anyone who announces a system of philosophy as his own work says in effect that before this philosophy there was none at all. For if he were willing to admit that there had been another (and a true) one, there would then be two different and true philosophies on the same subject, which is self-contradictory.

Synergistic model as a new true philosophy
1. **If** the synergistic model is a new true philosophy, **then** all previous philosophies are false. 2. The synergistic model is a new true philosophy.
:. 3. **Therefore:** All previous philosophies are false. (*MP 1 and 2)

[3:13]

* Modus Ponens—MP is defined as follows:
1. **If** p **then** q 2. p
:. 3. **Therefore:** q

[3:14]

Kant's Argument
1. **If** a new philosophy is true, **then** it is *not* the case that there has been a previous true philosophy. 2. There has been a previous true philosophy. 3. A new philosophy is true.
:. 4. **Therefore:** it is *not* the case that a new philosophy is true (MP on premises 1 and 3, or * MT on premises 1 and 2) :. 5. **Therefore:** A new philosophy is true **AND** it is *not* the case that a new philosophy is true.(* CJ of 3 and 4) **CONTRADICTION**

[3:15]

Modus Tollens—T is defined as follows: ("~" means not, or it is not the case)
1. **If** p **then** q 2. ~q
:. 3. **Therefore:** ~p

[3:16]

* Conjunction—CJ is defined as follows:
1. p 2. q
:. 3. **Therefore:** p and q

[3:17] Kant's point is that it would be arrogant, conceited and belittling towards all the previous philosophers to claim that you have "discovered" the true philosophy, and thus everyone else before you has been wrong, even though you are still dependent on these previous philosophies for the development of your own philosophy.

[3:18] Kant does not argue that the moral law of duty is something newly discovered rather it is a new explanation of how rational beings do in fact make moral decisions.[40]

[3:1] In other words, Kant is arguing that everyone can determine what their moral duties are absolutely, whereas the determination of the consequences of actions can only be at best probable.

[3:20] Everyone is able to satisfy the categorical command of morality, i.e. to submit one's subjective maxim to the universal

---

[40] Kant, *Critique Of Practical Reason*, p. 53.

The commonest intelligence can easily and without hesitation see what, on the principle of autonomy of the will, requires to be done; but on supposition of heteronomy of the will, it is hard and requires knowledge of the world to see what is to be done. That is to say, what duty is, is plain of itself to everyone; but what is to bring true durable advantage, such as will extend to the whole of one's existence, is always veiled in impenetrable obscurity; and much prudence is required to adapt the practical rule founded on it to the ends of life, even tolerably, by making proper exceptions. But the moral law commands the most punctual obedience from everyone; it must therefore, not be so difficult to judge what it requires to be done, that the commonest unpracticed understanding, even without worldly prudence, should fail to apply it rightly.

It is always in everyone's power to satisfy the categorical command of morality; whereas it is but seldom possible and by no means so to everyone, to satisfy the empirically conditioned precept of happiness, even without regard to a single purpose. The reason is, that in the former case there is question only of the maxim, which must be genuine and pure; but in the latter case there is question also of one's capacity and physical power to realize a desired object. A command that everyone should try to make himself happy would be foolish, for one never commands anyone to do what he of himself infallibly wishes to do. We must only command the means, or rather supply them, since he cannot do everything that he wishes. But to command morality under the name of duty is quite rational; for, in the first place, not everyone is willing to obey its precepts if they oppose his inclination; and as to the means of obeying this law, these need not in this case be taught, for in this respect whatever he wishes to do he can do.

consistency test, however, not everyone is able to do that which is required to attain that which is desired by consequence. Lastly, it makes no sense to command everyone to be happy if everyone already wishes to be happy. However, a moral command does make rational sense since often times people's inclinations make it so that they are not willing to obey their self-legislative maxims.

D. Responses To Criticisms

1. Jack-of-all-trades and a master of none response

[3:21] The synergistic model is by no means a Jack-of-all-trades and a master of none; rather, it is the developmental process of a practical moral philosophy. It is true that the very existence of this model depends on all previous philosophical investigations both successful and unsuccessful. It is the synthesizing of these deep philosophical insights into a coherent whole that gives the "new" model its depth and insight. Synergism is not a watering down process that attempts to please everyone, rather it is a synergistic concentration of that which is true in philosophy into a whole that is greater than the sum of its parts.

2. A new true philosophy response

[3:22] The synergistic model does not claim to be a new philosophy. As the name suggests, the synergistic model is a synthesization of that which works best in the history of moral philosophy in an attempt to attain practical moral decision-making. This does not mean, however, that it is a "new" true philosophy in the sense that no previous true philosophy could have existed. Rather, this philosophy's very existence depends on the existence of previous philosophy. Just as the new scientific developments towards truth in chemistry and medicine are dependent on that which has preceded them so also are the new moral developments towards truth dependent on that which has preceded them.

[3:23] It could be argued that the synergistic model likewise excludes all other pure models, however, it does not do so in such a way as to detract from the merits of the earlier models. Even if this is true, the synergistic model is, as Kant describes, "the unity of the true principle which unifies the whole of philosophy into one system."[41]

E. Unified Collective Whole

1. Hermeneutical circle

[3:25] The synergistic model is analogous to the *hermeneutical* circle, which states that in order to understand the parts there must be an understanding of the whole, and in order to understand the whole there must be an understanding of the parts. The parts here would refer to theories, intuitions, and mid-level principles.[42] The whole would be the unified conception that transcends any of the individual parts.[43]

[3:26] True moral understanding, like Kant argued, is a unification of several modes of thought that ultimately can only be understood from the perspective of the unified collective whole.

[3:27] Using the term collective is not an arbitrary choice of words. Although the connection is not a direct one, the following examples from Mill and Kant will show how important the social collective concept is in both of their theories. Now surely the synergistic model is not referring to a social collective conscious-

---

[41] Ibid., p. 5, [6:207]

[42] Mid-level principles will be discussed in the next section.

[43] Kant, *Critique Of Practical Reason*, pp. 20 - 21.

When we have to study a particular faculty of the human mind in its sources, its content, and its limits: then from the nature of human knowledge we must begin with its *parts*, with an accurate and complete exposition of them; complete, namely, so far as is possible in the present state of our knowledge of its elements. But there is another thing to be attended to which is of more philosophical and *architectonic* character, namely, to grasp correctly the *idea of the whole*, and from thence to get a view of all those parts as mutually related by the aid of pure reason, and by means of their derivation from the concept of the whole. This is only possible through the most intimate acquaintance with the system; and those who find the first inquiry too troublesome, and do not think it worth their while to attain such an acquaintance, cannot reach the second stage, namely, the general view, which is a synthetical return to that which had previously been given analytically. It is no wonder then if they find inconsistencies everywhere, although the gaps, which these indicate, are not in the system itself, but in their own incoherent train of thought.

ness, rather, it is referring to a metaphysical abstraction of moral decision-making in which the theoretical, inductive, and mid-level principles, are to be conceived of as a collective whole, each part having its purpose and function and it is only as a unified collective whole that they form a moral decision-making model.

[3:28] Mill argued that conceiving oneself as part of a collective is the ultimate sanction of the greatest happiness morality. In the performance of any moral action it is natural to conceive oneself as part of a collective as all ends are not individual, but rather, all ends are to be identified with those of others.

> [3:29] "The social state is at once so natural, so necessary, and so habitual to man, that, except in some unusual circumstances or by an effort of voluntary abstraction, he never conceives himself otherwise than as a member of a body … This conviction is the ultimate sanction of the greatest happiness morality."[44]

[3:30] Mill in his last chapter of Utilitarianism argues that justice is a different kind of obligation in that they are perfect obligations that are the most absolute and imperative, of any other

---

[44] Mill, *Utilitarianism*, Chapter 8, [3:54-81].

The social state is at once so natural, so necessary, and so habitual to man, that, except in some unusual circumstances or by an effort of voluntary abstraction, he never conceives himself otherwise than as a member of a body; and this association is riveted more and more, as mankind are further removed from the state of savage independence. … Society between equals can only exist on the understanding that the interests of all are to be regarded equally. … In this way people grow up unable to conceive as possible to them a state of total disregard of other people's interests. … They are also familiar with the fact of cooperating with others and proposing to themselves a **collective**, not an individual, interest as the aim of their actions. So long as they are co-operating, their ends are identified with those of others; there is at least a temporary feeling that the interests of others are their own interests. … The good of others becomes to him a thing naturally and necessarily to be attended to, like any of the physical conditions of our existence. … In an improving state of the human mind, the influences are constantly on the increase which tend to generate in each individual a feeling of unity with all the rest; which, if perfect, would make him never think of, or desire, any beneficial condition for himself in the benefits of which they are not included. … [A] person in whom the social feeling is at all developed cannot bring himself to think of the rest of his fellow creatures as struggling rivals. … [O]ne of his natural wants [is] that there should be harmony between his feelings and aims and those of his fellow creatures. … This conviction is the ultimate sanction of the greatest happiness morality.

class of obligations, and therefore they are guarded by our natural sentiments. Justice, it would seem, is also closely connected to what Mill calls the collective.[45, 46]

[3:31] Mill argues that utilitarianism, or the greatest happiness principle, holds to the position that unless virtue is psychologically desired as an end in itself, the mind will not be in the most conducive state for happiness.

> [3:32] "[The utilitarian doctrine] maintains not only that virtue is to be desired, but that it is to be desired disinterestedly, for itself. ... Virtue, according to the utilitarian doctrine, is not naturally and originally part of the end, but it is capable of becoming so; and in those who love it disinterestedly it has become so, and is desired and cherished, not as a means to happiness, but as a part of their happiness. ... [T]he utilitarian standard, ... enjoins and requires the cultivation of the love of virtue up to the greatest

---

45 Mill, *Utilitarianism*, Chapter 8, [5:116].

The same superiority of intelligence, joined to the power of sympathizing with human beings generally, enables him to attach himself to the collective idea of his tribe, his country, or mankind in such a manner that any act hurtful to them raises his instinct of sympathy and urges him to resistance.

46 Mill, *Utilitarianism*, Chapter 8, [5:203,241].

[J]ustice is a name for certain moral requirements which, regarded collectively stand higher in the scale of social utility, and are therefore of more paramount obligation, than any others, though particular cases may occur in which some other social duty is so important as to overrule any one of the general maxims of justice. ... [W]e do not call anything justice which is not a virtue, we usually say, not that justice must give way to some other moral principle, but that what is just in ordinary cases is, by reason of that other principle, not just in the particular case.

strength possible, as being above all things important to the general happiness." [47]

[3:333] As stated above justice is a category of virtue and as a result of being virtuous those types of behaviors are more certain than any other types of actions. From desire, (the passive sensibility), comes the will, (the active phenomenon). However, because the will is amenable to habit there are two results that can occur, 1. because something is willed it is desired, and 2. something can be willed that is no longer desired giving certainty to the behavior, i.e. the action is determined by a habit or a virtuous trait.[48]

---

[47] Mill, *Utilitarianism*, Chapter 8, [5:24, 25, 30,53].

[The utilitarian doctrine] maintains not only that virtue is to be desired, but that it is to be desired disinterestedly, for itself. ... [T]hey not only place virtue at the very head of things which are good as means to the ultimate end, but they also recognize as a psychological fact the possibility of its being, to the individual, a good in itself, without looking to any end beyond it; and hold that the mind is not in a right state, not in a state conformable to utility, not in the state most conducive to the general happiness, unless it does love virtue in this manner—as a thing desirable in itself. ...Virtue, according to the utilitarian doctrine, is not naturally and originally part of the end, but it is capable of becoming so; and in those who love it disinterestedly it has become so, and is desired and cherished, not as a means to happiness, but as a part of their happiness. ... [T]he utilitarian standard, ... enjoins and requires the cultivation of the love of virtue up to the greatest strength possible, as being above all things important to the general happiness.

[48] Mill, *Utilitarianism*, Chapter 8, [4:65,70,76,78].

Will, the active phenomenon, is a different thing from desire, that state of passive sensibility. ... The distinction between will and desire thus understood is an authentic and highly important psychological fact; but the fact consists solely in this—that will, like all other parts of our constitution, is amenable to habit, and that we may will from habit what we no longer desire for itself, or desire only because we will it. It is not the less true that will, in the beginning, is entirely produced by desire. ... Will is the child of desire, and passes out of the dominion of its parent only to come under that of habit. ... Both in feeling and in conduct, habit is the only thing which imparts certainty; and it is because of the importance to others of being able to rely absolutely on one's feelings and conduct, and to oneself of being able to rely on one's own, that the will to do right ought to be cultivated into this habitual independence.

[3:34] Kant also argued for the concept of the collective in that every person's end is to be each individual's end also. Mill, of course, recognized this as well.[49]

[3:35] When Kant talks about the supreme principle of the doctrine of virtue the concept of the collective is clearly a part of it: "The supreme principle of the doctrine of virtue is: act in accordance with a maxim of ends that it can be a universal law for everyone to have."[50] In his Groundwork for the Metaphysics of Morals, Kant argued for the Kingdom of Ends in which people collectively would consider each person's end as their own end.[51]

[3:36] It cannot be stressed enough that the synergistic model is like the social arrangement of a unified collective whole in that the whole is greater than the sum of its parts. The parts can only be understood from the perspective of the whole, and the whole can only be understood from the perspective of the parts.

2. Hologram

[3:37] Another analogy for the synergistic model would be that of a hologram. If a hologram picture is cut it into little pieces, each little piece will contain the entire picture. When these distributed parts are viewed collectively they transcend the individual realm and become part of the collective realm.

---

[49] Mill, *Utilitarianism*, Chapter 8. [5:124,126].

When Kant (as before remarked) propounds as the fundamental principle of morals, "So act that the rule of conduct might be adopted as a law by all rational beings," he virtually acknowledges the interests of mankind collectively. ... To give any meaning to Kant's principle, the sense put upon it must be that we ought to shape our conduct by a rule which all rational beings might adopt *with benefit to their collective interests.*

[50] Kant, *The Metaphysics of Morals; Preface to Doctrine of Right*, pp. 157, [6:395].

The supreme principle of the doctrine of virtue is: act in accordance with a maxim of *ends* that it can be a universal law for everyone to have. – In accordance with this principle a human being is an end for himself as well as for others, and it is not enough that he is not authorized to use either himself or others merely as means; it is in itself his duty to make man as such his end.

[51] Immanuel Kant, *The Groundwork for the Metaphysics of Morals,* (1785), Translated by James W. Ellington, (Indianapolis: Hackett Publishing Company, 1981), [433]

[3:38] Analogies obviously do not prove particular objective facts, rather, they only illustrate certain similarities. It could be argued that the hologram is an illustration of a distributive process of identical elements and therefore could illustrate a counter-example of a pluralistic unifying process. Although this may be the case, the hologram is here being used as an illustration of a phenomenon in which the whole perception is greater than the perception of the parts. Because this holographic effect is a common experience, it serves well as a partial analogy of the synergistic process in which the pluralistic parts participate in the larger unified collective whole.

[3:39] The hermeneutical-circle and the holographic process are analogies that illustrate how the synergistic model is a never ending, interrelated process, within a unified collective whole, i.e., a unified philosophy.

IV. Mid-Level Principles and The Synergistic Model

A. Synergistic Model

1. Development Of Mid-Level Principles

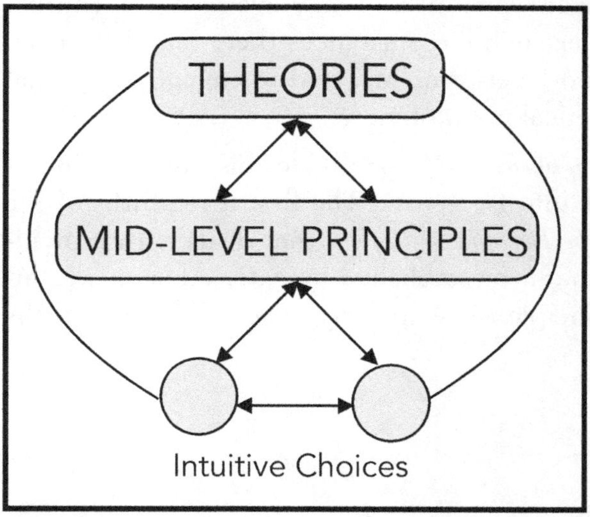

[4:1] When adopting this synergistic model, there is a natural development of "mid-level principles." These are abstract principles that are justified by both the theory model and the intuition model. These mid-level principles will be either derivable from, consistent with, or at least not in conflict with the theory(ies) and/or intuition(s). These mid-level principles are partial substantive developments of abstract or ethereal theories, and the partial theory development of practical or intuitional choices resulting in principles that are easily accessible on a regular basis.

[4:2] Mid-level principles may be likened to that of Mill's secondary principles. Mill believed that people live most of their lives by appealing to secondary principles. It is only when there are conflicting secondary principles that there is ever the need to appeal to the primary principle of utility—the greatest happiness principle.

> [4:3] "We must remember that only in these cases of conflict between secondary principles is it requisite that first principles should be appealed to. There is no case of moral

obligation in which some secondary principle is not involved." [52]

[4:4] In other words, Mill's position is that individuals can usually appeal to established rules or guidelines for the making of most moral decisions. However under unique and novel circumstances, situations may arise in which the established rules or guidelines are no longer coherent and may even start to conflict with each other. Under such circumstances there may be a need to depart from the mid-level principles and to engage in rational analysis from a theoretical point of view.

[4:5] Kant in his *Metaphysics of Morals* divides his investigation of the doctrine of duties into two parts. The first three-fifths of the book is devoted to *The Doctrine of Right*[53] that deals with individual rights, or duties that are established by external laws, i.e., judicially using the principle of reciprocity. The second two-fifths

---

[52] Mill, *Utilitarianism*, Chapter 8, [2:195].

[53] **Doctrine of right:** For Kant the "Doctrine of Right," is concerned only with "duties of outer freedom", i.e. narrow duties–the manner in which one person's behavior affects others, as in the fulfillment of contracts. External constraint is morally possible, i.e., duties the state coerces by using punitive prudential incentives. (Right behaviors are also moral duties that should all be done from an ethical motive.) Doctrine of Right deals with the *'formal* condition of outer freedom (the consistency of outer freedom with itself if its maxim were made universal law.' One begins with the end and then seeks out the maxim of action in conformity with duty, i.e., to adopt maxims on empirical grounds. Kant, *Metaphysics of Morals, p. xi,146,* [6:380].

of the book is devoted to The Doctrine of Virtue[54] that deals with ethics or duties that cannot be given by external laws. The following quotes show how the differences between the doctrine of right and the doctrine of virtue really is a matter of the approach that is taken when using the synergistic model, i.e., whether the approach is from the 'top-down' or the 'bottom-up.'

> [4:6] "One can think of the relation of end to duty in two ways: one can begin with the end [particular intuitive choices][55] and seek out the *maxim* of actions [general mid-level principles] in conformity with duty [*a priori* theory] [bottom-up or intuitive approach] or, on the other hand, one can begin with the maxim of actions [general *a priori* mid-level principles] in conformity with duty [*a priori* theory] and seek out the end [free choice] that is also a duty [*a priori* theory] [top-down or theory approach]. –The *doctrine of right* takes the first way [bottom-up]. What end anyone wants to set for his action is left to his free choice. The maxim of his action, however, is determined *a priori*, namely, that the freedom of the agent could coexist with the freedom of every other in accordance with a universal law.

---

[54] **Doctrine of virtue:** Kant defines the "Doctrine of Virtue" or "ethics," as "the science of how one is under obligation without regard for any possible external lawgiving." And "the part of the general doctrine of duties that brings inner, rather than outer, freedom under laws." 'the supreme principle of the doctrine of virtue is: act in accordance with a maxim of *ends* that it can be a universal law for everyone to have. – In accordance with this principle a human being is an end for himself as well as for others, and it is not enough that he is not authorized to use either himself or others merely as means; it is in itself his duty to make man as such his end.' Ethics 'provides a *matter* (an object of free choice), and end of pure reason which it represents as an end that is also objectively necessary, that is, an end that, as far as human beings are concerned, it is a duty to have. –For since the sensible inclinations of human beings tempt them to ends (the matter of choice) that can be contrary to duty, lawgiving reason can in turn check their influence only by a moral end setup against the ends of inclination, an end that must therefore be given *a priori*, independently of inclinations.' One begins with the maxim of actions in conformity with duty and then seeks out the end that is also a duty. Only *an end that is also a duty* can be called a duty of virtue. Duty of virtue is based on free self-constraint. (For finite holy beings, who could never be tempted to violate duty, there would be no doctrine of virtue but only a doctrine of morals. … Thus human morality in its highest stage can still be nothing more than virtue.) The ends that are also duties are *one's own perfection* and *the happiness of others*. Kant, *Metaphysics of Morals*, p. *xi, 146-8*, [6:381-383].

[55] Bracketed text is interpretive additions not found in the text.

> [4:7] But *ethics* takes the opposite way [top-down]. … Hence in ethics the *concept of duty* [*a priori* theory] will lead to ends [freely chosen] and will have to establish *maxims* [*a priori* mid-level-principles] with respect to ends we *ought* to set ourselves [*a priori* theory], grounding them in accordance with moral principles. … Only *an end that is also a duty* can be called a **duty of virtue**. …
>
> [4:8] What essentially distinguishes a duty of virtue from a duty of right is that external constraint to the latter kind of duty is morally possible, whereas the former is based only on free self-constraint." [56]

[4:9] The mid-level principles from the doctrine of right are those rights and liberties that are considered to be necessary for the maximization of all citizens' freedoms in conformity with the end of perpetual peace.

[4:10] In a pluralistic environment in which agents are making social decisions, each of which are holding to different theories and/or intuitions, it is common, for example, in the United States, to appeal to the Constitution, which can be thought of as mid-level principles. The Constitution thus consists of basic rights and liberties that most "participants" find either derivable from, compatible with, or at least not in conflict with their theories and/or intuitions as they relate to the freedom of all citizens.[57]

---

[56] Kant, *Metaphysics of Morals; The Doctrine of Virtue,* p. 147-148, [6:382-383].

[57] Kant, *Metaphysics of Morals; The Doctrine of Right*, p. 95, [6:319].

A law that is so holy (inviolable) that it is already a crime even to call it in doubt *in a practical way,* and so to suspend its effect for a moment, is thought as if it must have arisen not from human beings but from some highest, flawless lawgiver; and that is what the saying "All authority is from God" means. This saying is not an assertion about the *historical basis* of the civil constitution; it instead sets forth an idea as a practical principle of reason: the principle that the presently existing legislative authority ought to be obeyed, whatever its origin.

[4:11] The doctrine of virtue consists of those ends that are also duties that establish a law for the maxims of actions.[58] 'They are *one's own perfection*[59] and *the happiness of others*.'[60]

[4:12] These mid-level principles are mutually constraining in that each principle limits the exercise of the other principles because of coherency, through the process of weighing and balancing, and specification.

[4:13] When persons do find themselves having to act from a motive of duty, it still may be the case that they will not have to appeal to their theory or first principle. During the whole past duration of the human species, mankind has already determined many positive beliefs as to what are moral actions and have de-

---

[58] Kant, *Metaphysics of Morals; The Doctrine of Virtue,* p. 152, [6:389].

Only the concept of an *end* that is also a duty, a concept that belongs exclusively to ethics, establishes a law for maxims of actions by subordinating the subjective end (that everyone has) to the objective end (that everyone ought to make his end). The imperative "You ought to make this or that (e.g., the happiness of others) your end" has to do with the matter of choice (an object). Now no free action is possible unless the agent also intends an end (which is the matter of choice). Hence, if there is an end that is also a duty, the only condition that maxims of actions, as means to ends, must contain is that of qualifying for a possible giving of universal law.

[59] **One's own perfection:** Kant says that this is an end that is also a duty, along with the happiness of others. He argues that 'The word *perfection* is open to a good deal of misinterpretation. Perfection is sometimes understood as a concept belonging to transcendental philosophy, ... Then again, as a concept belonging to *teleology,* it is taken to mean the harmony of a thing's properties with an end. Perfection in the first sense could be called quantitative (material) perfection, and in the second, qualitative (formal) perfection. The quantitative perfection of a thing can be only one. But one thing can have several qualitative perfections, and it is really qualitative perfection that is under discussion here. The duty of one's own perfection is to cultivate one's faculties, the highest being understanding, the faculty of concepts and of one's will in which the law becomes also the incentive to his action that conforms with duty and he obeys the law from duty. Kant, *Metaphysics of Morals; The Doctrine of Virtue,* p. 150, [6:387].

[60] **Happiness of others:** Kant says this is one of the ends that is also a duty, along with one's own perfection. 'When it comes to my promoting happiness as an end that is also a duty, this must therefore be the happiness of *other* human beings, whose (permitted) end I thus make my own end as well. It is for them to decide what they count as belonging to their happiness; but it is open to me to refuse them many things that they think will make them happy but that I do not, as long as they have no right to demand them from me as what is theirs.' Kant, *Metaphysics of Morals; The Doctrine of Virtue,* p. 151, [6:388].

veloped these mid-level principles by which actions can be determined. As Roger J. Sullivan says in the introduction to the *Metaphysics of Morals*:

> [4:14] "When faced with a difficult decision, a person will already have adopted a number of these very general rules, [i.e., mid-level principles] and his or her decision about how to act will then be a problem for judgment, i.e., for deciding which rule is most relevant in this particular case and exactly how to follow it." [61]

Mill also talks directly about this:

> [4:15] "People talk as if … at the moment when some man feels tempted to meddle with the property or life of another, he had to begin considering for the first time whether murder and theft are injurious to human happiness. … [M]ankind must by this time have acquired positive beliefs, [i.e., mid-level principles] …
>
> [4:16] To consider the rules of morality as improvable is one thing; to pass over the intermediate generalization entirely and endeavor to test each individual action directly by the first principle [theory] is another. It is a strange notion that the acknowledgment of a first principle [theory] is inconsistent with the admission of secondary ones [mid-level principles].
>
> [4:17] Mill argues that "there exists no moral system under which there do not arise unequivocal cases of conflicting obligation, [mid-level principles]. These are the real difficulties, the knotty points both in the theory of ethics and in the conscientious guidance of personal conduct. [When there are] moral laws, [mid-level principles], all claiming independent authority, there is no common umpire entitled to interfere between them; their claims to precedence one over another rest on little better than

---

[61] Kant, *The Metaphysics of Morals*, Introduction by Roger J. Sullivan, p. x.

When faced with a difficult decision, a person will already have adopted a number of these very general rules, [i.e., mid-level principles] and his or her decision about how to act will then be a problem for judgment –for deciding which rule is most relevant in this particular case and exactly how to follow it. Finally, it is the role of character also to motivate a person actually to act on that judgment of what is the right thing to do. Just knowing the categorical imperative and the right moral principles will not make a person virtuous. Good character depends both on an initial commitment to obey those norms and a conscientious adherence to that commitment.

> sophistry, and, unless determined, … [they] afford a free scope for the action of personal desires and partialities. We must remember that only in these cases of conflict between secondary principles [mid-level principles] is it requisite that first principles, [Theory], should be appealed to. There is no case of moral obligation in which some secondary principle [mid-level principle] is not involved." [62]

[4:18] In addition to having secondary or mid-level principles by which we can conduct most of our moral lives, it is also the case that many of our decisions are not either moral or immoral but rather they are nonmoral decisions. Kant argues that those individuals that make nonmoral activities of life into "moral" ones are fanatics in which if their fanatical approach to life were to be considered virtuous, "virtue" would then become tyranny.[63]

[4:19] Mill believes that people are also mistaken when they claim that the utilitarian standard, for example, is too "exacting" in that utilitarianism mandates that all actions must be done with "all of society in mind."

[4:20] The mistake is that these individuals are confusing the motive or end of morality; "The greatest happiness principle for all of society"—motive, with that of the mid-level principles—rules of action. The fact of the matter is that almost all of our actions are not done because of the motive of moral duty—the greatest happiness principle for all of society, but rather because of some other motive, say mid-level principles.

[4:21] This is permissible as long as those mid-level principles, for example, do not violate "the greatest happiness principle for all of society.

> [4:22] The objectors to utilitarianism cannot always be charged with representing it in a discreditable light. On

---

[62] Mill, *Utilitarianism*, Chapter 8, [2:171-196].

[63] Kant, *Metaphysics of Morals; Doctrine of Virtue*, p. 167, [6:409].

Someone who allows *nothing to be morally indifferent* and strews all his steps with duties, as with mantraps; it is not indifferent to him whether I eat meat or fish, drink beer or wine, supposing that both agree with me. Fantastic virtue is concerned with petty details which, were it admitted into the doctrine of virtue, would turn the government of virtue into tyranny.

the contrary, those among them who entertain anything like a just idea of its disinterested character sometimes find fault with its standard as being too high for humanity. They say it is exacting too much to require that people shall always act from the inducement of promoting the general interest of society. But this is to mistake the very meaning of a standard of morals and confound the rule of action with the motive of it. It is the business of ethics to tell us what are our duties, or by what test we may know them; but no system of ethics requires that the sole motive of all we do shall be a feeling of duty; on the contrary, ninety-nine hundredths of all our actions are done from other motives, and rightly so done if the rule of duty does not condemn them." [64]

2. Fragmentation Of Decision-Making

[4:24] Within the scientific or objective world, there exists fragmentation. That is, "reality" cannot be known by using just one theory or approach. For example, sense perceptions alone are not enough in determining whether the sun goes around the earth—geocentric, or whether the earth goes around the sun—heliocentric. If vision alone were to be used, then it would seem reasonable to conclude that the universe is geocentric. However, most people are aware of the fact that their senses can be deceiving.[65] As a result, science has incorporated a pluralistic approach in which rationality, logic, and sense data are all used in differing degrees for different determinations. For example, Euclidian geometry is appropriate for everyday plane geometry; however, for some astronomical applications, it is necessary to use Einstein's General Theory of Relativity. Science is pluralistic in how and when it uses various models for determining the nature of reality. This fragmentation of science has in no way made it any less reliable; in fact, if anything it has only made it more reliable.

[4:25] In like fashion, the making of moral decisions is also pluralistic. What theories, intuitions, mid-level principles, or combi-

---

64 Mill, *Utilitarianism*, Chapter 8, [2:120-124].

65 Consider the art of magic, i.e., the art of illusions and deceptions.

nations thereof are used depends on what is being deliberated. Sometimes the use of one approach is more appropriate than using another approach. Other times it could be more appropriate to use several approaches resulting in the process of reflective-equilibrium.

[4:26] The analogy of the scientific approach is being used to illustrate the need for checks and balances in knowledge acquisition, along with the necessity for varied decision-making models depending upon the circumstances.

[4:27] One major difference between the first principles of science and the first principles of morality is that for morality the general theoretical test of what is right or wrong must precede the particular truths or objective actions, whereas, for science the objective experience precedes the general theory.[66]

3. Weighing And Balancing

[4:28] Theories, mid-level principles, and intuitions are often times composed of many *prima facie* "rights and liberties" that have to be weighed and balanced. This weighing and balancing process is an attempt to maximize all competing rights and liberties.

[4:29] All rights and liberties exist in a reciprocal relationship that is mutually constraining resulting in the necessity to balance. For example, no one could rationally hold to the view that freedom of speech is an absolute right in the sense that all persons have the liberty to yell "FIRE" in a crowded theater if they so desired even if there is no fire. In other words, the right of free-

---

[66] Mill, *Utilitarianism*, Chapter 8, [1:7-11].

The truths, which are ultimately accepted as the first principles of a science, are really the last results of metaphysical analysis. ... Though in science the particular truths precede the general theory, the contrary might be expected to be the case with a practical art, such as morals or legislation. All action is for the sake of some end, and rules of action, it seems natural to suppose, must take their whole character, and color from the end to which they are subservient. When we engage in pursuit, a clear and precise conception of what we are pursuing would seem to be the first thing we need, instead of the last we are to look forward to. A test of right and wrong must be the means, one would think, of ascertaining what is right or wrong, and not a consequence of having already ascertained it.

dom of speech needs to be weighed and balanced with the right of safe assembly.[67] As a result, no rights and/or liberties are absolute, rather they must be specified and balanced with all other competing rights and/or liberties considered.[68]

[4:30] Under the section above on the Development Of Mid-Level Principles it was shown that Mill emphasized this point stating:

> [4:31] "that only in these cases of conflict between secondary principles [mid-level principles] is it requisite that first principles, [Theory], should be appealed to. There is no case of moral obligation in which some secondary principle [mid-level principle] is not involved." [69]

[4:32] Kant argued that sometimes the certain use of freedom, (like freedom of speech), can actually become a hindrance to other freedoms in accordance with universal law, (like freedom of safe assembly). Coercion against those who try to exercise the hindering freedoms is therefore authorized.

> [4:33] "… Now whatever is wrong is a hindrance to freedom in accordance with universal laws. But coercion is a hindrance or resistance to freedom. Therefore, if a certain use of freedom is itself a hindrance to freedom in accordance with universal laws (i.e., wrong), coercion that is opposed to this (as a *hindering of a hindrance to freedom*) is

---

67 As the old saying goes; "the right for me to swing my fists ends at the tip of your nose."

68 Mill, *Utilitarianism*, Chapter 8, [2:189,191].

There exists no moral system under which there do not arise unequivocal cases of conflicting obligation. … They are overcome practically, with greater or with less success, according to the intellect and virtue of the individual.

69 Mill, *Utilitarianism*, Chapter 8, [2:195-196].

consistent with freedom in accordance with universal laws, that is, it is right." [70]

[4:34] The question can now be raised as to whether this idea of mid-level principles as not being absolute is contrary to Kant's moral conception of absolutes. After all Kant did argue that there could never be any conflict of obligations, whereas Mill argues that conflict of obligations will arise under any moral system. With regard to conflicting duties Kant said:

[4:35]

Conflict of Duties: A relation such that one duty would cancel out another duty (wholly or in part). However,
1. Since duty and obligation are concepts that express the objective practical necessity of certain actions.
2. Since two rules opposed to each other cannot be necessary at the same time.
3. If it is a duty to act in accordance with one rule, then to act in accordance with the opposite rule is not a duty but even contrary to duty.
:. 4. **Therefore:** a collision of duties and obligations is inconceivable. [71]

[4:36] "However, a subject may have, in a rule they have prescribed, two grounds of obligation, one or the other of which is not sufficient to put the subject under obligation, so that one of them is not a duty. –When two such grounds

[70] Immanuel Kant, *The Metaphysics of Morals; The Doctrine of Right,* (1785), Translated by Mary Gregor, (New York: Cambridge University Press, 1996), pp. 25-26, [6:231-232].

... Now whatever is wrong is a hindrance to freedom in accordance with universal laws. But coercion is a hindrance or resistance to freedom. Therefore, if a certain use of freedom is itself a hindrance to freedom in accordance with universal laws (i.e., wrong), coercion that is opposed to this (as a *hindering of a hindrance to freedom* is consistent with freedom in accordance with universal laws, that is, it is right. Hence there is connected with right by the principle of contradiction an authorization to coerce someone who infringes upon it.

... [For example], coercion which constrains everyone to pay his debts can coexist with the freedom of everyone, including that of debtors, in accordance with a universal external law. Right and authorization to use coercion therefore mean one and the same thing.

> conflict with each other, practical philosophy says, not that the stronger obligation takes precedence, but that the stronger ground of obligation prevails."[71]

[4:37] It should be noticed that what Kant is talking about here and what is being expressed with the concept of mid-level principles is totally compatible. The mid-level principles do not conflict in the sense that one principle, for example, says that persons have freedom of speech and another principle says that persons do not have freedom of speech. Rather, the weighing and balancing has to do with, for example, freedom of speech in combination with freedom of safe assembly. Therefore, ethical duties are wide obligations in which various duties mutually constrain each other, e.g., love of one's neighbor in general by love of one's parents.

[4:38] The maxims of actions, or mid-level principles, prescribe not actions themselves, rather it leaves a playroom for free choice to do the action for an end that is also a duty.[72]

[4:39] Kant argues that there are certain duties that are indirect duties rather than direct duties. Indirect duties would be those duties that are done for the sake of preventing or warding off temptations to violate one's duty. Seeking prosperity, for example, may be an indirect duty so as to prevent poverty, which can

---

[71] Kant, *The Metaphysics of Morals; Doctrine of Right*, pp. 16-17, [6:224].

[72] Ibid., p. 153, [6:390].

… if the law can prescribe only the maxim of actions, not actions themselves, this is a sign that it leaves a playroom for free choice in following (complying with) the law, that is, that the law cannot specify precisely in what way one is to act and how much one is to do by the action for an end that is also a duty. – But a wide duty is not to be taken as permission to make exceptions to the maxim of actions but only as permission to limit one maxim of duty by another (e.g., love of one's neighbor in general by love of one's parents), by which in fact the field for the practice of virtue is widened. – The wider the duty, therefore, the more imperfect is a man's obligation to action.

be a temptation to vice.[73] This also is an exercise of weighing and balancing.

[4:40] Kant later presents casuistic questions to the reader asking whether there are cases and situations in which doing an action, which is normally impermissible, is permissible if it is done in order to prevent a greater violation.

> [4:41] "Nature's end in the cohabitation of the sexes is procreation, that is, the preservation of the species. Hence one may not, at least, act contrary to that end. But is it permitted to engage in this practice (even within marriage) *without taking this end into consideration?*
>
> [4:42] If, for example, the wife is pregnant or sterile (because of age or sickness), or if she feels no desire for intercourse, is it not contrary to nature's end, and so also contrary to one's duty to oneself, for one or the other of them, to make use of their sexual attributes –just as in unnatural lust? Or is there, in this case, a permissive law of morally practical reason, which in the collision of its determining grounds makes permitted something that is in itself not permitted (indulgently, as it were), in order to prevent a still greater violation? –At what point can the limitation of a wide obligation be ascribed to *purism* (a pedantry regarding the fulfillment of duty, as far as the wideness of the obligation is concerned), and the animal inclinations be allowed a latitude, at the risk of forsaking the law of reason?" [74]

[4:43] Another example of how Kant used this weighing and balancing concepts is in his discussion on punishment when he ar-

---

[73] Kant, *The Metaphysics of Morals; The Doctrine of Virtue*, p. 152, [6:388].

Adversity, pain, and want are great temptations to violate one's duty. It might therefore seem that prosperity, strength, health, and well-being in general, which check the influence of these, could also be considered ends that are duties, so that one has a duty to promote *one's own* happiness and not just the happiness of others. –But then the end is not the subject's happiness but his morality, and happiness is merely a means for removing obstacles to his morality –a *permitted* means, since no one else has a right to require of me that I sacrifice my ends if these are not immoral. To seek prosperity for its own sake is not directly a duty, but indirectly it can well be a duty, that of warding off poverty insofar as this is a great temptation to vice. But then it is not my happiness but the preservation of my moral integrity that is my end and so my duty.

[74] Ibid., pp. 179-180., [6:426].

gues that the purpose of punishment is not to just correct the harm that was done but also to avenge the crime. But punishment, he goes on to say, is a court decision not a personal one. He then presents an interesting argument on a person's duty to forgive and how that duty must be weighed and balanced with a person's duty not to let others "trample" on their rights.[75]

As Kant said earlier:

[4:44] "Be no man's lackey. –Do not let others tread with impunity on your rights. ... But one who makes himself a worm cannot complain afterwards if people step on him."[76]

4. Specification

[4:46] Specification is the process in which theories and mid-level principles are developed conceptually and shaped normatively, so that they can be applied to particular circumstances. Each new decision, within new circumstances, generally requires that

---

[75] Kant, *The Metaphysics of Morals; The Doctrine of Virtue,* pp. 207-208, [6:460-461].

The sweetest form of malice is the *desire for revenge.* Besides, it might even seem that one has the greatest right, and even the obligation (as a desire for justice), to make it one's end to harm others without any advantage to oneself.

Every deed that violates a humans being's right deserves punishment, the function of which is to *avenge* a crime on the one who committed it (not merely to make good the harm that was done). But punishment is not an act that the injured party can undertake on his private authority but rather an act of a court distinct from him, which gives effect to the law of a *supreme authority* over all those subject to it; and when (as we must in ethics) we regard human beings as in a rightful condition but *in accordance only with laws of reason* (not civil laws), then no one is authorized to inflict punishment and to avenge the wrongs sustained by them except him who is also the supreme moral lawgiver, and he alone (namely God) can say "Vengeance is mine; I will repay." It is, therefore, a duty of virtue not only to refrain from repaying another's enmity with hatred out of mere revenge but also not even to call upon the judge of the world for vengeance, partly because a human being has enough guilt of his own to be greatly in need of pardon and partly, and indeed especially, because no punishment, no matter from whom it comes, may be inflicted out of hatred. –It is therefore a duty of human beings to be *forgiving.* But this must not be confused with *meek toleration* of wrongs, renunciation of rigorous means for preventing the recurrence of wrong by others; for then a human being would be throwing away his rights and letting others trample on them, and so would violate his duty to himself.

[76] Ibid., p. 188, [6:436-437].

our abstract theories and/or mid-level principles be interpreted in terms of how they can and/or should be applied to practical life.

[4:47] Kant argued that the doctrine of right, which has to do only with narrow duties, is mathematically precise in what it does, i.e., no specification. However, virtue is concerned with wide duties which does not dictate what must be done rather the appeal is to maxims of actions, that leave a wide playroom, for how one chooses to act in accordance with the duties of self-perfection, and the happiness of others. In other words, the broad and general mid-level principles of maxims need to be specified for particular circumstances. Therefore virtue is casuistry, which has no part with regard to civil rights.[77] With civil rights you have mathematical exactitude. With virtue you have room for exceptions.[78]

[4:48] Mill also argued that it is not because of a "fault" in the mid-level principles that moral agents must recognize exceptions, rather it is because of the complexities of the moral life that make

---

[77] Ibid., pp. 168-169, [6:411].

The doctrine of right has to do only with narrow duties, whereas ethics has to do with wide duties. Hence the doctrine of right, which by its nature must determine duties strictly (precisely), has no more need of general directions (a method) as to how to proceed in judging than does pure mathematics; instead, it certifies its method by what it does.–But ethics, because of the latitude it allows in its imperfect duties, unavoidably leads to questions that call upon judgment to decide how a maxim is to be applied in particular cases, and indeed in such a way that judgment provides another (subordinate) maxim (and one can always ask for yet another principle for applying this maxim to cases that may arise). So ethics falls into a casuistry, which has no place in the doctrine of right.

[78] Kant, *The Metaphysics of Morals; The Doctrine of Right,* p. 26, [6:233].

The doctrine of right wants to be sure that *what belongs* to each has been determined (with mathematical exactitude). Such exactitude cannot be expected in the doctrine of virtue, [ethics], which cannot refuse some room for exceptions.

it impossible not to have exceptions in order to accommodate for the peculiarities of a variety of circumstances.[79]

[4:49] As reasonable as this may sound, Mill has been criticized for presenting a flippant philosophy in which there are no absolutes and as a result most any action could be justified as long as it resulted in the greatest amount of happiness, i.e., critics argue that Mill's moral approach would allow the performing of "immoral" or "unjust" actions as long as they resulted in the greatest amount of happiness.

[4:50] Mill of course anticipated such simplistic criticisms and argued that usually when an immoral action is considered expedient, the expediency is only an immediate or temporary end and when you consider the expediency in the long run, and its effect not only on the agent's long term character but also its long term influence on society as a whole, then such violations are not ex-

[79] Mill, *Utilitarianism*, Chapter 8, [2:187].

It is not the fault of any creed, but of the complicated nature of human affairs, that rules of conduct cannot be so framed as to require no exceptions, and that hardly any kind of action can safely be laid down as either always obligatory or always condemnable. There is no ethical creed which does not temper the rigidity of its laws by giving a certain latitude, under the moral responsibility of the agent, for accommodation to peculiarities of circumstances.

pedient and they move into the category of becoming even one of societies worst enemies.[80]

Later on Mill argues that:

> [4:51] "Justice implies something which is not only right to do, and wrong not to do, but which some individual person can claim from us as his moral right."[81]
>
> [4:52] "To have a right, then, is, I conceive, to have something which society ought to defend men in the possession of."[82]

[4:53] Mill presents five universal *principles* of justice and injustice that he believed were as close to being absolute as is possible. They were the following:

> [4:54] "1. unjust to deprive anyone of his personal liberty, his property, or any other thing which belongs to him by law. …

---

[80] Mill, *Utilitarianism*, Chapter 8, [2:159-164].

Again, utility is often summarily stigmatized as an immoral doctrine by giving it the name of "expediency." … But the expedient, in the sense in which it is opposed to the right, generally means that which is expedient for the particular interest of the agent himself. … When it means anything better than this, it means that which is expedient for some immediate object, some temporary purpose, but which violates a rule whose observance is expedient in a much higher degree. The expedient, in this sense, instead of being the same thing with the useful, is a branch of the hurtful. Thus it would often be expedient, for the purpose of getting over some momentary embarrassment, or attaining some object immediately useful to ourselves or others, to tell a lie. But inasmuch as the cultivation in ourselves of a sensitive feeling on the subject of veracity is one of the most useful, and the enfeeblement of that feeling one of the most hurtful, things to which our conduct can be instrumental; and inasmuch as any, even unintentional, deviation from truth does that much toward weakening the trustworthiness of human assertion, which is not only the principal support of all present social well-being, but the insufficiency of which does more than any one thing that can be named to keep back civilization, virtue, everything on which human happiness on the largest scale depends—we feel that the violation, for a present advantage, of a rule of such transcendent expediency is not expedient, and that he who for the sake of convenience to himself or to some other individual, does what depends on him to deprive mankind of the good, and inflict upon them the evil, involved in the greater or less reliance which they can place in each other's words, acts the part of one of their worst enemies.

[81] Mill, *Utilitarianism*, Chapter 8, [5:101].

[82] Mill, *Utilitarianism*, Chapter 8, [5:142].

> 2. legal rights of which he is deprived may be rights which *ought* not to have belonged to him. …
>
> 3. considered just that each person should obtain that (whether good or evil) which he *deserves,* and unjust that he should obtain a good or be made to undergo an evil which he does not deserve. …
>
> 4. unjust to *break faith* with anyone: to violate an engagement, ether express or implied, or disappoint expectations raised by one's own conduct. …
>
> 5. inconsistent with justice to be *partial*—to show favor or preference to one person over another in matters in which favor and preference do not properly apply.[83]
>
> [4:55] Justice is a name for certain classes of moral rules which concern the essentials of human well-being more nearly, and are therefore of more absolute obligation, than any other rules for the guidance of life; and the notion which we have found to be of the essence of the idea of justice—that of a right residing in an individual—implies and testifies to this more binding obligation." [84]

This is in total accord with what Kant had to say about conflicting obligations when he said:

> [4:56] "When two such grounds conflict with each other, practical philosophy says, not that the stronger obligation takes precedence, but that the stronger *ground of obligation* prevails. …
>
> A principle that makes certain actions duties is a practical law. A rule that the agent himself makes his principle on subjective grounds is called his *maxim;* hence, different agents can have very different maxims with regard to the same law.
>
> The categorical imperative, which as such only affirms what obligation is, is: act upon a maxim that can also hold as a universal law." [85]

---

[83] Mill, *Utilitarianism,* Chapter 8, [5:39].

[84] Mill, *Utilitarianism,* Chapter 8, [5:203].

[85] Kant, *The Metaphysics of Morals; Preface to Doctrine of Right,* pp. 16-17, [6:224-225].

[4:57] For example, suppose the moral end was to be in good physical shape. The maxim might be to go for a one-hour walk every day at 3:00 pm. Another individual may have a very different maxim such as to ride a bike to work four times a week. Both maxims are very different and both move the individual towards the moral end of good physical shape.

[4:58] One of the most important concepts in the understanding of Kant's philosophy of ethical duties is that the moral law can only prescribe maxims of actions not actions. In fact in his book, *The Metaphysics of Morals The Doctrine of Virtue,* he has an entire section entitled, "**Ethics Does Not Give Laws for *Action (Right Does That)*, but Only for *Maxims* of Actions**" devoting sections

VI-IX to this subject.[86, 87, 88,]

---

[86] Ibid., p. 153, [6:390].

... if the law can prescribe only the maxim of actions, not actions themselves, this is a sign that it leaves a playroom for free choice in following (complying with) the law, that is, that the law cannot specify precisely in what way one is to act and how much one is to do by the action for an end that is also a duty. – But a wide duty is not to be taken as permission to make exceptions to the maxim of actions but only as permission to limit one maxim of duty by another (e.g., love of one's neighbor in general by love of one's parents), by which in fact the field for the practice of virtue is widened. – The wider the duty, therefore, the more imperfect is a man's obligation to action; as he, nevertheless, brings closer to *narrow* duty (duties of right) the maxim of complying with wide duty (in his disposition), so much the more perfect is his virtuous action.

[87] Ibid., p. 155, [6:392].

At first sight this looks like a *narrow* obligation, and the principle of duty seems to prescribe with the precision and strictness of a law not only the *legality* but also the *morality* of every action, that is, the disposition. But in fact the law, here again, prescribes only the *maxim of the action*, that of seeking the basis of obligation solely in the law and not in sensible impulse (advantage or disadvantage), and hence not the *action itself*.

[88] Ibid., p. 156, [6:393].

... duty is only a *wide* one; the duty has in it a latitude for doing more or less, and no specific limits can be assigned to what would be done. – The law holds only for maxims, not for determinate actions.

89

[4:59] Kant talks directly about the concept of specification at the end of his discussion of the elements of virtue. Whenever you take noumenal or *a priori* mid-level concepts of morality and put them in particular practice in the phenomenal or material world there will be incompleteness. How do you treat, for example, human beings who are pure vs. depraved, cultivated vs. crude, learned vs. unschooled, academic scholars vs. specialists, or peo-

---

[89] Ibid., pp. 167-168, [6:410].

… first, in terms of what is formal, … the conditions that serve to distinguish … the doctrine of morals. …(1) that duties of virtue are duties for which there is no external lawgiving; (2) that since a law must yet lie at the basis of every duty, this law in ethics can be a law of duty given, not for actions, but only for the maxims of actions; (3) that (as follows in turn from this) ethical duty must be thought of as wide, not as narrow, duty.

… second, in terms of what is *material*, present the doctrine of virtue not merely as a doctrine of duties generally but also as a *doctrine of ends*, so that a human being is under obligation to regard himself, as well as every other human being, as his end.

Third, with regard to the distinction of the material from the formal in the principle of duty, it should be noted that not every *obligation of virtue* is a duty of virtue … there is only *one* obligation of virtue, whereas there are *many* duties of virtue; for there are indeed many objects that it is also our duty to have as ends, but there is only one virtuous disposition, the subjective determining ground to fulfill one's duty. – Hence all the *divisions* of ethics will have to do only with duties of virtue

ple who differ in rank, age, sex, health, or wealth?[90] Answer: with casuistic judgments that allows playroom for differing circumstances and conditions.

[4:60] Both Mill and Kant would agree and approve of the concept of mid-level principles and how they are principles that need to be specified, and weighed and balanced, for particular actions.

5. Weighing And Balancing Is Not A Separate Process From Specification

[4:61] Weighing and balancing is not a process that can be separated from specification, and specification is not a process that can be separated from weighing and balancing. These fine distinctions are necessary for understanding the process of moral

---

[90] Kant, *The Metaphysics of Morals; The Doctrine of Virtue,* pp. 214, [6:468-469].

These (duties of virtue) do not really call for a special chapter in the system of pure ethics. ... They are only rules modified in accordance with differences of the *subjects* to whom the principle of virtue (in terms of what is formal) is *applied* in cases that come up in experience (the material). Hence, like anything divided on an empirical basis, they do not admit of a classification that could be guaranteed to be complete. ... How should one behave, for example, toward human beings who are in a state of moral purity or depravity? Toward the cultivated or the crude? Toward the learned or the unschooled, and toward the learned in so far as they use their science as members of polite society or outside society, as specialists in their field (scholars)? Toward those whose learning is pragmatic or those in whom it proceeds more from spirit and taste? How should people be treated in accordance with their differences in rank, age, sex, health, prosperity or poverty, and so forth? These questions do not yield so many different kinds of ethical *obligation* (for there is only *one,* that of virtue as such), but only so many different ways of *applying* it (corollaries). Hence they cannot be presented as sections of ethics and members of the *division* of a system (which must proceed *a priori* from a rational concept), but can only be appended to the system.

thinking but it would be absurd to try and keep them distinct, as they also are part of the unified collective whole.[91, 92]

B. Testing Out the synergistic Model

1. Should A Person Help Others Who Are In Need—Beneficence?

[4:64] In testing out the synergistic model, the following simple moral inquiry will be addressed: "A person should help others who are in need."

a. Assume the opposite

[4:65] From the several approaches available, the agent needs to inspect their culturally accepted moral commitments, i.e., intuitions, to get a "feel" for what they ought to do. Let's assume that their intuitions tell them: "a person should help others who are in need." Using the *Reductio ad absurdum*,[93] a common and acceptable

---

[91] Mill, *Utilitarianism*, Chapter 8, [5:135-238].

All persons are deemed to have a *right* to equality of treatment, except when some recognized social expediency requires the reverse. And hence all social inequalities which have ceased to be considered expedient assume the character, not of simple inexpediency, but of injustice, and appear so tyrannical that people are apt to wonder how they ever could have been tolerated—forgetful that they themselves, perhaps, tolerate other inequalities under an equally mistaken notion of expediency, the correction of which would make that which they approve seem quite as monstrous as what they have at last learned to condemn. The entire history of social improvement has been a series of transitions by which one custom or institution after another, from being a supposed primary necessity of social existence, has passed into the rank of a universally stigmatized injustice and tyranny. So it has been with the distinctions of slaves and freemen, nobles and serfs, patricians and plebeians; and so it will be, and in part already is, with the aristocracies of color, race, and sex.

[92] Kant, *The Metaphysics of Morals; The Doctrine of Virtue*, p. 147, [6:383].

But virtue is not to be defined and valued merely as an *aptitude* and a long-standing *habit* of morally good actions acquired by practice. For unless this aptitude results from considered, firm, and continually purified principles, then, like any other mechanism of technically practical reason, it is neither armed for all situations nor adequately secured against the changes that new temptations could bring about.

[93] *Reductio ad absurdum*: is the logical technique that is used to prove that a deductive argument is valid by assuming the opposite and showing that it results in a logical contradiction.

approach in logic, the agent asserts the opposite, "a person should not help others who are in need," and then analyzes the argument to see if a contradiction arises either with 1) the other intuitions that they hold to, or 2) the mid-level principles, or 3) the moral theory(ies). If a contradiction arises in one or more of these, then the opposite proposition is in fact the case, i.e. "a person should help others who are in need."

b. Evaluate intuitions

[4:66] The agent evaluates the "opposite" proposition "a person should not help others who are in need," with their other intuitive choices to see if a contradiction arises. In other words, the agent needs to make sure that all their intuitions equilibrate with each other. If they have another, or several other intuitions that contradict the proposition of "a person should not help others who are in need," then the agent will logically have to either abandon the proposition and assume the opposite, "a person should help others who are in need," or change all of their previously held conflicting intuitions. Some conflicting intuitions might be ones such as the following: it is morally right to help others in need; or, it is morally wrong not to help others in need. Changing a person's collective moral intuitions that have come together over a lifetime so as to not contradict "a person should not help others who are in need," is a highly improbable conclusion. As a result, by *Reductio ad absurdum* "a person should help others who are in need."

[4:67] However, just for argument sake, let us assume that the agent was able to equilibrate their lifetime intuitions with the proposition "a person should not help others who are in need," so that another check and balance—mid-level principles, can also be considered.

c. Evaluate mid-level principles

[4:68] The agent now compares the proposition "a person should not help others who are in need," with their other mid-level principles to see if a contradiction arises. The agent could have gone straight to their theory(ies) for the comparison, but the mid-level principles are less abstract and easier to use since they are a compilation of the essential agreements between their pluralistic theories and they have been established through the experience of history. These mid-level principles are mutually constraining in that each principle limits the exercise of the other principles through the process of weighing and balancing, and specification.

[4:69] If the new mid-level principle conflicts with the other *established* mid-level principles then there are two choices; 1) the agent can either change all their conflicting established mid-level principles so that they conform with the new mid-level principle or 2) they can change their new mid-level principle to conform with the established mid-level principles. The latter will be most probable as generally the established mid-level principles come about through the integration of numerous synergistic experiences, while this new mid-level principle has not gone through that process. If there is an established mid-level principle such as beneficence (do good), then it would seem that the agent would be obliged to either change that provision of beneficence or go back and reconsider their new mid-level principle of "a person should not help others who are in need." When considering whether or not the mid-level principle of beneficence (do good), ought to be modified or rejected the agent would most likely have to consider the following specifications of beneficence: people ought to help others in need when the personal costs of helping others is small in comparison to the benefit; people ought to help others in need because people are ends in themselves and all persons deserve dignity; people ought to help others in need because someday they may need some help; people ought to help others in need because it is just the right thing to do; and so on and so forth. However, because of the multitude, weight, and strength of these it is very unlikely that the mid-level principle of beneficence could or would be rejected, rather it seems clear that the agent would be rationally obligated to reject the proposition of: "a person should not help others who are in need" as the statement is in direct contradiction with the principle of beneficence. As a result, by *Reductio ad absurdum* "a person should help others who are in need."

[4:70] However, once again, just for argument sake, let us assume that the agent was able to equilibrate their lifetime development of mid-level principles with the proposition "a person should not help others who are in need," so that another check and balance—theory(ies) can also be considered.

d. Evaluate theory(ies)

[4:71] The agent now compares the proposition "a person should not help others who are in need," with their theory or theories of choice to see if a contradiction occurs, and if it does, then the opposite proposition is affirmed, "a person should help others in need." Three moral theories that are usually of interest are a) religion, b) utilitarianism, and c) deontology.

1) Religion

[4:72] The moral theory of religion clearly contradicts the proposition that "a person should not help others who are in need." The Golden rule is one such religious rule that is clearly a universal principle in the theory of religion.

- **Christianity:** Do unto others as you would have them do unto you. Matthew 7:12
- **Confucianism:** Do not do to others what you would not like yourself. Then there will be no resentment against you, either in the family or in the state. Analects 12:2
- **Buddhism:** Hurt not others in ways that you yourself would find hurtful. Udana-Varga 5,1
- **Hinduism:** This is the sum of duty; do naught onto others what you would not have them do unto you. Mahabharata 5,1517
- **Islam:** No one of you is a believer until he desires for his brother that which he desires for himself. Sunnah
- **Judaism:** What is hateful to you, do not do to your fellowman. This is the entire Law; all the rest is commentary. Talmud, Shabbat 3id
- **Taoism:** Regard your neighbor's gain as your gain, and your neighbor's loss as your own loss. Tai Shang Kan Yin P'ien

- **Zoroastrianism:** That nature alone is good, which refrains it from doing to another what is not good for itself. Dadisten-I-dinik, 94,5

2) Utilitarianism

[4:73] The moral theory of utilitarianism also clearly contradicts the proposition that "a person should not help others who are in need." Utilitarian happiness is not just the agent's own happiness but that of all concerned. To such an extent that utilitarianism requires the agent to be totally impartial like a benevolent spectator, i.e., a spectator that wishes the best interest or the maximization of the happiness of others. Mill argues that the ideal perfection of utilitarianism is the golden rule, do unto others as you would have them do unto you, and love your neighbor as you love yourself.[94]

[4:74] The motive of the action may not determine the consequences of an action, but for the utilitarian it has a lot to do with the moral worth of the agent. Virtue is of vital importance for the utilitarian as virtuous dispositions assures the promotion of beneficial ends probably more than any other character trait.[95]

3) Deontology

[4:75] The deontological moral theory of Kant also clearly contradicts the proposition that "a person should not help others who are in need." Three quotes should suffice to establish this determination.

> [4:76] "Undoubtedly in this way also are to be understood those passages of Scripture which command us to love our neighbor and even our enemy. For love as an inclination cannot be commanded; but beneficence from duty, when no inclination impels us and even when a natural and un-

---

[94] Mill, *Utilitarianism*, Chapter 8, [2:114-117].

The happiness which forms the utilitarian standard of what is right in conduct is not the agent's own happiness but that of all concerned. As between his own happiness and that of others, utilitarianism requires him to be as strictly impartial as a disinterested and benevolent spectator. In the golden rule of Jesus of Nazareth, we read the complete spirit of the ethics of utility. "To do as you would be done by," and to "love your neighbor as yourself," constitute the ideal perfection of the utilitarian morality.

[95] Mill, *Utilitarianism*, Chapter 8, [2:125-126].

The motive has nothing to do with the morality of the action, though much with the worth of the agent. He who saves a fellow creature from drowning does what is morally right, whether his motive be duty or the hope of being paid for his trouble.

> conquerable aversion opposes such beneficence, is practical, and not pathological, love. Such love resides in the will and not in the propensities of feeling, in principles of action and not in tender sympathy; and only this practical love can be commanded.[96]

> [4:77] I should never act except in such a way that I can also will that my maxim should become a universal law.[97]

> [4:78] A fourth man finds things going well for himself but sees others (whom he could help) struggling with great hardships; and he thinks what does it matter to me? … I shall take nothing from him nor even envy him; but I have no desire to contribute anything to his well-being or to his assistance when in need. … Even though it is possible that a universal law of nature could subsist in accordance with that maxim, still it is impossible to will that such a principle should hold everywhere as a law of nature. For a will which resolved in this way would contradict itself, inasmuch as cases might often arise in which one would have need of the love and sympathy of others and in which he would deprive himself, by such a law of nature springing from his own will, of all hope of the aid he wants for himself." [98]

2. A Person Should Help Others Who Are In Need—Beneficence

[4:79] The synergistic model does an excellent job in describing how people do in fact make moral determinations and it also showed itself as an effective model for prescribing how people ought to act morally. The conclusion with the above exercise was that "a person should help others who are in need—beneficence" regardless of whether the evaluative focus was on intuitions, mid-level principles, and or theory(ies). This convergence of conclusions from all three categories strengthens the probability of the correctness of the above conclusion.

---

96 Immanuel Kant, *The Groundwork for the Metaphysics of Morals,* (1785), Translated by James W. Ellington, (Indianapolis: Hackett Publishing Company, 1981) p. 12, [399].

97 Ibid., p. 14, [402].

98 Ibid., p. 32, [423].

Conclusion

[4:80] This section has investigated the five major problems or considerations with the pure theory model, (i.e., gray areas, intuitions are used, metaphysical disagreements, infinite regress, and criterion), and the three major problems or considerations with the pure intuition model, (i.e., theories are used, theories would not be needed, and disagreements would be unresolvable). It then synthesized these two models forming the synergistic model. After examining the model's strengths and weaknesses, it was argued that the synergistic model was a model that is able to unify moral philosophy into one collective whole. Mid-level principles were then shown to be a natural development in the practical usage of this model and the synergistic model was then justified pragmatically through the use of codes of ethics, Mill's utilitarianism, and rationally through the use of Kant's deontological ethics. Finally, the synergistic model was presented with a simple test case to see how one might practically use such a model.

[4:81] The synergistic model unifies moral philosophy into one collective whole. As a result, the synergistic model not only provides a clearer philosophical understanding of how moral decisions are in fact made, but, more importantly, it helps in the understanding of how moral agents ought to make moral decisions both individually and as members of a pluralistic society.

***

III. MORAL THEORY

Overview

[i:1]

This section focuses on the justifications for the development of mid-level principles both pragmatically and rationally. The pragmatic justification of mid-level principles will be made by appealing to how pluralistic groups do in fact make moral decisions focusing on codes of ethics and consequential evaluations. The rational justification of mid-level principles will be made by appealing to John Rawls' political framework and Immanuel Kant's *a priori* justifications.

[i:2] The fact that there are intersubjective cognitive agreements on the broad and general universal values of mid-level principles, makes it possible for pluralistic decision-making to occur even though there may be great differences in the beliefs of the individual members of the group.

I. Pragmatic Justifications Of Mid-Level Principles

A. Codes of ethics

[1:1] A pragmatic justification of mid-level principles is easiest to illustrate by discussing how pluralistic groups, or societies, do in fact make moral decisions. Since, by definition, it is impossible for pluralistic groups, or societies to come to an agreement on what is the appropriate "worldview," often times there will be a "code of ethics" upon which all participants will agree.

[1:2] The content of these "codes" will usually be mid-level principles that are either derivable from, consistent with or at least not in conflict with, every member's worldview. For example, it is not uncommon for a medical ethics committee to be composed of a multi-disciplinary and interprofessional team of doctors, nurses, social workers, psychologists, clergy, lay community persons, and even philosophers. Every one of these members has varying interests and concerns, and it would be futile to try to make everyone adopt a single worldview. However, by adopting a code of ethics, like Principlism, they find that there can be a very strong consensus on those principles that are essential for decision-making, or as Mill states, "human affairs which are classed, by universal or widely spread opinion, as just or as unjust."[1] Medical codes of ethics, for example, are now understood as the converging of various mid-level principles.

[1:3] Mill indicates that those who use different rationales can come to the same conclusion much like, for example, what happens when a pluralistic group adopts a code of ethics. Utilitarians, for example, have generally put more value on the "higher capacities" of the mind than on the physical or "lower capacities." Regardless of whether the value is based on the intrinsic nature of the "higher capacities" or their circumstantial advantages such as permanency, safety, uncostliness, etc. Either way, the utilitarians have proved their case whether using only quantitative distinctions, or by using both quantitative and qualitative distinc-

---

[1] Mill, *Utilitarianism,* Chapter 8; [5:16].

tions. The bottom line is that the rational for the choice of the mental pleasures over the bodily pleasures can be argued from either prudential advantages or because of its higher intrinsic value, i.e., different rationales can come to the same conclusion.[2]

[1:4] Once the pluralistic group has accepted the mid-level principles they are then able to start the process of specification, and weighing and balancing. Weighing and balancing being the process that attempts to establish the various rights and liberties; specification is the process in which mid-level principles are developed conceptually and shaped normatively so that they can be applied to the particular circumstance at hand.

B. Utilitarianism

1. Teleology

[1:5] Teleology as a descriptive doctrine argues that all of nature that includes intentional agents are goal directed or functionally organized and as such have moral consideration. Now this isn't to be confused with the theory of evolution that manifests itself in the non-teleological process of natural selection. Although it can be argued that all sentient beings respond or act in a teleological fashion, it does not follow that the behavior of sentient beings is in anyway in contradiction with the overall process of the non-purposive natural selection.

[1:6] One moral theory that falls under the category of teleology is utilitarianism. Utilitarianism is a consequential moral theory that aims at maximizing the end.

---

[2] Mill, *Utilitarianism,* Chapter 8; [2:22-24].
It must be admitted, however, that utilitarian writers in general have placed the superiority of mental over bodily pleasures chiefly in the greater permanency, safety, uncostliness, etc., of the former—that is, in their circumstantial advantages rather than in their intrinsic nature. And on all these points, utilitarians have fully proved their case; but they might have taken the other and, as it may be called, higher ground with entire consistency. It is quite compatible with the principle of utility to recognize the fact that some kinds of pleasure are more desirable and more valuable than others.

2. Defining the end before the right

[1:7] Utilitarianism holds that the defining of the end comes before the defining of right actions or rules. In other words, the end is defined independently from the right, and the right is then defined as that which maximizes the end. Therefore, if a person wishes to determine right actions, then they would have to first know what the end is that they are trying to pursue, then they would need to determine if the action that is being considered does in fact promote that end. For example, if the end is "the greatest amount of happiness for the greatest amount of people" then the right would be those actions or rules that would in fact result in the maximizing of the greatest amount of happiness for the greatest amount of people.

[1:8] An added complexity with utilitarianism is that the end can be maximized by the addition of quantitative and qualitative hedons, or units of pleasure.

a. Quantitative ends

[1:9] Quantitative ends are those pleasures or satisfactions—hedons, that maximize the total number of hedons in order to maximize the end of happiness.

b. Qualitative ends

[1:10] Qualitative ends are those ends that a person cannot have too much of. They are qualitative pleasures, that a person would not trade for any number of quantitative pleasures when maximizing the end of happiness.

Jeremy Bentham's utilitarianism argued for only quantitative pleasures. In contrast, John Stuart Mill's utilitarianism argued for both quantitative and qualitative pleasures.

3. Jeremy Bentham (1748-1832)

[1:11] In 1789 Bentham was enquiring as to what are the legitimate criteria for the acquiring of social rights? He argued that certainly the color of a person's skin does not distinguish a difference of kind between one human being and another. Even the degree of cognitive development does not distinguish a difference in kind as everyone will recognize that a full-grown horse or dog certainly has more cognitive development and communications than a young child. Bentham argued, and Mill continued to hold to this point of view, that the question is not whether or not a creature can reason or talk, rather the question is whether or not a creature can suffer. Moral considerations are not just for humans rather, moral considerations are for all sentient beings that can experience feelings.[3]

[1:12] Utilitarian morality in Bentham's view was quantitatively hedonistic. In other words, the moral rightness or wrongness of an action or rule he believed could be calculated using a hedonistic calculus, i.e., by simply summing up the pleasures and pains produced. If more pleasures were produced then the action tended towards moral rightness. If more pains were produced then the action tended towards moral wrongness. Some additional considerations that he thought may be necessary to consider were as follows:

[1:13]

1. **Intensity:** How strong would the pleasure or pain be?

2. **Duration:** How long would the pleasure or pain last?

3. **Propinquity or remoteness:** How soon would the pleasure or pain occur?

4. **Certainty or uncertainty:** What is the probability that the pleasure or pain would in fact occur?

---

[3] Bentham, *An Introduction to The Principles of Moral and Legislation,* 311n. The day may come when the rest of the animal creation may acquire those rights which could never have been witholden from them but by the hand of tyranny. The French have already discovered that the blackness of the skin is no reason why a human being should be abandoned without redress to the caprice of a tormentor. It may come one day to be recognized, that the number of legs, the villosity of the skin, or the termination of the *os sacrum,* are reasons equally insufficient for abandoning a sensitive being to the same fate. What else is it that should trace the insuperable line? Is it the faculty or reason, or, perhaps, the faculty of discourse? But a full-grown horse or dog is beyond comparison a more rational, as well as a more conversable, animal, than an infant of a day, or a week, or even a month, old. But suppose the case were otherwise, what would it avail? The question is not, *Can they reason?* Nor, *Can they talk?* But, *Can they suffer?*

5. **Fecundity:** What is the probability that the pleasure or pain would be followed by additional sensations of the same kind?

6. **Purity:** What is the probability that the pleasure or pain would be followed by additional sensations of the opposite kind?

4. John Stuart Mill, (1806-1873)

[1:15] John Stuart Mill, in contrast, held that there are not only quantitative pleasures but that there were also qualitative pleasures as well. A qualitative pleasure is a pleasure that an agent would not trade for any amount of a quantitative pleasures. The qualitative pleasure is preferable in kind, apart from the question of intensity. Mill held that the higher faculties of the mind were such qualitative pleasures. As Mill famously said,

> [1:16] "It is better to be a human being dissatisfied than a pig satisfied; better to be Socrates dissatisfied, than a fool satisfied. And if the fool, or the pig, are of a different opinion, it is because they only know their own side of the question. The other party to the comparison knows both sides." [4]

[1:17] Mill then argued that quantitative means are capable of becoming qualitative ends and that it is this psychological propensity of change in states that actually makes life interestingly diverse.

[1:18] Even power, money, and fame, which are clearly quantitative means, can become qualitative ends. However, unlike character traits such as virtue, which someone cannot have too much of, the other quantitative means that become qualitative ends must be limited. Take money for example, whose worth is solely based on its ability to satisfy a persons desire for material goods. After a period of time it is possible for money, that was once desired as an instrument for the attaining of happiness, to become desirable as an end in and of itself. In other words, acquiring money becomes part of the person's happiness or end. It is this psychological propensity for an action or activity that is a means to an end to become an end in and of itself, that gives life its in-

---

[4] Mill, *Utilitarianism,* Chapter 8; [2:38-40].

terest and variety. Purpose and meaning in life, becomes whatever meaning and purpose each individual develops as their end. However, Mill believed that there were some types of happiness that were more advantageous for both the individual and society such as virtue. The disinterested love of virtue is one such end, that no one can have too much of, whereas a person can have too much power, money and fame.[5]

[1:19] From this perspective, a person's quantitative use of "nature," for example, could be transformed into a conception of "nature" that is qualitative. Such transformations become a person's good or end, i.e., a person's meaning and purpose in life. An "end" is established when there is no answer to the question "why." In other words, the "end" is not a means to anything further, rather the end is an end in and of itself. To illustrate:

[1:20]

Q: Why do you go to school?
R: To get a degree.

Q: Why do you want a degree?
R: To get a job.

Q: Why do you want a job?
R: To make money.

Q: Why do you want to make money?
R: To provide for my family.

5 Mill, Utilitarianism, Chapter 8; [4:34-52].
Money's worth is solely that of the things to which it can buy … but money is, in many cases, desired in and for itself; the desire to possess it is often stronger than the desire to use it. … What was once desired as an instrument for the attainment of happiness has come to be desired for its own sake. In being desired for its own sake it is, however, desired as part of happiness. What was once desired as an instrument for the attainment of happiness has come to be desired for its own sake. … Life would be a poor thing, very ill provided with sources of happiness, if there were not this provision of nature. … Virtue is a good of this description. … The difference between virtue and the love of money, power, or fame is that they may, and often do, render the individual noxious to the other members of society to which he belongs, whereas there is nothing which makes him so much a blessing to them as the cultivation of the disinterested love of virtue.

Q: Why do you want to provide for your family?
R: Because it makes me happy.

Q: Why do you want to be happy?
R: Because I want to be happy … motivations go no further than happiness.

[1:21] There is no "reason" for happiness as happiness is not a means to anything else. Happiness is the end.

[1:22] Utilitarianism can also be thought of as having two major divisions: 1) act utilitarianism, and 2) rule utilitarianism.

[1:23] Act utilitarianism is the view that an act is morally obligatory to the extent that particular acts, maximizes the good or end. Since it is necessary to define the end before the right action can be determined and if the end is the maximizing of pleasure and the minimizing of pain, then the act that maximizes pleasure and minimizes pain will then be the morally correct action. Acts are not right or obligatory because of their inherent character, their underlying motives, or their relation to divine or social dictates, rather actions are morally right to the extent that they maximize pleasures and minimize pains.

[1:24] Rule utilitarianism, like all consequentialists, also defines the end prior to that of the right. However in this view, the rightness of an action depends on the consequences not of the action itself, but on the consequences of various sets of rules or principles of action. As Mill argues, the focus for the utilitarian is to universally maximize both quantitative and qualitative pleasures to the greatest extent possible, not just for mankind, but also for all sentient beings universally.[6]

[1:25] Many Utilitarians, such as John Stuart Mill, use a combination of Act and Rule Utilitarianism. Mill's Rule Utilitarianism is manifested in his principles of justice such as personal liberty, property, desert, good faith, impartiality, and equality.

[1:26] Like Hobbs, for example, Mill argues that personal security is the most vital of all social interests, and this security interest is something that no "fellow creature" can do without. The strong feelings associated with being secure, psychologically makes the end of safety, not a matter of degree, rather safety as an end becomes a real difference in kind, i.e., one which not just ought rarely if ever be violated but one which should never be violated, i.e., security as an end is absolute in nature for all fellow

---

[6] Mill, *Utilitarianism*, Chapter 8; [2:62-63].

According to the greatest happiness principle, as above explained, the ultimate end, with reference to and for the sake of which all other things are desirable—whether we are considering our own good or that of other people—is an existence exempt as far as possible from pain, and as rich as possible in enjoyments, both in point of quantity and quality; the test of quality and the rule for measuring it against quantity being the preference felt by those who, in their opportunities of experience, to which must be added their habits of self-consciousness and self-observation, are best furnished with the means of comparison.

This, being according to the utilitarian opinion the end of human action, is necessarily also the standard of morality, which may accordingly be defined "the rules and precepts for human conduct," by the observance of which an existence such as has been described might be, to the greatest extent possible, secured to all mankind; and not to them only, but, so far as the nature of things admits, to the whole sentient creation.

creatures.[7] Mill continues to argue that justice is based on two things, rules of conduct, and sentiments that sanction the rules which make the rules of justice different in kind from rules of social utility.[8] Justice collectively has a much higher scale of social utility than other moral considerations and therefore rarely if ever is overridden. But ultimately, under very improbably circumstances, the overriding of general maxims of justice could be justified.[9]

---

[7] Mill, *Utilitarianism*, Chapter 8; [5:145-150].

The interest involved is that of security, to everyone's feelings the most vital of all interests.

All other earthly benefits are needed by one person, but not needed by another; and many of them can, if necessary, be cheerfully foregone or replaced by something else; but security no human being can possibly do without; on it we depend for all our immunity from evil and for the whole value of all and every good, beyond the passing moment, since nothing but the gratification of the instant could be of any worth to us if we could be deprived of everything the next instant by whoever was momentarily stronger than ourselves.

Our notion, therefore, of the claim we have on our fellow creatures to join in making safe for us the very groundwork of our existence gathers feelings around it so much more intense than those concerned in any of the more common cases of utility that the difference in degree (as is often the case in psychology) becomes a real **difference in kind**.

The claim assumes that character of absoluteness, that apparent infinity and incommensurability with all other considerations which constitute the distinction between the feeling of right and wrong and that of ordinary expediency and inexpediency.

The feelings concerned are so powerful, and we count so positively on finding a responsive feeling in others (all being alike interested) that *ought* and *should* grow into *must*, and recognized indispensability becomes a moral necessity, analogous to physical, and often not inferior to it in binding force.

[8] Mill, *Utilitarianism*, Chapter 8, [5:127].

… justice supposes two things—a rule of conduct and a sentiment which sanctions the rule.

[9] Mill, *Utilitarianism*, Chapter 8, [5:239-241].

Justice is a name for certain moral requirements which, regarded collectively, stand higher in the scale of social utility, and are therefore of more paramount obligation, than any others, though particular cases may occur in which some other social duty is so important as to overrule any one of the general maxims of justice. Thus, to save a life, it may not only be allowable, but a duty, to steal or take by force the necessary food or medicine, or to kidnap and compel to officiate the only qualified medical practitioner. In such cases, as we do not call anything justice which is not a virtue, we usually say, not that justice must give way to some other moral principle, but that what is just in an ordinary case is, by reason of that other principle, not just in the particular case.

[1:27] The argument can easily be made that security is of vital interests not just to human beings, rather security is a vital interest to all sentient-beings that can experience such a sentiment. Much like all sentient beings avoid pain and pursue pleasure so also the lack of security is avoided as a kind of pain, and security is pursued as a kind of pleasure.

a. Criticisms Against Utilitarianism

[1:29] Some of the most common objections made against the utilitarian hedonistic calculus are 1) aggregate utility criticism, 2) average utility criticism, 3) justice criticism, and 4) motive criticism.

1) Aggregate Utility Criticism:

[1:30] The aggregate utility criticism is that if the hedonistic calculus is primarily concerned with the total summation of pleasure, then there could arise a moral mandate to decrease the total amount of pleasure each individual experiences as long as that action or rule is compensated by increasing the total number of individual experiencers. For example, suppose we have 10 individuals who each experience 10 hedons of pleasure for a total of 100 hedons. Using aggregate utility, if an action or rule would decrease each individual's experience to 8 hedons of pleasure but the population was increased to 13 then the total amount of hedons experienced would be 104 hedons justifying the action or rule. In fact, using the aggregate utility to the extreme, it would be justifiable to decrease each individual's experience to 1 hedon of pleasure as long as the population was increased to 101, for a total amount of hedons experienced being 101.

[1:31] The aggregate utility criticism argues that the hedonistic calculus could result in unacceptable low levels of experienced pleasures as long as it was compensated by an increase in population of the experiencing group.

[1:32] This type of thinking could, for example, easily justify the current methods used for factory farming, especially if pain and suffering is not considered.

2) Average Utility Criticism:

[1:33] The average utility criticism could be used as a response to the aggregate utility criticism. Average utility argues that what is important is not the total amount of hedons experienced, rather the hedonistic calculus needs to determine what action or rule produces the greatest average utility for the hedonistic experiencers. However, unlike the aggregate utility criticism where increasing the number of experiencers of hedons seems to be more important than increasing each individual's total amount of hedons, average utility results in focusing the importance of decreasing the total amount of experiencers so as to maximize the average number of hedons the remaining members experience. For example, suppose like above we have 10 individuals who each experience 10 hedons of pleasure for a total of 100 hedons. Using average utility, if an action or rule would increase each individual's experience to 12 hedons of pleasure but the population was decreased to 9 then the total amount of hedons experienced would be 108 hedons justifying the action or rule. In fact, using the average utility to the extreme, it would be justifiable to increase an individual's experience to 101 hedons of pleasure even if it resulted in the extermination of all but one individual, as the total amount of hedons experienced would be 101.

[1:34] The average utility criticism argues that the hedonistic calculus could, for example, result in mass exterminations of groups or species, or could result in actions that would eliminate those whose happiness is below average.

3) Justice Criticism:

[1:35] The justice criticism builds on the aggregate utility criticism and the average utility criticism arguing that the hedonistic calculus could justify unjust distributions of pleasures. For example, suppose like above there are 10 individuals who each experience 10 hedons of pleasure for a total of 100 hedons. However, if an action or rule would increase 6 individuals pleasure to 11 hedons yet decrease each of the other 4 individual's experience to 9 hedons of pleasure then the total amount of hedons experienced would be 102 hedons justifying the action or rule. In fact, going to the extreme, it would be justifiable, or at least neutral, to increase the 6 individual's pleasures to 16 hedons even if it meant decreasing each of the remaining 4 individual's experience to 1 hedon of pleasure resulting in a total amount of hedons experienced being 100 or the same aggregate of the initial distribution.

[1:36] The justice criticism may not result in increases or decreases of populations, though those issues are also arguably justice topics, rather in this instance the argument is that the hedonistic calculus could result in unequal and unfair distributions of pleasure and pain within the group for no apparent rational or fair reasons.

[1:37] The justice criticism argues that utilitarianism could result in the justification of unjust actions such as enslaving 10% of the population for the greater benefit of 90% of the population, i.e., the "greatest good for the greatest amount of people."

[1:38] Suffering of a limited amount of animals, for the amusement of a much larger number of spectators, such as what occurs in rodeo's, could possibly be justified under such a hedonistic calculus so the criticism claims.

4) Motive Criticism:

[1:39] The motive criticism argues that if in utilitarianism it is the end result that determines the moral rightness or wrongness of an action, such as the greatest happiness principle, or some other positive consequence, then the motive of the agent becomes totally irrelevant in the determination of the morality of the action. Someone could "push the red button" with the intent of polluting or destroying the world, yet if the opposite happened because of some unforeseeable causes then that action would be a morally praiseworthy action even though the motive was abominable. This criticism argues that certainly morality must include the agent's motive and to the extent that utilitarianism does not do so, and only focuses on the consequences, so also utilitarianism fails to be a sufficiently comprehensive moral theory.

b. Responses to the Utilitarian Criticisms

[1:40] The aggregate utility criticism, average utility criticism, justice criticism, and motive criticism are all "straw-man" fallacies of logic.

1) Jeremy Bentham

[1:41] Jeremy Bentham would have categorized the aggregate and average utility problems as a problem of justice and that social justice does in fact result in significant increases in pleasure and reductions of pain. In other words, Bentham would have said that if the hypothetical results presented seem unfair, unjust, or just plain "wrong" then more than likely those hypothetical scenarios are not probable and a correct hedonistic calculus of the scenario would have come up with a totally different calculus.

[1:42] Just as individuals can make mathematical errors, so also individuals can make hedonistic calculus errors. Possible counter examples do not necessary result in probable counter examples.

2) John Stuart Mill

[1:43] John Stuart Mill's response would also be that the aggregate utility, average utility, and justice problems are all "straw-man" fallacy arguments. John Stuart Mill clearly would have argued that there are quantitative and qualitative distinctions of pleasures and pains and that they need to be taken into account when making a hedonistic calculus. Justice, for John Stuart Mill qualitatively outweighs any number of quantitative pleasures. Mill argues in chapter five of *Utilitarianism* that rules of justice are more absolute than any other considerations and that the rules of justice are no longer a matter of degree but become absolute in nature as a matter of kind, a type of qualitative pleasure. Therefore, if an action or rule would ultimately violate the qualitative ends of justice, then that action or rule would be considered to be immoral.[10]

[1:44] Therefore the criticism made against utilitarianism that the theory could result in the justification of unjust actions such as enslaving 10% of the population for the greater benefit of 90% of the population, i.e., the "greatest good for the greatest amount of people" certainly is a misrepresentation of John Stuart Mill's Utilitarianism. Mill would argue that personal liberty of everyone is as close to an absolute rule as you can get and is essentially a necessary element for social structure, or social contract, and that the above criticism is therefore a straw-man argument. Principles of justice, such as a constitution, are such absolute rules that are very rarely over-ridden and if they are it is not on the basis of justification of unjust actions, rather what is just in one circumstance may be unjust in a different circumstance.

[1:45] Mill argues that these "absolute" rules of justice are in fact the necessary qualitative components for the "greatest good for the greatest amount of people," or in this context the "greatest good for the greatest amount of sentient beings."

[1:46] Lastly, with regard to the "bad motive" but "good consequences" criticism, here are just a couple of quotes from Mill that addresses this "straw-man" fallacy. This first quote accentuates the importance of equal consideration, of all sentient beings.

> [1:47] "As between his own happiness and that of others, utilitarianism requires him to be as strictly impartial as a disinterested and benevolent spectator. In the golden rule of Jesus of Nazareth, we read the complete spirit of the ethics of utility. "To do as you would be done by," "to love

---

[10] Mill, *Utilitarianism*, Chapter 8, [5:246].
Justice remains the appropriate name for certain social utilities which are vastly more important, and therefore more absolute and imperative, than any others are as a class (though not more so than others may be in particular cases); and which, therefore, ought to be, as well as naturally are, guarded by a sentiment, **not only different in degree, but also in kind**; distinguished from the milder feeling which attaches to the mere idea of promoting human pleasure or convenience at once by the more definite nature of its commands and by the sterner character of its sanctions.

your neighbor as yourself," constitute the ideal perfection of utilitarian morality."[11]

[1:48] Bentham and Mill argued that all sentient beings ought to be given moral consideration not just in terms of good consequences but also with regard to motives as well. In fact it is very difficult to separate the motive of the action from the action itself. For example, Mill argues that the golden rule of do unto others as you would have them do unto you and to love your neighbor as you love yourself, is the complete spirit, or motive of the ethics of utility.[12] Perhaps this is because virtue or motive does in fact have significant consequential results or maybe it is because virtue or motive is a qualitative end. However, whatever utilitarian argument you make based on quantitative or qualitative arguments you will still come to the same universal conclusion of the golden rule.[13]

[1:49] Mill then goes on to address the complaint that this utilitarian requirement is way too rigorous and demanding to be practical. Mill agrees that the motive does not determine the morality of the action, yet also clearly states that the motive does determine the worth of the agent, which is very important, espe-

[11] Mill, *Utilitarianism*, Chapter 8, [2:115].

[12] Mill, *Utilitarianism*, Chapter 8, [2:115].
As between his own happiness and that of others, utilitarianism requires him to be as strictly impartial as a disinterested and benevolent spectator. In the golden rule of Jesus of Nazareth, we read the complete spirit of the ethics of utility. "To do as you would be done by," "to love your neighbor as yourself," constitute the ideal perfection of utilitarian morality.

[13] Mill, *Utilitarianism*, Chapter 8, [2:22].
It must be admitted, however, that utilitarian writers in general have placed the superiority of mental over bodily pleasures chiefly in the greater permanency, safety, uncostliness, etc., of the former—that is, in their circumstantial advantages rather than in their intrinsic nature. And on all these points, utilitarians have fully proved their case; but they might have taken the other and, as it may be called, higher ground with entire consistency. It is quite compatible with the principle of utility to recognize the fact that some kinds of pleasure are more desirable and more valuable than others.

cially if you are the agent or you are part of the society that depends on the behavior of the agent.[14]

[1:50] Most actions are done for the benefits of individuals that comprise the world at large, thus making utilitarianism a very practical moral theory. In other words, very rarely are there any individuals that will be in a position to act in such a way that will consequentially have a significant influence to the world at large.

[1:51] If individuals are most effective in their moral actions with regard to those who are in a closer relationship with them, then utilitarianism concludes that in those circumstances, they have a higher moral obligation to maximize those individual relational benefits rather than focusing on their ineffective abilities to influence the world at large.

[1:52] The world at large is in fact composed of individual parts, in which all individual interactions are a significant part of the collective whole." [15]

[1:53] Although there may be other criticisms made against various types of consequentialistic and utilitarian moral theories, it is clear that the aggregate, average, justice, and motive criticisms fail as "straw-man" fallacies when addressed towards classic utilitarians such as Jeremy Bentham and John Stuart Mill.

---

[14] Mill, *Utilitarianism*, Chapter 8, [2:125].
... utilitarian moralists have gone beyond almost all others in affirming that the motive has nothing to do with the morality of the action, though much with the worth of the agent.

[15] Mill, *Utilitarianism*, Chapter 8, [2:126-128].
He who saves a fellow creature from drowning does what is morally right, whether his motive be duty or the hope of being paid for his trouble; he who betrays the friend that trusts him is guilty of a crime, even if his object be to serve another friend to whom he is under greater obligations.
But to speak only of actions done from the motive of duty, and in direct obedience to principle: it is a misapprehension of the utilitarian mode of thought to conceive it as implying that people should fix their minds upon so wide a generality as the world, or society at large.
The great majority of good actions are intended not for the benefit of the world, but for that of individuals, of which the good of the world is made up; and the thoughts of the most virtuous man need not on these occasions travel beyond the particular persons concerned, except so far as is necessary to assure himself that in benefiting them he is not violating the rights, that is, the legitimate and authorized expectations, of anyone else.

C. Universalizability

[1:55] Universalizability is usually associated with the classic deontologist Immanuel Kant. Kant, in his Doctrine of Right, argues for the universal principle of autonomy:

> [1:56] "Any action is right if it can coexist with everyone's freedom in accordance with a universal law, or if on its maxim the freedom of choice of each can coexist with everyone's freedom in accordance with a universal law." [16]

Kant, in his Doctrine of Virtue, argues that:

> [1:57] "The supreme principle of the doctrine of virtue is: act in accordance with a maxim of ends that it can be a universal law for everyone to have." [17]

[1:58] The principle of universalizability is also clearly evident with John Stuart Mill's utilitarianism. Mill, in his book *Utilitarianism* argues for the universal principle or rule of nonmaleficence in the following:

> [1:59] "In the case of abstinences indeed—of things which people forbear to do from moral considerations, though the consequences in the particular case might be beneficial—it would be unworthy of an intelligent agent not to be consciously aware that the action is of a class which, if practiced generally, would be generally injurious, and that this is the ground of the obligation to abstain from it. … [E]very systems of morals … enjoin to abstain from whatever is manifestly pernicious to society." [18]

[1:60] Mill also argues for the universal principle of beneficence in the following:

> "In the golden rule of Jesus of Nazareth, we read the complete spirit of the ethics of utility. 'To do as you would be done by,' and 'to love your neighbor as yourself,' constitute the ideal perfection of utilitarian morality." [19]

---

[16] Kant, *The Metaphysics of Morals; Doctrine of Right*, p. 24, [6:230].

[17] Kant, *The Metaphysics of Morals; Doctrine of Virtue*, p. 157, [6:395].

[18] Mill, *Utilitarianism*, Chapter 8, [2:131-132].

[19] Mill, *Utilitarianism*, Chapter 8, [2:116-117].

[1:61] Principlism with its universality and its resultant concepts of equality is clearly represented by both Kant and Mill. Whether or not this agreement gives Principlism more regard is another issue. However, it does show that mid-level principles are clearly recognized as derivable from, consistent with, or at least not in contradiction with some of the most significant western moral systems of morality.

II. Rational Justification Of Mid-Level Principles

A. John Rawls

[2:1] John Rawls' social political framework is a theoretical model that clearly supports the development of mid-level principles as presented in his books, *A Theory of Justice,*[20] and *Political Liberalism.*[21]

1. Diagram

[2:2]

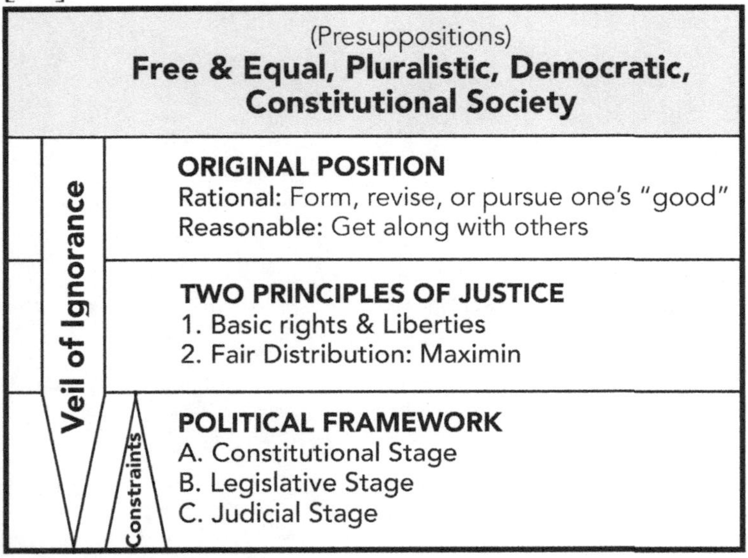

a. Presuppositions

[2:3] Rawls puts forth a hypothetical scenario in which he presupposes that there are individuals who live within a pluralistic, free and equal, democratic, constitutional society.

b. Rational and Reasonable Citizens

[2:4] He further presupposes that all the individuals in this hypothetical society are persons, that are rational and reasonable, (*ra-*

---

[20] John Rawls, *A Theory of Justice,* …

[21] John Rawls, *Political Liberalism,* …

tional meaning the ability to form, revise, or pursue one's "good," i.e., one's "purpose and meaning of life," and reasonable meaning having the ability to get along with others). Rawls then presents us with the task of determining what principles of justice should be adopted for the citizens of this society if we were to be their representatives.

c. Veil of Ignorance

[2:5] To make sure that we do this fairly, Rawls puts us, or the representatives, behind a "veil of ignorance," called the "original position," in which all that is known is that the individual(s) that are represented are rational and reasonable as above defined. The task is to make sure that the citizen(s) have the "basic goods" that would be necessary for the continuation or development of their rational and reasonable states.

d. Two Principles of Justice

[2:6] Rawls argues that from this original position, it would be logically consistent to construct principles of justice that would ensure those necessary "basic goods." Rawls comes up with the following *Two Principles of Justice*, which are in hierarchical order. (Hierarchical order meaning; that 1. the first principle of justice must be established before establishing the second principle of justice, and 2. the first principle of justice can never be violated or infringed upon by the second principle of justice, or anything else lower in hierarchy). The *Two Principles of Justice* is summarily given as follows: 1. The establishment of basic rights and liberties through the process of reflective-equilibrium,[22] and 2. If there is going to be any unequal distribution it must benefit all, or at minimum the least well off, i.e., maximization of the minimal condition—maximin. These two complementary principles of justice can be interpreted as being a type of mid-level principles.

[2:7] The first principle of justice comes about by a.) looking at what rights and liberties have historically worked well for

---

[22] Rawls is the author of the term reflective-equilibrium.

democracy, b.) intuitions,[23] and c.) trial and error. These rights and liberties are then justified through a process of reflective-equilibrium—a back and forth process between theory, mid-level principles, intuitions, and practical application. Through this process of reflective-equilibrium, the specific rights and liberties become established and they mutually constrain each other.

[2:8] The second principle of justice is the distributive principle that utilizes the maximin principle, i.e., maximizes or improves the worse-off condition. In doing this, Rawls is not a "pure" egalitarian in that he does allow unequal distributions of "social goods" as long as it benefits all, especially the least well off. However, because of the hierarchical order, the distribution cannot violate any of the basic rights or liberties under the first principle of justice when implementing the distributive principles of the second principle of justice.

e. Political Framework

[2:9] Once the two principles of justice are established, Rawls believes that it is then logical to construct a just political framework that would be composed of the *Constitutional Stage, the Legislative Stage,* and the *Judicial Stage*. The *Constitutional Stage* is responsible for the specifying and balancing of the basic rights and liberties of the first principle of justice. The *Legislative Stage* is responsible for the specifying and balancing of the distributive aspects of the second principle of justice. Lastly the *Judicial Stage* would apply all of the above to actual specific situations. All the steps are in hierarchical order and the veil of ignorance gets thinner as one goes from the constitutional stage to the legislative stage and finally to the judicial stage where there is no veil. This "thinning" of the veil of ignorance is essential as the situations become more and more specific at each successive stage and therefore more knowledge is required. Also as the veil of ignorance thins, the additive constraints of the political framework increases. The resultant hierarchical ordering is a protective mechanism that makes sure that the basic rights and liberties that

[23] Rawls actually talks about "lucky guesses" which is a "type" of intuition.

are the necessary "goods" for the development of rational and reasonable citizens are not infringed upon.

[2:10] Rawls begins his political framework with certain presuppositions, and from there constructs the two principles of justice, constitution stage, legislative stage, and judicial stage using essentially the synergistic model. It is also important to note that Rawls' political framework is not "*the* framework" but only one of many possible frameworks that can be constructed through the use of this synergistic model.

2. Mid-level Principles

[2:11] Through this process of building this just political framework, it seems that Rawls' two principles of justice can be considered to be a type of mid-level principles. These mid-level principles are then to be specified and balanced using a process analogous to the synergistic model and implemented by the three branches of government.

B. Deontological Ethics

[2:13] Deontological ethics are moral theories according to which certain acts must or must not be done because it is one's duty to do so.

[2:14] Deontological theories either specify the good or end independently from the right, or deontological theories do not interpret the right as necessarily maximizing the end. In contrast, utilitarianism starts with determining the end and then the right is that which promotes or maximizes the end.

[2:15] For deontological theories you determine the right by *a priori* reasoning and the moral agent then has a duty to perform such actions or maxims of actions independently of the end.

[2:16] Deontological theories come in a variety of forms depending on what "formal criteria" is being used for its development. Some classic examples of formal criteria that have been used for deontological theories are; 1. intuitions, 2. divine command, 3. universal law, and 4. contractarianism.

1. Intuitionism:

[2:17] Axiomatic system of self-evident truths using not only first principles of a deductive system but also using principles whose truth can be seen immediately upon reflection. Like the mathematical axioms of addition, subtraction, multiplication, division, and equality, which cannot be proven but are known to be true based on being self-evident, so also duties may likewise be self-evident.

[2:18] Just as mathematics which uses unprovable axioms as first principles has not diminished the reliability of mathematics so also morality that is based on unproven self-evident duties or intuitions is not diminished in reliability because of its unproven first principles.

2. Divine Command:

[2:19] Moral principles are taken to be laws issued by God to humanity, and their authority thus derives from God's supremacy.

3. Universal Law:

[2:20] Moral principles are based on the formal criteria of either universal freedom for the social political context of rights, or universal maxims of actions for the personal context of virtue.

4. Contractarianism:

[2:21] Moral principles represent the ideal terms of social cooperation for people who live together in fellowship, and regard each other as "equals"—sociological fairness. Authority is based on group consensus.

C. Kantian Morality:

[2:23] Immanuel Kant, 1724–1804, is the most famous of the deontological ethicists.

Kant wrote three treatises on ethics:

1. Groundwork of the Metaphysics of Morals, 1785
2. Critique of Practical Reason, 1788
3. Metaphysics of Morals, 1797

[2:24] Depending on the subject being addressed, it appears that Kant appeals to each of the varieties of deontological theories as presented above.

[2:25] In the *Metaphysics of Morals,* Kant's latest and most mature work on ethics, he divides his text into two parts: Doctrine of Right, and the Doctrine of Virtue. He argues that in ancient times there was just morality in general. However as time progressed it was considered helpful to divide up the single category of morality into two divisions: civil rights, that focuses on external laws and coercion, and virtue, that focuses on all that is not based on civil rights, i.e., not based on external laws and coercion.[24]

1. The Doctrine of Right

[2:26] The Doctrine of Right is Kant's social and political position on how the formal criteria of universal freedom, or autonomy ought to be used in the development of civil laws in order to attain the final end of social peace, as determined by reciprocity, and motivated by external coercion. That which is civilly wrong is that which hinders the universal freedom or autonomy, i.e., social rights, and that which is civilly right is that which hinders the hindering of universal freedom or autonomy, i.e., external coercion. This *a priori* structure of civil rights is necessary no matter how developed or perfected a society becomes as there

---

[24] Kant, *The Metaphysics of Morals; Doctrine of Virtue,* p. 145, [6:379].
In ancient times "ethics" signified the doctrine of morality in general, which was also called the doctrine of duties. Later on it seemed better to reserve the name "ethics"[or virtue] for one part of moral philosophy, namely for the doctrine of those duties that do not come under external laws. Accordingly, the system of the doctrine of duties in general is now divided into the system of the doctrine of right, which deals with duties that can be given by external laws, and the system of the doctrine of virtue/ethics, which treats of duties that cannot be so given.

will always be legitimate conflicts of interests because there will always be limited resources and a need for arbitration.[25]

[2:27] In other words, even if civil beings were to be "perfected" there would still be a need for a public lawful condition enforced by the application of external coercion. Beings, no matter how perfected, must leave the individual state of nature and bind themselves to the social civil condition. If beings do not leave this individual state of nature, it may not necessarily be an unjust arrangement, yet it would at the very minimum be a state devoid of justice, which is an unacceptable condition as there will always arise legitimate conflicts of rights even in a perfected state of nature. Therefore it is permissible to force all citizens to create a social contract and then make the citizens conform or abide to the social contract mandates by coercion if necessary.[26]

[2:28] The civil condition is thought of by pure rational concepts alone—*a priori* and the teleological end, "the entire final end" is "perpetual peace" which is the only state that secures what is mine and what is yours in a constitutional state. Regardless of whether or not perpetual peace is real or fiction, society needs to construct the political framework in such a way that it promotes perpetual peace putting an end to the heinous waging of war.

---

[25] Kant, *The Metaphysics of Morals; Doctrine of Right*, pp. 89-90, [6:312].
It is not experience from which we learn of human beings' maxim of violence and of their malevolent tendency to attack one another before external legislation endowed with power appears. On the contrary, however well disposed and law abiding men might be, it still lies *a priori* in the rational idea of such a condition that before a public lawful condition is established individual human beings, peoples and states can never be secure against violence from one another, since each has its own right to do what seems right and good to it and not to be dependent upon another's opinion about this. … [individual beings] must leave the state of nature, in which each follows its own judgment, unite itself with all others, subject itself to a public lawful external coercion … determined by law, … i.e. … a civil condition

[26] Ibid., p. 90, [6:312].
It is true that the state of nature need not, just because it is natural, be a state of injustice, of dealing with one another only in terms of the degree of force each has. But it would still be a state devoid of justice, in which when rights are in dispute, there would be no judge competent to render a verdict having rightful force. Hence each may impel the other by force to leave this state and enter into a rightful condition. …

[2:29] Peace is not just part of civil rights it is the entire final end. In order to attain the end of peace, in a society in which people live in close proximity with each other requires a constitutional framework.[27]

[2:30] In the Doctrine of Right using rational—*a priori* moral reasoning it is a logically self-evident principle that an action or rule is right if it can coexist with everyone's freedom.[28]

[2:31] And when dealing with the doctrine of right, or civil law, the motivation for compliance is coercion.[29] Civil law is not meant to teach virtue but only to determine what is right.

[2:32] When legislating laws and punishment for noncompliance, it is not a contradiction of universal freedom to take away the freedom of an individual that violates other individual's freedoms. In fact society has a moral obligation to coerce violators of

---

[27] Ibid., p. 123, [6:354].
Now morally practical reason pronounces in us its irresistible veto: there is to be no war. ...The question is no longer whether perpetual peace is something real or a fiction, ... Instead, we must act as if it is something real, though perhaps it is not; we must work toward establishing perpetual peace and the kind of constitution that seems to us most conducive to it in order to bring about perpetual peace and put an end to the heinous waging of war...For this is our duty, ...
It can be said that establishing universal and lasting peace constitutes not merely a part of the doctrine of right but rather the entire final end of the doctrine of right within the limits of reason alone; for the condition of peace is the only condition in which what is mine and what is yours are secured under laws for a multitude of human beings living in proximity to one another and therefore under a constitution.

[28] Kant, *The Metaphysics of Morals; Doctrine of Right*, p. 24, [6:230].
Any action is right if it can coexist with everyone's freedom in accordance with a universal law, or if on its maxim the freedom of choice of each can coexist with everyone's freedom in accordance with a universal law.

[29] Ibid., p. 25, [6:231].
When one's aim is not to teach virtue but only to set forth what is right, one may not and should not represent that the law of right as itself the incentive to action. ... [coercion is].

the law based on the principle of universal freedom.[30] Having civil rights and having the authorization to use coercion are one and the same thing.[31] Freedom that is compatible with the freedom of others is the only original right belonging to all.[32]

[2:33] And in terms of civil rights, if someone has never affected the civil rights of others then that person has not done anyone any civil wrong.[33] The underlying principle in civil law is the principle of reciprocity or social contract. If someone violates someone else's civil rights then that person loses his or her civil rights. Reciprocity arises from a universal rule.[34]

[2:34] Kant in his Doctrine of Right argues for the necessity of a civil constitution, based on universal freedom, reciprocity, and

---

[30] Ibid., p. 25, [6:231].
Resistance that counteracts the hindering of an effect promotes this effect and is consistent with it. Now whatever is wrong is a hindrance to freedom in accordance with universal laws. Therefore, ... coercion that is opposed to this is consistent with freedom in accordance with universal law, that is, it is right. Hence there is connected with right by the principle of contradiction an authorization to coerce someone who infringes upon it.

[31] Ibid., pp. 25-26, [6:232].
Strict right rests on the principle of its being possible to use external constraint that can coexist with the freedom of everyone in accordance with universal laws. ... Right and authorization to use coercion therefore mean one and the same thing.
The law of a reciprocal coercion necessarily in accord with the freedom of everyone under the principle of universal freedom is, as it were, the construction of that concept.

[32] Ibid., p. 30, [6:237].
Freedom, insofar as it can coexist with the freedom of everyone in accordance with a universal law, is the only original right belonging to every man by virtue of his humanity.

[33] Ibid., p. 30, [6:238].
...before [a human being] performs any act affecting rights he has done no wrong to anyone; being authorized to do to others anything that does not in itself diminish what is theirs.

[34] Ibid., pp. 44-45, [6:255-6:256].
I am therefore not under obligation to leave external objects belonging to others untouched unless everyone else provides me assurance that he will behave in accordance with the same principle with regard to what is mine. This assurance does not require a special act to establish a right, but is already contained in the concept of an obligation corresponding to an external right, since the universality, and with it the reciprocity, of obligation arises from a universal rule.

external coercion, establishing that the sole and final end is peace.

2. The Doctrine of Virtue

[2:36] Kant in his Doctrine of Virtue goes beyond the Doctrine of Right by arguing that *a priori* reasoning results in ends as duties that must be freely chosen, without any external coercion as motivation. Those ends that are also duties are one's own perfection and the happiness of others.[35]

[2:37] With civil rights others can be constrained to perform certain actions. With virtue constraint is not a part, as virtue deals with the duty of choosing moral ends, and choice of moral ends cannot be coerced rather they can only be freely chosen.[36]

[2:38] In the Doctrine of Right, or civil rights, the legislative end is peace by the promotion of universal freedoms. Citizens are allowed the freedom to use their free choice to choose whatever end(s) they wish to pursue as long as the citizens conform to the law even if coercion is necessary. Conversely, in the Doctrine of Virtue there is never any external coercion used for compliance.

---

[35] Kant, *The Metaphysics of Morals; Doctrine of Virtue*, p. 146, [6:380].
The doctrine of right dealt only with the formal condition of outer freedom (the consistency of outer freedom with itself if its maxim were made into a universal law), that is, with right. But ethics goes beyond this and provides an object of free choice, an end of pure reason which it represents as an end that is also objectively necessary, that is, an end that, as far as human beings are concerned, it is a duty to have.

[36] Ibid., p. 146, [6:381].
I can indeed be constrained by others to perform actions that are directed as means to an end, but I can never be constrained by others to have an end: only I myself can make something my end. ...That ethics contain duties that one cannot be constrained by other to fulfill follows merely from its being a doctrine of ends, since coercion to ends is self-contradictory.

Rather self-constraint by awe of ones freedom is the only motive that has any moral worth.[37]

[2:39] Civil law starts with peace as the social end and then creates a framework of justice with legislation that maximizes the universal freedom of all citizens by particular actions. What ends a citizen holds to, is left totally up to the individual's free choice, as long as it is compatible with the freedom of others.[38]

[2:40] Virtue starts with *a priori* maxims of actions, or general mid-level principles, then from there the moral agent derives ends that moral agents have a duty to seek out.

[2:41] Kant argues that choosing a good or end is an activity of freedom, and as such, ends can never be coerced. You can force someone to conform to actions such as civil laws, but you can never force someone to adopt a moral end. But even more interesting is that in the Doctrine of Virtue there must be some ends that are not practical, ends that can be recognized by pure *a priori* reasoning if there is to be a categorical imperative. And the ends that are also duties, are self-perfection and the happiness of others.[39]

[2:42] There is no duty to perfect others as self-perfection is an individual act of freedom and so it is impossible to perfect another. This self-perfection will be manifested as the agent diminishes

---

[37] Ibid., p. 147, [6:382].
One can think of the relation of an end to a duty in two ways: One can begin with the end [perpetual peace] and seek out the maxim of actions in conformity with duty or on the other hand, one can begin with the maxim of actions in conformity with duty and seek out the end that is also a duty. In the doctrine of right, what end anyone wants to set for his action is left to his free choice. The maxim of his action, however, is determined *a priori*, namely, that the freedom of the agent could coexist with the freedom of every other in accordance with a universal law.

[38] Ibid., p. 148, [6:383].
But ethics takes the opposite way.
... what essentially distinguishes a duty of virtue from a duty of right is that external constraint to the latter kind of duty is morally possible, whereas the former is based only on free self-constraint.

[39] Ibid., p. 150-151, [6:386-6:357].
What Are the Ends That Are Also Duties?
They are one's own perfection and the happiness of others.

their ignorance and as they cultivate a pure virtuous disposition. There is also no duty for one's own happiness, only for the happiness of others, as individuals already pursue their own happiness by the inclinations of nature.[40]

[2:43] What does the end of self-perfection entail? Self-perfection is the harmony of the agent's properties with an end. Self-perfection of the mental faculties would entail the maximization of understanding and the minimization of ignorance. Self-perfection of the will would be the development of the purest virtuous disposition in which the motivation for compliance to the moral agents' self-legislation is the sublime awe of recognizing that they themselves are not only the source of the moral legislation but that they have the ability to self-legislate, independently of inclination, i.e., by pure *a priori* determination.[41,42]

---

[40] Ibid., p. 149, [6:384-6:385].
An end is an object of free choice. ... Every action, therefore, has its end; and since no one can have an end without himself making the object of his choice into an end, to have any end of action whatsoever is an act of freedom on the part of the acting subject, not an effect of nature. But because this act which determines an end is a practical principle that prescribes the end itself, not the means, it is a categorical imperative of pure practical reason. ... Since there are free actions there must also be ends to which, as their object these actions are directed. But among these ends there must be some that are also duties.— For were there no such ends, then all ends would hold for practical reason only as means to other ends; and since there can be no action without an end, a categorical imperative would be impossible. This would do away with any doctrine of morals.

[41] Ibid., p. 150, [6:386].
One's own perfection...[qualitative (formal) perfection] as a concept belonging to teleology, it is taken to mean the harmony of a thing's properties with an end. ... cultivating one's faculties, the highest of which is understanding. At the same time this duty includes the cultivation of one's will. ... A human being (1) has a duty to diminish his ignorance, and (2) carry the cultivation of his will up to the purest virtuous disposition, in which the law becomes also the incentive to his actions that conform with duty and he obeys the law from duty. This disposition is inner morally practical perfection.

[42] Ibid., p. 152, [6:389].
Only the concept of an end that is also a duty, a concept that belongs exclusively to ethics, establishes a law for maxims of actions by subordinating the subjective end (that everyone has) to the objective end (that everyone ought to make his end). ... No free action is possible unless the agent also intends an end (which is the matter of choice.)

[2:44] The Doctrine of Virtue is also very different from the Doctrine of Right in that in the Doctrine of Right legislation prescribes precisely what the action that is being legislated is and the penalties for violation.

[2:45] In the Doctrine of Virtue, only the maxim of actions—not actions, or broad general principles, are being prescribed and how an individual fulfills the maxim is determined by the agent's judgment giving the moral agent playroom for free choice in following the ethical law.

[2:46] Take beneficence (do good), for example. There may be an obligation to be charitable but how an agent is to be charitable with regard to time, labor, or money is self-determined and to whom the agent is to be charitable to is also left to the agent's judgment. This is defined as an imperfect duty in that duties of virtue do not specify what actions are to be done and to whom those actions should be directed.

[2:47] These imperfect duties of virtue also require that the moral agent not only specify the broad moral principles or maxims of actions, but that the agent also balance those principles with regard to other maxims of actions or principles, such as love of one's neighbor with love of one's parents.[43]

[2:48] With perfect duties the individual knows exactly what action they are required to perform, and to whom the action is to be directed towards.

[2:49] Perfect duties are duties of civil rights. Imperfect duties are duties of virtue.[44] "The supreme principle of the doctrine of

---

[43] Ibid., p. 153, [6:390].
...[Ethical] laws can prescribe only the maxim of actions, not action themselves, this is a sign that it leaves a playroom for free choice in following (complying with) the [ethical] law, that is, that the law cannot specify precisely in what way one is to act and how much one is to do by the action for an end that is also a duty.—But a wide duty is not to be taken as permission to make exceptions to the maxim of actions but only as permission to limit one maxim of duty by another (e.g., love of one's neighbor in general by love of one's parents)... The wider the duty, therefore, the more imperfect is man's obligation to action. ...

[44] Ibid., p. 157, [6:395].
Imperfect duties are, accordingly, only duties of virtue.

virtue or ethics is: act in accordance with a maxim of ends that it can be a universal law for everyone to have."[45]

[2:50] In conclusion, Kant's moral theory is divided into two parts; The Doctrine of Right, and The Doctrine of Virtue. The Doctrine of Right is the construction of a constitutional government using the formal criteria of universal freedom of all for attaining the sole and final end of perpetual peace mandated by specific legal actions that are motivated by coercion, i.e. narrow duties. The Doctrine of Virtue are those ends that must be chosen freely and thus cannot be mandated by coercive law. Two wide duties that all have by virtue of *a priori* reasoning are one's own perfection and the happiness of others. A moral agent does not have a duty for their own happiness as everyone already pursues their own happiness by nature of their desires. A moral agent also does not have a duty to perfect others as self-perfection is by definition a personal free choice of ends and thus an activity that cannot be coerced. However, moral agents can freely choose to perfect themselves and they can freely choose to help others attain ends that others have determined will make them happy. How a moral agent attains this self-perfection and happiness of others is going to be different for every person and different for every circumstance and thus ethics is a practice of casuistry, i.e., judgment and a process of seeking truth.[46]

[2:51] In both the doctrine of right and the doctrine of virtue there are clearly defined ends. The end is "Peace" for the doctrine of right, and the ends that all rational beings ought to have

---

[45] Ibid., p. 157, [6:395].

[46] Ibid., p. 169, [6:411].
The doctrine of right has to do only with narrow duties, whereas ethics has to do with wide duties. Hence the doctrine of right, which by its nature must determine duties strictly (precisely), has no more need of general direction (a method) as to how to proceed in judging than does pure mathematics; instead, it certifies its method by what it does.—But ethics, because of the latitude it allows in its imperfect duties, unavoidably leads to questions that call upon judgment to decide how a maxim is to be applied in particular cases, and indeed in such a way that judgment provides another (subordinate) maxim. So ethics falls into a casuistry which has no place in the doctrine of right. ... Casuistry ... is not so much a doctrine about how to find something as rather a practice in how to seek truth.

as rational moral agents in the doctrine of virtue are 1. Self-perfection and 2. The happiness of others. With the doctrine of right, or the political realm, Kant starts out with the end of "Peace" and then determines what will in fact promote such peace in a pluralistic world that is composed of individuals that have various ends, or purposes and meanings of life. The rubric used in the doctrine of right in order to accomplish this is the compatibility of legislation/rights and liberties, with universal freedom along with the concept of reciprocity. Kant's Doctrine of Right is therefore teleological in that the "good/end" of "Peace" was first determined or established as a political axiom or first principle, then through the process of *a priori* analysis using universal freedom and reciprocity Kant determines the social laws/ rights and liberties. The motivation for compliance to the established political rights and liberties is coercion as based on the judicial principle of reciprocity.

[2:52] Kant's Doctrine of Virtue is also teleological, in that the "good/ends" of the moral duties of self-perfection and the happiness of others, are *a priori* duties that all rational beings ought to choose to pursue. However, in the doctrine of virtue, the moral ends are the result of *a prior* reasoning, whereas in the doctrine of right "Peace" is the axiomatic starting point and the social contracts are derived through *a prior* reasoning using the principles of universality and reciprocity. The moral or virtuous maxims of actions, or the broad and general principles, provide the playroom and variability for agency and freedom the necessary conditions for virtue and/or moral worth. The motivation for compliance to these broad and general maxims is the sublime awe that the agent experiences when the agent recognizes that they are not being determined by outside forces, rather they are freely self-legislating through the process of *a priori* reasoning establishing a good will.

3. Diagram of the Metaphysics of Morals

[2:53] The following is a diagram that outlines the component parts of the Doctrine of Right and the Doctrine of Virtue as described in the preceding section on Kant's *Metaphysics of Morals*.

METAPHYSICS OF MORALS	
Doctrine of Right	**DOCTRINE OF VIRTUE**
Civil Rights/Outer Freedom	**Personal Ethics/Ends**
Formal Criteria/Reciprocity/*a priori*/Categorical Imperative/ Universal Command/Law of the Collective Will: Universal Freedom	Formal Criteria/*a priori*/Categorical Imperative/ Universal Command / Law of Our Own Will: Universal Maxims of Actions/Ends
Rational End: Duty to Others—Social Peace/ Outer Freedom; Not Happiness—Empirical Not Moral Autonomy—Ethics/ Virtue	Rational Ends: Rational beings have an obligation to pursue: 1. Self-Perfection and 2. Happiness of Others
Perfect/Narrow Duties: 1. Specific Actions and 2. Specific Punishment for Non-compliance	Imperfect/Wide Duties: 1. General rules "playroom" 2. No coercion for noncompliance
Motive for compliance: Inclination/Coercion /Force: "Rights" extend only in so far as there is effective coercion	Motive for compliance: Rationality/Duty/Awe
Process: Good/end determined before right 1. Start with the rational social end—Peace 2. Then rationally derive the specific rights and liberties based on universal freedom for all citizens—Negative Commands or principles such as nonmaleficence—do no harm. A. Private Rights—Natural Rights *a priori* B. Public Rights—Civil Rights: secures what is mine or yours by public laws	Process: Right determined before good/end 1. Start with universal maxims of actions 2. Then derive the following rational ends: A. Duty to Oneself: Self-Perfection (knowledge and good will) B. Duty to Others: Happiness of Others (Help others accomplish their ends). Positive Commands or principles such as beneficence—do good.
The aim of juridical law is to prevent individuals from compelling others to perform actions that are not a means to their own ends and vice versa, i.e., negative rights. Teleology—Good/End: PEACE	The aim of Ethics, or the Duty Of Ends is: 1. Self-Perfection—self-chosen ends, and 2. The Happiness Of Others—their self-chosen ends. Teleology—Good/End: 1. Self-perfection and 2. Happiness of Others

a. Criticisms Against Immanuel Kant

[2:55] Three of the most common objections made against Immanuel Kant are:

1) anthropocentric criticism,

2) absolutist criticism, and

3) motive criticism.

1) Anthropocentric Criticism:

[2:56] This criticism claims that Kant is anthropocentric in that he only gives regard to rational human beings and does not consider all sentient beings as a class in his moral discussions. Kant and the philosophical traditions associated with Kant typically argue that any duties that rational beings may have towards non-rational animals, humans or not, are duties that are only "indirect." It is claimed that Kant's categorical imperative: "Act in accordance with a maxim of ends that it can be a universal law for everyone to have" can only be exercised and/or applied by rational moral agents who can understand the categorical imperative and the social rules and contractual agreements that result. The criticism is also that to the degree to which Kant failed to provide direct rights to those who are not rational is the degree to which his moral theory fails.

2) Absolutist Criticism:

[2:57] This criticism claims that Immanuel Kant's moral duties requires that moral agents do their moral duties regardless of the consequences. If a person's moral duty is to "push the red button," and the consequence is that the world would be destroyed, then you would still be morally obliged to "push the red button" as consequences are not relevant considerations. Certainly something is wrong with such a moral system.

3) Motive Criticism:

[2:58] This criticism claims that Immanuel Kant's moral duties requires that moral agents do their moral duties as pure *a priori* determinations independent of motives or "feelings." Thus, if a spouse provides flowers for their mate because of their love, then the action has no moral praise. If a spouse has no love and no desire whatsoever to give flowers to their spouse, but does so purely because of duty then the action is praiseworthy. Certainly something is wrong with such a moral system that disregards what many if not most moral agents would consider to be one of the most important aspects of moral conduct.

b. Responses to the Criticisms About Immanuel Kant

1) Anthropocentric Criticism Response:

[2:59] Kant's moral system is in fact anthropocentric and he does argue that rational beings have only indirect duties towards non-rational beings. However, both the Doctrine of Right and the Doctrine of Virtue are easily modified to take into account all sentient beings. Kant argues that there is only one innate right, i.e. freedom or independence from another's choice insofar as it can coexist with the freedom of others. This innate freedom also involves innate equality by the principle of universality.[47]

[2:60] Suppose Kant were to change his position of who has innate freedom from that of humanity to that of all sentient beings? When Kant was writing the *Metaphysics of Morals* he was primarily concerned with the epistemological justification of political rights and moral responsibilities of human agents. Today, Kant would have clearly extended his position beyond that of the rational public just as he was extending the moral positions of his time. As a result, it would be reasonable to conclude that Kant would have addressed the issue of sentient beings if he were writing today.

[2:61] If moral agents were to recognize all sentient beings as having the innate right of freedom, then certainly the sociological consequences would be quite significant. It would mean that all

---

[47] Kant, *The Metaphysics of Morals; Doctrine of Right*, p. 30, [6:237].
There is Only One Innate Right
Freedom (independence from being constrained by another's choice), insofar as it can coexist with the freedom of every other in accordance with a universal law, is the only original right belonging to every person by virtue of their humanity. This principle of innate freedom involves innate equality, that is, independence from being bound by others any more than someone can in turn bind them.

sentient beings freedom would have to be recognized under the doctrine of right and no law would be justified unless innate equality was allowed for all sentient beings disallowing the restriction of freedom of any and all sentient beings when it did not conflict with other's freedom. It seems that such recognition of freedom would, on the one hand, result in the restriction of meat eating for those whom the eating of meat is not a necessary nutritional requirement, and a discontinuing of current animal farms or feed lots that unnecessarily restrict animal freedoms that are being raised for the purpose of consumption. Carnivorous animals and their prey, on the other hand, could still be allowed in areas of conservation where the "circle of life" would still be the most desirous for those involved.

[2:62] Kant's doctrine of virtue, with regard to personal responsibility would require little or no modification at all since it is rational beings that have the moral responsibility to promote the happiness of others. Virtue is a personal responsibility in which individuals have an *a priori* duty to choose the ends of self-perfection and the happiness of others as a duty of ends. The difference would be that the happiness of others would now include not just human interests but all sentient beings' interests.

[2:63] Most sentient beings under the Doctrine of Virtue would in fact easily fulfill the moral responsibility of self-perfection, such as hunting skills, satisfactions etc. and indirectly promotes the happiness of others, by living harmoniously in the web of life.

2) Absolutist Criticism Response:

[2:64] The absolutist criticism is a "straw-man" argument. Under the doctrine of right it is true that motivation that is considered for compliance is coercion and that the teleological end is peace. However, Kant time and again states that citizens ends are not determined and can be anything an agent chooses as long as they comply with the law that is based on the universal maxim of freedom for all. Legislative political laws are perfect or narrow duties that would require specific actions and punishment for noncompliance yet the framework still allows for any number of choices of personal ends that rational beings may pursue. It is true that many sentient beings would not be able to understand and comply with such narrow duties and specific laws, nor would they be able to exercise reciprocity and it is because of such differences in abilities that would put those who are more rational into greater positions of stewardship towards the promotion and care of other sentient beings interest in freedom. As long as there is no violation of universal freedom, then citizens are allowed to behave and to choose any ends they wish which is the exact opposite of the absolutist criticism.

[2:65] Under the doctrine of virtue, there is also, once again, the allowance of all matters of choice of actions and ends. Imperfect wide duties by definition are not absolute which is once again the exact opposite position of the absolutist criticism.

3) Motive Criticism Response:

[2:66] The motive criticism is also a "straw-man" argument. It is true that in the Doctrine of Right the motive of coercion is referred to. Yet even here the ideal would be compliance to the law because of motives other than coercion. However, under the Doctrine of Virtue motive is of paramount importance to such an extent that it is in fact the motive of the action itself that gives virtue its moral worth. The sublime recognition that moral agents are in fact the authors of there own legislation is the awe-inspiring motive which is also the perfected will. Once again the motive criticism is the exact opposite of what Kant actually proposed.

Conclusion

[2:67] This section has justified mid-level principles pragmatically: through the use of codes of ethics and Mill's utilitarianism, and rationally: through the use of Rawls' theory of justice and Kant's deontological ethics.

[2:68] This synergistic model successfully unifies moral philosophy into a collective whole. This occurs not because diverse groups have agreed upon beliefs because, by the very definition of what "diversity" is, they do not. Rather the interesting fact, is that like intersubjective agreements, such as the experiences of "color," diverse groups of people, and even diverse species, can and do have intersubjective cognitive agreements on broad and general universal mid-level principles. Recognition of such general values, as presented as Principlism, will help pluralistic societies come to decision-making agreements.

***

IV. PRINCIPLISM

Overview

[i:1]

Principlism focuses on the broad and general intersubjective agreements of autonomy (informed consent), beneficence, (r do good), nonmaleficence, (do no harm), and justice (be fair). This section will present the historical background of the development and implementation of Principlism as legal criteria both nationally and internationally. Then each of the principles will be investigated individually in order to understand what each principle represents so that the activity of specification and balancing can be implemented effectively. Such implementation will result in a morally progressive society that respects and values pluralism and diversity.

I. Principlism's Origin: The Belmont Report

[1:1] Principlism was first formalized as a moral decision-making approach by the National Commission for the Protection of Human Subjects of Biomedical and Behavioral Research in a document called the Belmont Report on April 18, 1979. The Commission came into existence on July 12, 1974 when the National Research Act (Pub. L. 93-348) was signed into law. After four years of monthly deliberations, the Commission met in February 1976 at the Smithsonian Institution's Belmont Conference Center and presented a statement of the basic ethical principles that ought to be considered for biomedical and behavioral research: autonomy, or informed consent, beneficence (do good), and justice (be fair). The Commission recommended that the Belmont Report be adopted in its entirety as a statement of the Department's policy for the Secretary of Health, Education, and Welfare.

[1:2] The Belmont Report's cause of origin can be traced back to December 9, 1946 when the American Military Tribunal started criminal proceedings against 23 German physicians and administrators for war crimes and crimes against humanity. During the trials, the Nuremberg Code was drafted for the establishment of standards for judging individuals who conducted biomedical experiments on concentration camp prisoners. The Nuremberg Code in its final form was established in 1948 and was the first international document that advocated voluntary informed consent for participants of research on human subjects.

[1:3] Although the Nuremberg Code was an international document, that advocated voluntary informed consent, it did not carry the force of law in the United States or any other country for that matter. As a result both for profit private enterprises and national governments blatantly violated the Nuremberg Code on numerous occasions.

A. Thalidomide Case

[1:4] An example of for profit private enterprise violation of informed consent is the Thalidomide Case. In the 1950's the drug thalidomide, which was an approved sedative in Europe but not an approved sedative in the United States, was being advertised by pharmaceutical companies and prescribed by physicians for controlling sleep and nausea throughout pregnancy. Most patients that were taking this drug had not given an informed consent for this drug as they had not been informed of the risks involved nor had they been informed that the Federal Drug Administration—FDA had not approved thalidomide for human use. In fact, the FDA actually had denied its approval six times. In Europe an estimated 8,000 to 12,000 infants were born with deformities caused by thalidomide, and of those only about 5,000 survived beyond childhood. Even though the drug did not have FDA approval 2.5 million tablets had been given to more than 1,200 American doctors and nearly 20,000 patients received thalidomide tablets, including several hundred pregnant women. In the end, 17 American children were born with thalidomide-related deformities, such as abnormally short limbs with toes sprouting from the hips and flipper-like arms, and an estimated 40,000 people developed drug-induced peripheral neuropathy. Public outcry resulted in U.S. senate hearings passing the Kefauver Amendments into law in 1962. This law forced drug manufacturers to prove their products safety and effectiveness to the FDA before they would be allowed to bring them to market. Legislation was necessary as for profit drug companies were not going to abide by the international Nuremberg Code if money could be made and if there were no legal penalties for not abiding by international rules.

[1:5] (On May 26, 2006, the U.S. Food and Drug Administration—FDA granted approval of thalidomide for the treatment of leprosy with sales of $300 million per year)

B. Syphilis Study at Tuskegee

[1:6] An example of the United States government violation of informed consent is the Syphilis Study at Tuskegee (1932-1972). In this case the U.S. Pubic Health Service recruited 600 low-income African-American males from Tuskegee Alabama. 400 of the men were infected with syphilis. They were told that they would be given free medical care, lunches, and transportation to and from the healthcare facilities each month. However, the subjects were never informed that they had the communicable disease of syphilis. As a result many of the subjects sexual encounters and wives were infected with syphilis and many of those women also gave birth to children having congenital syphilis.

[1:7] The cure for syphilis, a simple administration of penicillin, was readily available in the 1950's yet the United States Government continued to keep the Tuskegee patients uninformed as to their condition, denied treatment, and/or lied to the patient by saying that they were being treated for syphilis when in reality they were only being given a placebo with no medical benefits. If by chance a subject was diagnosed as having syphilis by another physician the U.S. Government researchers would intervene to prevent treatment.

[1:8] In 1966, Peter Buxtun, Public Health Services—PHS venereal disease investigator questioned the morality of the experiment by sending a letter to the director of the Division of Venereal Diseases. The Center for Disease Control—CDC supported the Syphilis Study at Tuskegee and even had the support from the local chapters of the National Medical Association who represented African American physicians. After six years of unsuccessful influence Peter Buxtun decided to expose the Syphilis Study at Tuskegee to the media through the Washington Star on July 25, 1972. The New York Times then published the story the next day as front-page news. Because of the resultant public outcry an *ad hoc* advisory panel was put together and they determined that the Syphilis Study at Tuskegee was medically unjustified and the United States Department of Health, Education, and Welfare—DHEW finally stopped the study in 1973.

[1:9] The National Association for the Advancement of Colored People—NAACP filed a class action lawsuit against the study resulting in a 9 million dollar settlement and free healthcare for the surviving participants and their family members who were infected with syphilis as a consequence of the government study. However, it wasn't until May 16, 1997 that a public apology was finally given by the U.S. government to the eight remaining study subjects and their families by President Clinton.

> [1:10] "To the survivors, to the wives and family members, the children and the grandchildren, I say what you know: No power on Earth can give you back the lives lost, the pain suffered, the years of internal torment and anguish. What was done cannot be undone. But we can end the silence. We can stop turning our heads away. We can look at you in the eye and finally say on behalf of the American people, what the United States government did was shameful, and I am sorry. ... To our African American citizens, I am sorry that your federal government orchestrated a study so clearly racist. That can never be allowed to happen again. ... Since the study was halted, abuses have been checked by making informed consent and local review mandatory in federally-funded and mandated research." https://www.cdc.gov/tuskegee/clintonp.htm

[1:11] The following is the letter from the Macon County Health Department recruiting black males from Tuskegee Alabama to participate in the syphilis study without their knowledge.

Macon County Health Department

ALABAMA STATE BOARD OF HEALTH AND U.S. PUBLICH HEALTH SERVICE COOPERATING WITH TUSKEGEE INSTITUTE

Dear Sir:

Some time ago you were given a thorough examination and since that time we hope you have gotten a great deal of treatment for bad blood. You will now be given your last chance to get a second examination. This examination is a very special one and after it is finished you will be given a special treatment if it is believed you are in a condition to stand it.

If you want this special examination and treatment you must meet the nurse at ______________________ on ____________________at ___________________ M. She will bring you to the Tuskegee Institute Hospital for this free treatment. We will be very busy when these examinations and treatments are being given, and will have lots of people to wait on. You will remember that you had to wait for some time when you had your last good examination, and we wish to let you know that because we expect to be so busy it may be necessary for you to remain in the hospital over one night. If this is necessary you will be furnished your meals and a bed, as well the examination and treatment without cost.

REMEMBER THIS IS YOUR LAST CHANCE FOR SPECIAL FREE TREATMENT. BE SURE TO MEET THE NURSE.

Macon County Health Department

This letter is reproduced from an educational website at the University of Illinois's Poynter Center for the Study of Ethics and American Institutions (http://poynter.indiana.edu/sas/lb/facts.html.)

[1:12] "Bad blood" was the euphemism used for syphilis in order to keep them from knowing what was being discussed. The "special free treatment" was the term used for documenting the progression of the syphilis infected research subjects. Deception, harm and unjust selection of subjects was clearly the intent of the letter and those ends were successfully accomplished. The United States Center for Disease Control—CDC and the National Medical Association supported the tragic forty-year study that never resulted in any significant new medical knowledge. Of course, even if it had resulted in significant medical advances, that still would not have justified the deceptive study.

[1:13] Oddly enough, it appears that the researchers and supportive organizations were insensitive and unaware of their own moral violations. This reoccurring phenomena of individuals and groups being unaware or blind of their own discretions, is why it is now federal law that Institutional Review Boards—IRBs, are composed of pluralistic interdisciplinary members who have no involvement in the research being evaluated, and if a vulnerable population is being studied, a representative of that population should also present.

C. Belmont Report And Its Three Core Principles

[1:14] Principlism is the name that has been adopted when referring to the principles as presented by the Belmont Report. The Belmont report lists the following three principles: 1. Respect for persons, 2. Beneficence, and 3. Justice. Principlism refers to four principles 1. Autonomy (informed consent), 2. Beneficence (do good), 3. Nonmaleficence (do no harm), and 4. Justice or be fair. Principlism is the same moral approach as presented in the Belmont Report except that Principlism refers to four principles whereas the Belmont Report refers to only three principles. The Belmont Reports reduction of principles is because it combines both beneficence and nonmaleficence under the single principle of beneficence.

[1:15]

BELMONT REPORT	
PRINCIPLES	**APPLICATIONS**
Respect for Persons 1. Individuals should be treated as autonomous agents. 2. Persons with diminished autonomy are entitled to protection.	**Informed Consent** 1. Information a. Procedures b. Purpose c. Risks and benefits d. Alternatives e. Opportunity to ask questions and to withdraw at any time. 2. Comprehension 3. Voluntariness
Beneficence 1. Human subjects should not be harmed. 2. Research should maximize possible benefits and minimize possible harms.	**Assessment of Risks and Benefits** 1. The nature and scope of risks and benefits. 2. The systematic assessment of risks and benefits.
Justice The benefits and risks of research must be distributed fairly.	**Selection of Subjects** There must be fair procedures and outcomes in the selection of research subjects both individually and socially.

II. Principlism: General

A. Principlism As A Practical Approach

1. Intersubjective agreements

[2:1] Principlism has evolved into a practical approach for ethical decision-making that focuses on the common ground, or socially agreed upon values, or moral principles, of: autonomy (informed consent), beneficence (do good), nonmaleficence (do no harm), and justice (be fair). Even though humanity has great diversity with regard to moral justification, there still seems to be universal consensus on the broad moral principles. This social moral consensus is what is referred to as Principlism. The practicality of this approach is that Principlism can is derivable from, consistent with, or at the very least not in conflict with a multitude of ethical, theological, and social approaches towards moral decision-making.

[2:2] Descriptively, Principlism is much like pleasure, how people generate pleasure may differ, yet the human experience of pleasure is more similar than different. Perhaps a better analogy might be how humans experience color. Empirically, we know through colorblind testing that most individuals experience color more similarly than dissimilarly. This agreement in subjective experiences between others is referred to as intersubjective agreements even though there may be disagreements as to the origin, nature, and justification of those principles. Principlism is therefore a very effective means towards moral discussion as it bypasses the epistemic differences as to the origin, nature, and justification of morality and focuses instead on intersubjective agreements of morality. In public discourse, these intersubjective agreements on morality are often times referred to as basic human rights.

2. Nonnormative and normative morality

[2:3] Principlism is a social political construct in that humans have descriptively found themselves organized in societies with certain social actions being considered permissible and certain social actions being considered impermissible. These permissible and impermissible social agreements are defined as common morality. Common morality has two major subdivisions, nonnormative and normative.

[2:4] Nonnormative morality is descriptive in nature in that it describes how people do in fact act. Nonnormative morality is an empirical evaluation in that it uses scientific techniques to study how people do in fact reason and act not how they ought or ought not to act. Nonnormative morality is usually associated with the approaches of anthropologists, sociologists, psychologists, and historians. Their objective, as empirical scientists, is not to establish what ethically ought to be the case rather they are mainly concerned about what factually or conceptually is the case. Principlism fits this descriptive criterion.

[2:5] Normative morality is prescriptive in nature in that it prescribes how people ought or ought not to act. Failure to behave in such a particular way is then defined as acting or not acting morally. Normative morality can also be an empirical evaluation using scientific techniques, but in contrast to nonnormative morality, the focus is not on how people do in fact reason and act, but how they ought to act based on scientific cause effect relationships. In addition to the empirical scientific approach normative morality can also base its obligations on *a priori*, or pure rational determinations. Normative morality is usually associated with the approach of most moral theologians and many moral philosophers. Their objective, as empirical scientists and rationalists, is not to establish what moral decisions agents actually make, rather they are mainly concerned about what moral decisions they ought to make. Principlism fits this prescriptive criterion as well.

[2:6] In other words, Principlism is both descriptive and prescriptive in nature, in that it describes not only how people do in fact make moral decisions, but Principlism also prescribes how people ought to make moral decisions.

3. Principlism as grammar

[2:7] Grammar of language is a good analogy of how Principlism works in that grammar first describes how communicators do in fact construct a language, next the grammatical terms are analyzed, and finally the grammar then prescribes how speakers ought to construct language for the practical purpose of communication. Principlism, like grammar, describes how moral agents do in fact make moral decisions and then how they ought to make moral decisions if they are to be logically consistent.

[2:8] Principlism, as a pluralistic approach, is effective when making moral decisions institutionally, pedagogically, and in the community as pluralistic interdisciplinary groups by definition cannot agree on particular moral theories or their epistemic justifications. However, pluralistic interdisciplinary groups can and do agree on intersubjective principles.

[2:9] In the development of a principlistic moral framework it is therefore not a necessary condition that the epistemic origins and justifications of these principles be established. Rather the sufficient condition is that most individuals and societies, would agree that both descriptively and prescriptively there is wide agreement with the existence and acceptance of the general values of autonomy (informed consent), beneficence (do good), nonmaleficence (do no harm), and justice (be fair).

B. Specifying and Balancing

[2:10] Once these principles have been established the practical activity then becomes that of specifying how the principles are to be used in specific situations and balancing the principles with the other relevant moral principles.

1. Two types of moral dilemmas

[2:11] With Principlism a moral dilemma is when either one or both of the following dilemmatic categories occurs.

a. Single principle dilemma (Specification)

[2:12] With the single principle dilemma a decision is both morally right and wrong using a single principle, i.e., "damned if you do and damned if you don't ."

[2:13] This first form of a moral dilemma exists when an agent is both morally right and morally wrong when fulfilling a single moral principle. This is where specification comes into play. Specifying is when you take a general principle, such as autonomy (informed consent), and determine how it relates or ought to relate to a particular circumstance or situation. However, this also creates the situation in which there can arise individual and social disagreements as to what is the appropriate specification, to whom the principle should be applied to, as well as disagreements on factual information and evidence. The ideal in the use of Principlism is to avoid such internal conflicts by using good judgments in the specification of the principle in question.

b. Multiple principles dilemma (Balancing)

[2:14] With the multiple principle dilemma the decision has two or more relevant moral principles and the agent is not able to completely fulfill one or more moral principles without violating or competing with one or more other moral principles.

[2:15] This second form of a moral dilemma exists when an agent has two or more relevant moral principles that cannot be simultaneously fulfilled. Under such conditions the agent morally fulfills one or more moral principles, and is therefore acting morally, yet at the same time the agent morally fails to fulfill one or more other moral principles, and is therefore acting immorally at the same time. This is where balancing comes into play.

[2:16] Balancing is the analytic analysis of how two or more specified principles, that may seem to be competing with each other, ought to be weighed and/or balanced for a particular circumstance or situation. However, this also creates the situation in which there can arise individual and social disagreements as to what are the competing moral principles, and even if there is agreement as to what moral principles ought to apply, there still can arise disagreements as to what are or should be the appropriate weights of those competing moral principles, to whom they ought to apply, as well as disagreements on factual information and evidence. The ideal in the use of Principlism is to avoid such conflicts of multiple principles by using good judgments in the balancing of the various principles in question. It is not that various principles actually conflict with each other, rather it is an evaluative problem of determining which of the four moral principles are the most relevant moral principles for the particular circumstance.

2. Pluralistic social decision-making

a. Bill of Rights

[2:17] Dilemmatic decision-making is not unusual when making pluralistic social decisions. The Bill of Rights in the United States Constitution exemplifies this process. A citizen's freedom of speech, for example, does not allow someone to yell "FIRE" in a crowded theater when there is no fire as individual constitutional rights and liberties are constrained by other individual rights and liberties, such as freedom of assembly, and therefore they must be specified for particular situations and then balanced with the other inevitable competing principles. Rarely do all the justices of the Supreme Court agree unanimously with the court's decision further indicating the extent and depth of dilemmatic decision-making, both in the specification and balancing of the rights and liberties in the Constitution.

b. Formal criterion

[2:18] Principlism, presented as a formal criterion, is a description and prescription of moral decision-making that has a deep and rich heritage that has yet to be formalized for pluralistic interdisciplinary groups. Moral decision-making in pluralistic environments is possible as Principlism describes how diverse people do in fact make moral decisions and Principlism also prescribes how diverse people ought to make moral decisions based on the intersubjective agreements of common morality. Instead of focusing on the epistemic differences of various philosophical and religious perspectives, Principlism focuses on the intersubjective agreements, and that is why it works so effectively in interdisciplinary pluralistic environments.

[2:19] Principlism could be modified by adding or subtracting certain component principles yet practically the four principles of autonomy (informed consent), beneficence (do good), nonmaleficence (do no harm), and justice (be fair), are broad and comprehensive enough to sufficiently cover most cases and provides the necessary output power for making interdisciplinary moral decisions.

C. Incommensurable Beliefs

[2:20] Even though pluralistic groups will in large part have shared universal values—Principlism, it is still clearly recognized that there is and will be incommensurable beliefs as to how the specification and balancing procedures found in the principlistic approach ought to be implemented. However, Principlism has the advantage over most other moral approaches in that Principlism emphasizes the shared interdisciplinary universal values, or principles, and uses them in a systematic and transparent fashion resulting in shared understandings and/or compromise. Principlism has tremendous output power for the practice of interdisciplinary moral decision-making.

III. Principlism: Particular

[3:1] What follows is an analysis of each of the major principles of Principlism: autonomy (informed consent), beneficence (do good), nonmaleficence (do no harm), and justice (be fair).

A. Autonomy

1. Autonomy means: self-rule

[3:2] Autonomy is a broad moral concept found in common morality. Etymologically autonomy is derived from the Greek words *autos* meaning self and *nomos* meaning rule i.e., self-rule. Historically autonomy was exclusively used in reference to the sovereignty of a nation. In contemporary ethics, autonomy is primarily used in reference to individuals.

2. Autonomy's three necessary conditions

[3:3] All autonomous choices must meet the following three necessary conditions:

a. Intention:

[3:4] The agent must make a decision or choice.

b. Understanding:

[3:5] The agent must have substantial information or knowledge.

c. Freedom:

[3:6] The agent must not be substantially constrained by controlling influences.

[3:7] The first necessary condition of intention or choice is not a matter of degree. Rather, an agent either makes a choice or they don't make a choice. The other two criterions of understanding and freedom are a matter of degree as it is impossible for any agent to have complete understanding or to be totally free from all controlling influences. However, choices are considered to be autonomous as long as there is an intentional choice or decision along with substantial understanding and substantial freedom from controlling influences. What substantial means will need to be determined both by the type of agent and by the circumstances surrounding the judgment.

a. Intentionality / Consent / Choice

[3:8] When an agent chooses with substantial understanding and substantial freedom, then an autonomous decision has been made. How this autonomous consent is communicated to others can be of three varieties:

1) Express Consent

[3:9] When an autonomous agent conveys their decision by verbal or written form.

2) Implied Consent

[3:10] When an autonomous agent infers their decision by a gesture or action such as the lifting of an arm for a shot.

3) Tacit Consent

[3:11] When an autonomous agent infers their decision by not objecting, e.g., by being silent or passive.

[3:12] Once it is determined that an agent has or is able to intentionally make a choice, the next step is to determine if the other two criteria of understanding and freedom have been met.

b. Understanding / Acquisition of Knowledge

[3:13] In most decision-making processes, it is essential to acquire a certain amount of information in order for a decision to be considered autonomous, hence the term informed consent. What amount and type of information that would be in order to be considered sufficient or substantial will be dependent upon the agent's needs, the type of decision being made, and the circumstances surrounding the decision.

Understanding as a negative right

[3:14] Understanding as a negative right will emphasize the moral obligation of others to not interfere with the agent's acquisition of knowledge.

Understanding as a positive right

[3:15] Understanding as a positive right will emphasize the moral obligation of others to provide, or to make accessible, the necessary information for the agent to be considered substantially or sufficiently informed in order for the decision to be autonomous.

[3:16] Because society is becoming more complex and industrialized and because decision-making is becoming more complex there is an increased need to focus on the legal requirements and obligations of both providing information (positive rights) and not interfering with the acquisition of information (negative rights).

Increased complexity & competence

[3:17] The importance of autonomy (informed consent), is based on the ideal notion that an autonomous decision is the most effective means of promoting an agent's best interests. This may be the case for a competent agent that is making decisions within the limits of their abilities as determined by the complexity and difficulty of the decision. However, as society becomes more complex and decisions become more difficult the number of agents that are capable of being competent or able to make sound decisions that will in fact promote their best interests becomes smaller and smaller. Under those conditions it becomes imperative to appeal to a more paternalistic model of decision-making in which decision-making is deferred to those who do have the ability to make sound decisions with the best interests of the agent in mind.

[3:18] Interestingly, there has been a historic legal progression from the use of the more paternalistic professional practice standard to the more autonomous reasonable practice standard for information disclosure. This is somewhat of a paradox as this is occurring at the same time that the industrialization of many aspects of life, such as healthcare, food, economy, education, etc., is making decision-making much more complex and difficult resulting in fewer agent's that are actually competent enough to be able to make sound decisions that will maximize their best interests. In contradiction to best interests, it appears that as contemporary circumstances provide greater paternalistic justifications, the legal system at the same time is legislating more autonomous decision-making criteria. It is not that one model of information disclosure is correct and another is wrong, rather what needs to be recognized is that each is correct when applied to appropriate agents and appropriate circumstances and each can be wrong when applied to inappropriate agents and inappropriate circumstances.

[3:19] The following are the three standards of information disclosures that are either legally required and/or morally necessary. They are the professional practice standard, the reasonable person standard, and the subjective standard.

[3:20]

1) Professional Practice Standard

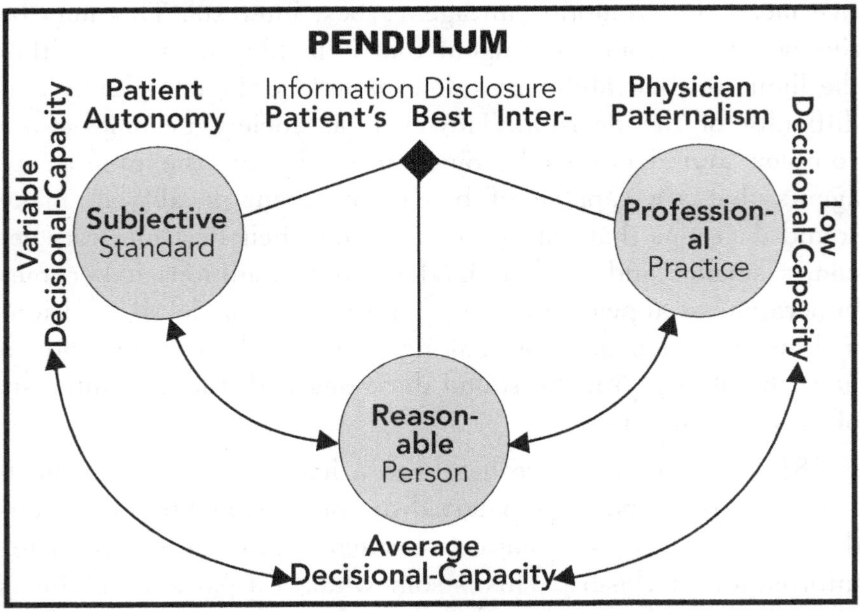

a) Strengths

[3:21] The professional practice standard holds to the belief that the proper amount and kinds of information necessary to disclose and withhold is that which the professionals in that field and community do in fact commonly disclose or withhold.[1] This reasoning is usually based on the beneficent and non-maleficent tra-

[1]Beauchamp and Childress, *Principles of Biomedical Ethics*, 2nd ed., p. 74.

dition. The reasoning is that it is the professionals who have the training, knowledge and experience necessary for the determination of just what amount and kinds of information are necessary to disclose and to withhold in order to benefit or to maximize the best interests of the agents whom they effect. The professional practice standard holds that the agents generally do not have the professional expertise, knowledge and experience, necessary to be able to a) determine what information is needed in order for them to make a decision and b) determine what action would in fact be in their best interests even if given all substantial information. In other words, autonomy (informed consent) is not the determining factor for the professional practice standard, rather the determining factor is the best interests of the agent. As a result, the only people who are able to determine whether there has been an improper amount of information disclosure to the agent, or an improper decision made for the benefit of the agent, are by the professionals themselves, not the agents. Historically, the professional practice standard has been the general legal standard for information disclosure.[2]

[3:22] This position asserts that the professional community's customary practice determines what is the appropriate type and amount of information disclosure. Some benefits of this standard is that a) it can paternalistically maximize the best interests of the agent, b) it can provide more efficiency of time and resources because of not having to deal with the lack of experience and capabilities of the agents fumbling decision-making, and c) it is an easy and effective way for the legal system to determine if the professional practice standard had been met or not. The legal system simply subpoenas a few expert witnesses—professionals, then under oath asks them what type of information disclosure they typically provide.

[3:23] The following criticisms are weaknesses in the professional practice standard that need to be considered.

---

[2]"Approximately seventy-five percent of the legal jurisdictions in the United States cling to the more traditional professional practice standard". Beauchamp and Childress, *Principles of Biomedical Ethics*, 2nd ed., p. 75.

b) Weaknesses

(1) Professional standards may not exist

[3:24] The professional practice standard can exist only if there are customary standards as to the amount and type of information that is to be disclosed or withheld. However, today's society is pluralistic and mobile and the homogeneity of personal, social and political viewpoints within communities is rare. Even if there were to be some consensus as to a standard of disclosure, the issue as to how much consensus would be needed for the establishment of such a standard would still need to be addressed.

(2) Professional standards may be inappropriate

[3:25] Inappropriate types and amounts of information disclosure could be justified. This complaint, even if it is only theoretical, is that pervasively negligent care *could* be perpetuated with impunity[3] if relevant professionals generally offer the same inferior level of information, whether through ignorance, as a genuine conviction, or for reasons of professional solidarity.[4]

(3) Professionals may not be able to determine ends for others

[3:26] Implicit in the professional practice standard is the assumption that the professionals, because of their knowledge, background, and experience, are in a better position to make decisions to effect individual ends, i.e., best interests, than the individuals themselves. This could be true in a homogenous society in which everyone has the same shared end or best interests, but it certainly is not true in a pluralistic society in which there are vast differences in individuals' subjective and objective beliefs and ends.

(4) Professional standards undermines autonomy

[3:27] The professional practice standard has the tendency to undermine autonomy. The specific informational needs of the agent are deemphasized and the paternalistic informational criteria of the professional are emphasized. However, it could be ar-

---

[3]Beauchamp and Childress, *Principles of Biomedical Ethics*, 2nd ed., p. 75.

[4]Faden and Beauchamp, *A History and Theory of Informed Consent*, p. 31.

gued that it is the promotion of autonomy, not beneficence or nonmaleficence that is the primary function and justification of the rules of informed consent.[5] The professional practice standard does not consider the agent's intersubjective, subjective and objective beliefs, fears, and hopes as having overriding authority.[6] As a result individual autonomy could be compromised for the sake of what the professional would consider beneficent or nonmaleficence. The reduction of an agent's autonomy for the sake of professional values needs to be clearly justified if implemented.

(5) Professional standards may not maximize the best interest of the agent.

[3:27] The professional practice standard may not always be in the agent's best interests. As professional aspirations, economic goals, and conflicts of interests increase, professionals may set aside the best interests of the agent for their own personal or professional gains or best interests. If a variety of good decisions

---

[5]Beauchamp and Childress, *Principles of Biomedical Ethics*, 2nd ed., p. 75.

[6]Objective: belonging to the object of thought rather than the thinking subject.

Subjective: belonging to the thinking subject rather than the object of thought.

Intersubjectivity: The property of holding in reference to more than one subject, rather than purely subjectively. For example, the proposition 'hydrogen sulfide smells like rotten eggs', may be said to hold intersubjectively because there is common agreement upon its truth. Anthony Flew, *A Dictionary of Philosophy*, Revised Second Edition (New York: St. Martin's Press, 1979), p. 177.

In a paper, entitled *Clinical Medicine as a Science*, delivered at the "Conference on Changing Values in Medicine", Cornell University Medical College, Ernan McMullin said "Since knowledge is by nature bipolar, involving both subject and object, there is a sense in which all knowledge is subjective, that is, it pertains to a knowing subject. It is likewise objective in the same broad sense, since it necessarily has an object even if that object should happen to be the product of imagination only. When philosophers speak of the "intentionality" of the knowledge-act, it is this peculiar duality that they are principally addressing. ... There are some complications here in the context of those theories of knowledge (those of Kant ...) where knowledge either inevitably or appropriately reflects the cognitive structures of the knower." This paper can be found in the anthology by Eric J. Cassell, Mark Siegler, *Changing Values in Medicine* (New York: University Publications of America, 1979), p. 168.

can be made that will maximize both the best interests of the agent, and those of the professional, then who's criteria ought to be considered in making such a determination? The professional practice standard would paternalistically say that the professionals are in the best position to make such a determination, and those who emphasize personal autonomy would say that the agent is in the best position to make such a determination.

(6) Professional standards may violate constitutional rights and liberties.

[3:29] For a competent agent the professional practice standard fails to promote certain constitutional rights and liberties. The professional practice standard has the potential to violate individual freedom and equality, freedom of thought, liberty of conscience and personal liberty. This constitutional violation is a result of the conviction that the proper moral role of the professional is to act in the agent's best interests as determined by the professional community rather than as determined by the individual agent.

(7) Professionals often times will not testify against each other

[3:30] Although the professional practice standard is easy to implement for the judicial system the professional practice standard is very difficult for the plaintiff to prove that a professional disclosure violation has occurred. The agent, as the effected individual, would have to have one or more professionals, usually from the local community, testify against one of their own professional colleagues. When there is strong professional solidarity and when professionals depend on each other for support and referrals the testimony often times becomes compromised because of conflicts of interests.

2) Reasonable Person Standard

[3:30]

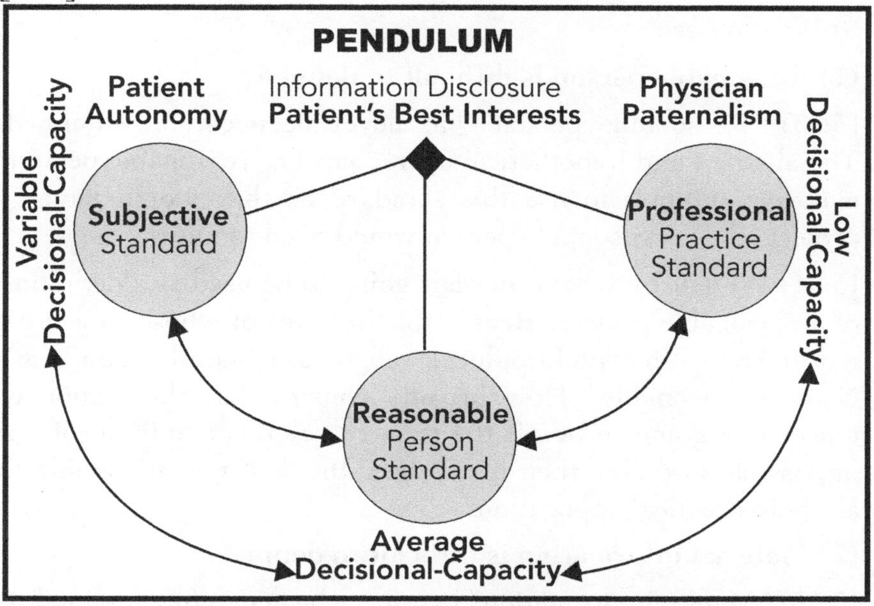

a) Strengths

[3:31] The reasonable person standard asserts that information disclosure is based on what a hypothetical "reasonable person" would consider as necessary "material information." Two benefits of this standard are: a) it shifts the right to decide what amount and type of information is relevant or necessary for an informed consent from the paternalistic professional practice point of view towards that of an autonomous reasonable person[7] point of view and b) it provides an easy and effective way for the legal system to determine if the standard has been met or not. The legal system simply creates and legislates a "grocery list" of information that must be disclosed and then goes through the list, point by point to determine if the standard has been met or not.

---

[7]Kenneth F. T. Cust, "Hypothetical Contractarianism and the Disclosure Requirement Problem in Informed Consent" *The Journal of Medical Humanities*, Vol. 12, No. 3, (1991), pp. 120-121.

[3:32] However, the reasonable person standard is not immune to its conceptual, moral, and practical difficulties either.[8]

b) Weaknesses

(1) Reasonable person is difficult to defined.

[3:33] "Reasonable person" has never been carefully defined. The abstract and hypothetical character of a "reasonable person" makes it difficult to use this standard as they would have to project what a reasonable person would need to know.

[3:34] Who or by what criteria is going to be used as a definition of a reasonable person? Reasonable in terms of whose subjective worldview? What philosophical, religious or moral grounds are deemed reasonable? How broadly construed is this notion of reasonable going to be? If the term reasonable is difficult if not impossible to define then it will be difficult if not impossible to apply in practical applications.

(2) Material information is difficult to define.

[3:35] "Material information" has never been carefully defined. If it is impossible to determine who or by what criteria the definition of a reasonable person is then it will also be impossible to determine what "material information" is necessary for a reasonable person.

[3:36] Again, if these terms are difficult if not impossible to define then these definitions will be difficult if not impossible to apply in practical applications.

[3:37] If living in a pluralistic society means living in a society that has a number of differing but reasonable beliefs, then it would seem that it would be exceedingly difficult if not impossible to disclose the relevant and reasonable information specific to each individual's subjective beliefs.

(3) Reasonable person's informational needs may differ

[3:38] The reasonable person standard determines the amount of information that a reasonable person would require in order to

---

[8]Beauchamp and Childress, *Principles of Biomedical Ethics*, 2nd ed., p. 77.

assess the risks and benefits of a proposed decision under particular circumstances. The problem is that the amount and type of information that one reasonable person might require might not be the same amount and type of information that is material or relevant for another reasonable person. In other words, the specific informational needs may differ from one reasonable person to another reasonable person and as a result, the reasonable person standard will not accomplish its purpose of providing the appropriate information criteria necessary for autonomous self-determination.[9]

(4) Reasonable person standard may not promote the agent's best interest

[3:39] Another objection to the reasonable person standard is that it may not always be in the agent's best interests to be provided the "material information." In other words, the value of autonomy and informed consent may come into conflict with not only the values of beneficence, nonmaleficence, and justice but could also come into conflict with the agent's best interests, the very foundation of Principlism. If an agent is given all relevant information to make an informed consent the individual may not make the right decision with respect to maximizing their own best interests as the paternalistic professional practice decision would have.[10] In order for the professional to act in the best interests of the agent it may be necessary not to comply with the reasonable person standard. But then the question arises as to whether or not there are a variety of reasonable decisions that can be made under particular circumstances. If so, then by what right can some reasonable decisions be considered better than other reasonable decisions?

---

[9]Cust, "Hypothetical Contractarianism and the Disclosure Requirement Problem in Informed Consent", p. 121.

[10]An example of the possible conflict between beneficence and "informed consent" is when the "proper" treatment involves the use of a placebo. A patient may think they need a pain killer when in fact the pain is psychogenic. Thus believing that it would be unreasonable to prescribe a pain killer the doctor prescribes a placebo instead. Obviously with a placebo you cannot disclose all information for "proper" medical treatment.

(5) Decisions are often made independent of information

[3:40] Ruth R. Faden[11] empirically determined that although 93% of patients surveyed said that the disclosed information they received was helpful, only 12% used that information in their decision for consent. In the end, the patients were either accepting the professional's recommendation without using the material information for weighing risks and benefits or patient's were making their decisions either independently of or prior to the information disclosure. This brings to question the extent to which material information is necessary or even used for actual decision-making.

(6) Reasonable person standard may violate constitutional rights and liberties.

[3:41] Because the reasonable person standard does not take into consideration pluralistic standards of reasonable, the reasonable person standard may violate constitutional rights and liberties such as freedom of thought, personal liberty, and liberty of conscience in pluralistic societies. The reasonable person standard assumes that it is possible to come up with a reasonable protocol or standard that can be applied to all agents because that protocol or standard is believed to be universally reasonable. The problem arises when differing agents have differing beliefs of what material information would be even under similar circumstances. The issue here is that what is unreasonable for one group of individuals might be quite reasonable for another group of individuals who as autonomous persons share differing beliefs. An example of this is the person who refuses to have a porcine heart valve put in because of the belief that pork is unclean, whereas another person accepts the porcine heart valve because they believe animals are here for their benefit and a third person

---

[11]Ruth R. Faden, "Disclosure and Informed Consent; Does It Matter How We Tell It?" *Health Education Monographs* 5 (1977): 198-215; Ruth R. Faden and Tom L. Beauchamp, "Decision-Making and Informed consent: A Study of the Impact of Disclosed Information," *Social Indicators Research* 7 (1980): 313-36; and, for an extension, Ruth R. Faden, et al., "Disclosure of Information to Patients in Medical Care," *Medical Care* 19 (July 1981): pp. 718-33.

who thinks that any use of a sentient animal for purposes that are not in the animal's best interests is immoral and wrong.

3) Subjective Standard

[3:42]

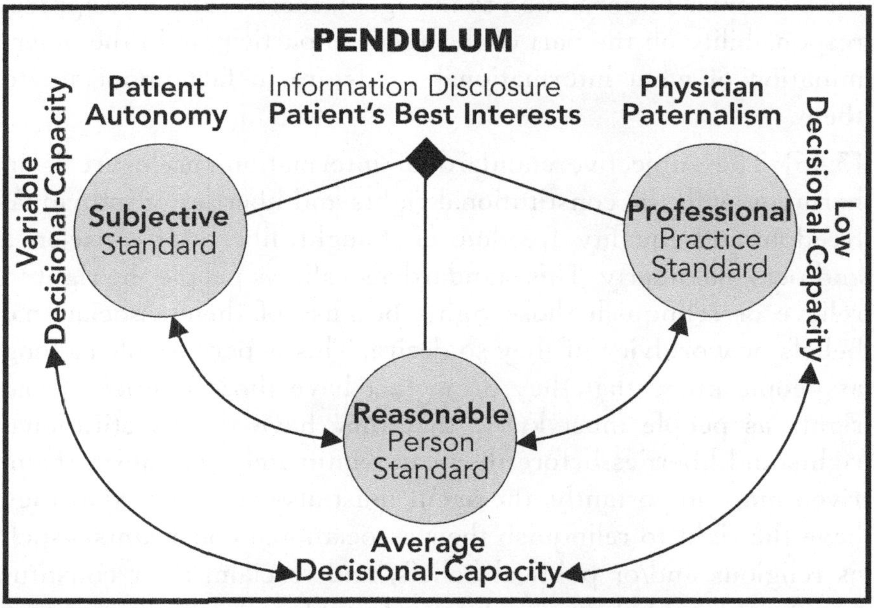

a) Strengths

[3:43] The subjective standard asserts that information disclosure is based on the specific informational needs of the person involved. The benefit of this standard is that it alone acknowledges a person's specific informational needs for determining the proper type and amount of information disclosure necessary for an agent to make an autonomous decision. It is assumed that an autonomous decision will in fact result in the best interests of the agent.

[3:44] The subjective standard is the most individually specific of the disclosure standards. Both the professional practice standard and the reasonable practice standard create objective information disclosure determinations. In contrast, the subjective standard is specific and unique to each agent both personally and circumstantially. This standard does not judge individual beliefs; rather it accepts them as a given and tries to individualize the information disclosure criteria for each individual and their situation so that they can make an informed autonomous decision that maximizes their best interests.[12]

[3:45] In addition to the professional responsibility to provide the customized information to the agent, there is also a reciprocal responsibility on the part of the agent to participate in the determination of what informational needs are in fact important to them.

[3:46] The subjective standard of information disclosure is in harmony with the constitutional rights and liberties of individual freedom and equality, freedom of thought, liberty of conscience and personal liberty. This standard also allows people the right to relieve or relinquish those rights because of their associational beliefs or worldview if they so desire. This is permissible as long as people know that they do in fact have those political social rights as people must know that they have the constitutional rights and liberties before they can legitimately relinquish them. Even more importantly, the agent must also recognize that they have the right to relinquish their associational constraints—such as religious and/or political beliefs, and to claim their constitutional rights and liberties as free and equal citizens.

[3:47] In the landmark case of *Canterbury v. Spence*:

"The root premise is the concept, fundamental in American jurisprudence, that "[e]very human being of adult years and sound mind has a right to determine what shall be done with his own

---

[12]Mill argues forcefully in his book *On Liberty*, "The traditions and customs of other people are, to a certain extent, evidence of what their experience has taught *them*; presumptive evidence, and as such, have a claim to his deference: but, in the first place, their experience may be too narrow; or they may not have interpreted it rightly. Secondly, their interpretation of experience may be correct, but unsuitable to him. Customs are made for customary circumstances, and customary characters: and his circumstances or his character may be uncustomary. Thirdly, though the customs be both good as customs, and suitable to him, yet to conform to custom, merely *as* custom, does not educate or develop in him any of the qualities which are the distinctive endowment of a human being. … The mental and moral, like the muscular powers, are improved only by being used. … He who lets the world, or his own portion of it, choose his plan of life for him, has no need of any other faculty than the ape-like one of imitation." Mill, "On Liberty", p. 307.

body…" True consent to what happens to one's self is the informed exercise of a choice, and that entails an opportunity to evaluate knowledgeably the options available and the risks attendant upon each."[13]

[3:48] However, the subjective standard also has its share of conceptual, moral, and practical difficulties. What is ideal is not necessarily practical in a non-ideal world.

b) Weaknesses

(1) Subjective standard is too demanding

[3:49] Even if a professional could determine what the agents specific informational needs are, it is not reasonably to expect professionals to do an exhaustive background and character analysis of each agent in order to make such determinations. The subjective standard unrealistically demands too much from the professional.

[3:50] Not only is it not clear with regard to what material information would be for the agent, it is also not clear just what the characteristics of the agent are other than that they are potentially autonomous.

(2) Subjective standard may be indeterminable

[3:51] If the agent does not know what their specific information needs are for their deliberations then it cannot be expected that the professional or someone else should be able to figure it out for the agent. It is unreasonable to expect professionals to determine what the goals and aspirations of agents are, when the agents themselves may not even know what their goals and aspirations are.

(3) Subjective standard may not promote the agent's best interests

[3:52] From a beneficent (do good) position it can be argued that it may not be in the individual's best interests to always be given the amount and type of information required by the subjective

---

[13] 464 F. 2d 772, 780 (D.C. Dir. 1972), quoting Schloendorff v. Society of New York Hosp., 211 N.Y. 125, 105 N.E. 92, 93 (1914).

standard in order for the agent to act autonomously. The individual may make an autonomous decision that will not promote their own best interests or the agent might intentionally make the wrong decision that may as a result violate the principles of beneficence (do good), nonmaleficence (do no harm) and/or justice (be fair). So if the professional knows that the disclosure of information will result in a decision that will not promote the agent's best interests, or will result in a wrong decision, then it would seem that there may be an obligation on the part of the professional not to provide such information. Autonomy (informed consent) is not the *summum bonum* or the ultimate good in all cases, rather autonomy (informed consent) is highly valued because it normally results in the maximization of the best interests of the agent. If autonomy (informed consent) does not promote the agent's best interests, under some conditions, then autonomy (informed consent) ought not to be promoted under those conditions. Under such circumstances perhaps the more paternalistic professional practice standard, or the objectively uniformed reasonable person standard, would be more appropriate.

(4) Subjective standard is legally problematic

[3:53] Legally a court would not be able to determine if or when the subjective information requirement had been met as the criteria would be different from person to person and from context to context. The legal system works best when there are written contracts that can be agreed upon and evaluated.

(5) Decisions are often made independent of information

[3:54] Empirical studies have shown that individuals often times make decisions prior to and/or independent of information disclosure and individuals often times accept professional recommendations without weighing the risks and benefits of the information carefully. Therefore, material information does not seem to be necessary when decisions are being made prior to and/or independently of the information.

4) Information nondisclosure

[3:55] Under some conditions full disclosure could diminish an agent's autonomy (informed consent) even to the point of making the agent incompetent, or it could result in more burdens than benefits, a violation of nonmaleficence (do no harm), or it could violate certain principles of justice (be fair). For example, within the healthcare system, a healthcare professional can legally proceed without providing full information disclosure under the following conditions:

a) Therapeutic privilege of nondisclosure

(1) emergency,

(2) incompetency

(3) waiver

[3:56] The therapeutic privilege of nondisclosure can only be invoked if there is an emergency which makes the disclosure impractical, or there is sufficient evidence to believe that disclosure of information would render the person incompetent to consent or to refuse treatment in order to maximize their best interests, or if the agent waives their right for material information.

[3:57] An example of a waiver is when a Jehovah's Witness, who has strict beliefs against having a blood transfusion, requests before surgery that if a blood transfusion is necessary for survival, then do it, but don't inform or disclose to them any information about the transfusion after the surgery. Such waivers are best done not individually, but by a group of professionals, such as a Bioethics Committee in order to avoid legal issues and potential abuse.

b) Therapeutic placebos nondisclosure

[3:58] In order for a therapeutic placebo to work, research and/or treatment must be conducted in such a way that the agent does not know if they are getting the treatment or the placebo. A study or treatment, such as this, is permissible as long as the benefits for the agent outweigh the burdens. If it is determined that the burdens of the placebo are greater than the benefits then the research or treatment must be stopped, or the professionals are obligated to provide the real drug or treatment instead of the placebo so as to promote the best interests of the agent. Once it is determined that the treatment arm is more beneficial than the placebo arm, then clinical equipoise has been broken making any continuance of the research ethically in violation of beneficence (do good), nonmaleficence (do no harm), and justice (be fair).

c) Research subjects: necessary conditions for nondisclosure

[3:59] Incomplete disclosures are permitted in research only if all of the following four necessary conditions are met:[14]

(1) Essential for Research

(2) No Substantial Risk To Agent

(3) Agent Informed of Incomplete Disclosure

(4) Agent Consents to Incomplete Disclosure

Information Disclosure Conclusion

[3:60] For informed consent, the politically ideal information disclosure standard for an ideally competent agent would be the subjective standard. However, it must be kept in mind that this is in the context of a well-ordered society in which citizens are in fact ideally competent. In the real world the complexity and difficulty of decision-making often times goes beyond the ability of the particular agent and therefore the agent is not ideally competent. In such situations the subjective standard might not be appropriate for them.

---

[14]Beauchamp and Childress, *Principles of Biomedical Ethics*, 2nd ed., p. 88. Discussion on withholding of information and permissible deception.

[3:61]

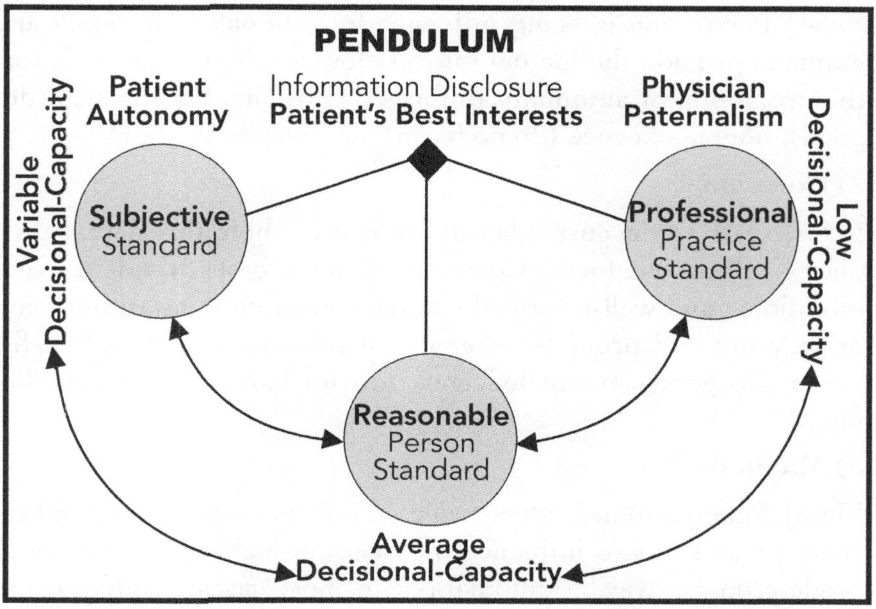

[3:62] As the pendulum of competency swings towards ideal competency the autonomous subjective standard becomes more and more appropriate. As the pendulum of competency swings towards non-ideal competency it swings through the reasonable person standard towards the paternalistic professional practice standard. Each disclosure standard has its appropriate use depending on the complexity and difficulty of the decision and the abilities of the agent.

c. Freedom: Controlling Influences By Others

[3:63] Substantial freedom from controlling influences is the third basic element of autonomy, competency and informed consent. The three categories of controlling influences by other persons are persuasion, coercion, and manipulation.[15]

---

[15]Ibid pp. 93-98.
Discussion on controlling influences.

1) Persuasion

[3:64] Persuasion is being influence by rationality. Rational arguments provide the factual information and logical analysis for the promotion of autonomy (informed consent), beneficence (do good), nonmaleficence (do no harm), and justice (be fair).

2) Coercion

[3:65] Coercion occurs when there is a credible threat that displaces self-directedness. Coercion, in most cases, renders even intentional and well-informed behavior nonautonomous, but may or may not still promote other moral principles such as beneficence (do good), nonmaleficence (do no harm), or justice (be fair).

3) Manipulation

[3:66] Manipulation is when selected information is presented in such a way so as to influence the decision-maker to decide in a predetermined way. Manipulation, in most cases, renders even intentional and well-informed behavior nonautonomous, but may or may not still promote other moral principles such as beneficence (do good), nonmaleficence (do no harm), or justice (be fair).

[3:67] Depending upon the agent and the circumstances persuasion, coercion, and manipulation may or may not be justified depending upon the relationship of the situation with the other principles of beneficence (do good), nonmaleficence (do no harm), or justice (be fair). Autonomy (informed consent) is a *prima facie* principle and is therefore not the *summum bonum* or ultimate end. However, it is not that under some circumstances that one principle may conflict or override another principle, rather it is that under some circumstances one or more principles may be more relevant than another principle.

3. Autonomy has *prima facie* standing

[3:68] The moral principles found in Principlism have *prima facie* standing, meaning that they are moral principles that ought to be followed, yet under certain circumstances the balancing process may determine that another principle has more relevance. For example, if an autonomous choice (informed consent) causes an undue burden to oneself, society or some other sentient being and if through the process of balancing it is determined that nonmaleficence (do no harm) is the more relevant principle in that particular situation, then the moral principle of nonmaleficence (do no harm) has more moral ground than that of autonomy (informed consent). It is not that there is a conflict of duties or obligation between the principles of autonomy (informed consent) and nonmaleficence (do no harm), rather it's that there is a higher ground of obligation of one principle or duty over the other principle or duty based on the situation. As Kant said:

> [3:69] "When two such grounds conflict with each other, practical philosophy says, not that the stronger obligation takes precedence, but that the stronger ground of obligation prevails."[16]

4. Autonomy as a basic human right

[3:70] Autonomy (informed consent) as a basic principle of individual and social morality falls under the category of being a basic human right. Human rights are socially constructed concepts in that all rights claims are also obligations of others claims. In other words, whenever there is a right others always have some type of reciprocal personal or social obligation. If someone claims to have a right, but cannot assert just what the obligation of others would in fact be, then they are not talking about a right.

[3:71] Rights are classified under two major categories; positive rights and negative rights.

a. Positive right

[3:72] When others in society have an obligation to provide something.

b. Negative right

[3:73] When others in society have an obligation to not interfere.

---

[16]Kant, *The Metaphysics of Morals; Doctrine of Right,* pp. 16-17, [6:224]

[3:74] The principle of autonomy (informed consent) as a civil right is composed of a combination of both positive and negative rights. The autonomous (informed consent) criteria of intentionality and freedom from controlling influences seem to be composed of negative rights where others individually or socially have an obligation of not interfering with the autonomous choice. The autonomous (informed consent) criterion of understanding seems to be both a negative and positive right. Understanding is a positive right when others individually or socially have an obligation either to provide or make accessible the information necessary for the making of a substantial informed autonomous decision, and understanding is a negative right when others individually or socially have an obligation of not interfering with the acquisition of information.

5. Autonomy requires competence

[3:75] Competence is a necessary condition for autonomy (informed consent) and is so closely associated that it shares the same three necessary conditions of intention, understanding and freedom.

[3:76] The difference is that competence is defined as the ability to perform a task and autonomy is defined as self-rule. Another difference is that competence is a social gate keeping function in that individuals are either considered legally competent or legally incompetent whereas autonomy (informed consent) is on a sliding scale. Even though there may technically be differing degrees or levels of competence—task-performing abilities, adult persons are socially categorized as being competent until proven to be incompetent.

[3:77] The threshold level for the determination of incompetence is based on the complexity or difficulty of the task or judgment being considered, not on the level of risk. Some easy tasks and judgments can be very risky and some very difficult tasks and judgments can have little if any risk at all. However, as the risk of a decision increases many laws have required a higher level of evidence for competence. The National Bioethics Advisory Commission, for example, has recommended a higher level of evidence for competence to consent to participate in research than to refuse participation in research.

6. Autonomy expressed as informed Consent

[3:78] Informed Consent is the legal term that is also very closely related to autonomy and competence as it also shares the same three necessary conditions of intention, understanding and freedom.

There are two general meanings of informed consent:

#1. Autonomous authorization

[3:79] An agent may give an informed consent by autonomously authorizing something—criteria #1 and still not fulfill the institutional—criteria #2. This is not considered a legal informed consent.

#2. Institutional authorization

[3:80] Conversely, an agent may give an informed consent by fulfilling the institutional—criteria #2 yet not give an autonomous authorization—criteria #1. This also is not considered a legal informed consent.

[3:81] A legal informed consent demands that there must be both an autonomous authorization and an institutional authorization.

[3:82] Regardless of whether the focus is on autonomy, competence, or informed consent, they all overlap on the necessary conditions of intentionality, understanding, and freedom.

B. Nonmaleficence

[3:83] Nonmaleficence is the principle of not harming others. It is generally considered a negative concept of intentionally refraining from harmful actions, i.e., the minimization of burdens.

[3:84] **Nonmaleficence:**

1. Perfect obligation.

a. Agent knows exactly what the refrainment in question is, e.g., 25 mph speed limit means do not go over 25 mph.

b. Agent knows exactly to whom the action is or is not to be directed towards, e.g., 25 mph is directed to drivers of vehicles.

2. Negative requirement of refrainment.

3. Agent must be impartial.

4. Failure to refrain often results in legal punishment.

C. Beneficence

[3:85] Beneficence is the principle of contributing to the welfare of others. It is generally considered a positive concept of intentionally acting for the benefit of others, i.e., the maximization of benefits.

[3:86] **Beneficence:**

1. Imperfect obligation.

a. Agent does not know exactly what the action in question is, e.g., charity can be in many forms.

b. Agent does not know exactly to whom it is or is not to be directed towards, e.g., charity can be directed to any number of persons or causes.

2. Positive requirement of action.

3. Agent need not be impartial.

4. Failure to act positively rarely results in legal punishment.

[3:87] The principles of beneficence (do good) and nonmaleficence (do no harm) are best understood as the maximization of benefits and the minimization of burdens. However, there still are some conceptual and moral difficulties with these distinctions. One of the most interesting difficulties is the distinction between quantitative and qualitative benefits and burdens.

Quantitative and qualitative benefits and burdens

[3:88] If there were no qualitative distinctions between benefits and burdens then it would be possible to implement a purely quantitative assessment. Under this quantitative rubric a person could just draw, for example, two columns listing benefits of a moral decision in the first column and burdens in the second column, sum up each column, and if the benefits outweigh the burdens then the person ought to go with the decision, if not then the person ought not to go with the decision.

[3:89] However, if one unit of measure differs qualitatively from another unit of measure then the whole process becomes nonsense as the agent will be comparing apples with oranges. For example:

QUALITATIVE ASSESSMENT
1. **If** an agent's spouse provides 100 units of benefits and 13 units of burdens for a total of 87 hedonic units. 2. **If** a pepperoni pizza provides 10 units of benefits and 3 units of burdens for a total of 7 hedonic units.
∴ 3. **Then:** it follows that, the agent should be willing to trade their spouse for 13 pepperoni pizzas for a total of 91 hedonic units or a total gain of 4 hedonic units.

[3:90] The problem with the above example is that either there was an under estimation of the quantitative units of the benefits of the spouse, or what is more probably the case, the quality of the relationship units is categorically different from that of the pizza units.

[3:91] Since qualitative values are subjective, but not necessarily relative, it shows the importance of autonomy (informed consent) determinations of benefits and burdens. Since qualitative values are also part of social contracts such as human rights values, it also shows the importance of justice (be fair) determinations when considering benefits and burdens.

[3:92] The principles of beneficence (do good) and nonmaleficence (do no harm) are an integral part of moral-decision making and understanding the distinction between quantitative and qualitative measurements fortifies the need for autonomy (informed consent) and justice (be fair) determinations.

D. Justice

[3:93] Justice (be fair) can be defined as the social protection of individual and social rights and liberties and the implementation of the fair distribution of benefits and burdens. Justice (be fair) is also the political realization of "peace" which is the absence of willful and systemic harm, and the presence of (roughly) equal real opportunities to realize our freedoms and capabilities.

[3:94] In this section the social protection of individual autonomy (informed consent) will be manifested to the degree that moral evaluations are socially determined or individually determined. The fair distribution of benefits and burdens will be manifested to the degree that the economic distributions of social goods are distributed fairly. Justice (be fair) will be described using the two criteria of 1. moral authority: government controlled morality vs. individual controlled morality, and 2. economic distribution: trickle-down economics vs. trickle-up economics.

[3:95]

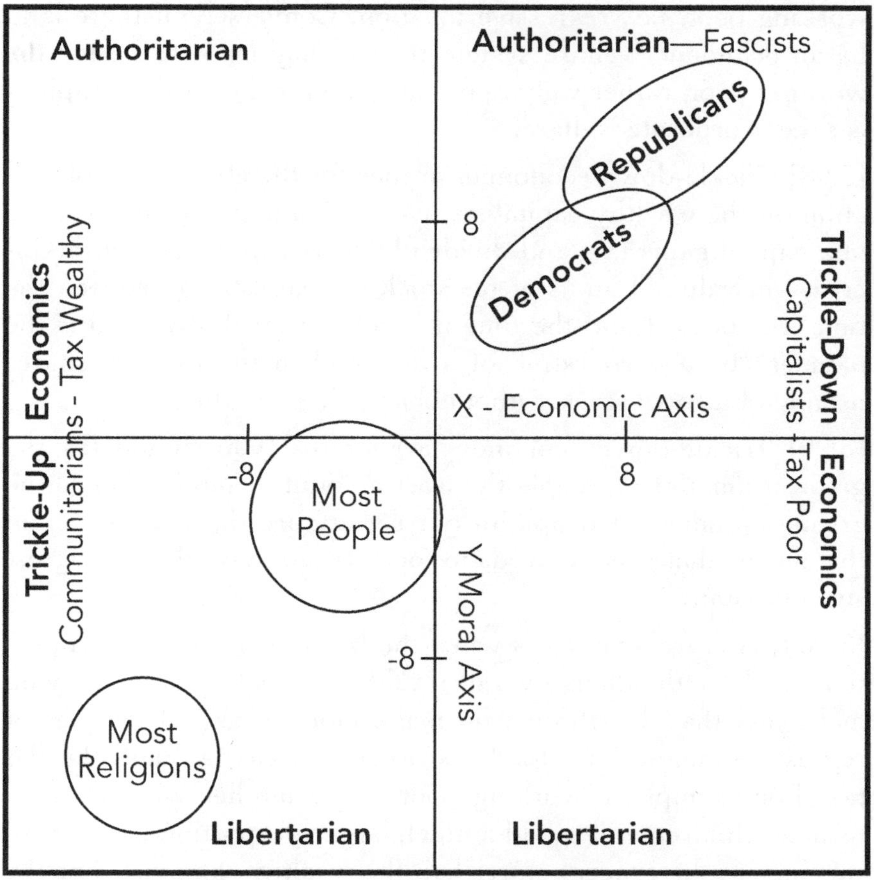

[3:96] The easiest way to understand the above diagram is by thinking of the x-axis and the y-axis independently. The x-axis is the economic line—right/left and the y-axis is the social morality line—up/down.

1. Economic x-Axis

a. Trickle-down economics (Right)

[3:97] The extreme right on the economic axis emphasizes trickle-down economics. Trickle-down economics is the viewpoint that money flows down from those who have capital wealth to the working poor. Since money flows from the top down this position holds that if there is to be any taxation then it ought not to tax capital wealth, rather it is better economically to tax the working poor, i.e., regressive taxation. Conversely, if there is to be an economic welfare system then it ought not to be for the working poor, rather welfare ought to be for the wealthy capitalists, i.e., corporate welfare.

[3:98] Trickle-down economics argues for the elimination of taxation on the wealthy capitalists by the elimination of inheritance tax, capital gains tax, and dividend tax. A capital gain is the increase in value of an asset (as stock or real estate) between the time it is bought and the time it is sold. A stock dividend is the payment by a corporation of a dividend in the form of shares usually of its own stock without change in par value.

[3:99] Trickle-down economics argues that you should tax the greatest amount of people the least amount of money. Since the greatest number of people in our society are the working poor, this means that society needs to focus taxation on them—regressive taxation.

[3:100] A regressive tax is when the burden of a tax, in proportion to the individuals overall wealth, is greater for those who make less than for those who make more. Classic examples of regressive taxation are food tax, sales tax, gas tax, and the flat tax. For example, a working poor single mother who has four teenage children will spend a much larger proportion of her total earnings at the grocery store than the wealthy capitalist. For the wealthy capitalist the food tax has little if any effect on their total wealth. Whereas for the working poor, the food-tax effectively is an additional tax on a very large proportion of their total income. Trickle-down economics is the viewpoint that economic responsibility results in the maximization of regressive taxation such as food tax and sales tax, and the minimization of progressive taxes such as capital gains, dividends, and inheritance taxes.

b. Trickle-up economics (Left)

[3:101] The extreme left on the economic axis emphasizes trickle-up economics. Trickle-up economics is the viewpoint that money flows up from the working class poor to those who have capital wealth. For example, workers are paid less than the value of their labor and the extra profits then trickle-up to those who do no work other than providing capital. Since there are relatively few individuals who are making very large sums of money and they are doing so without providing any labor, other than capital, this point of view thinks that this type of economic distribution is unjust and that there needs to be a process for redistributing the wealth more justly, i.e., progressive taxation.

[3:102] Since money flows up from the bottom then justice demands that taxation should be greater for the few rich than on the majority of the working poor. If the goal is to keep the economy as active as possible taxation of the poor should be minimized and taxation for the capitalists should be maximized. Trickle-up economics is the viewpoint that economic responsibility results in the maximization of progressive taxation such as capital gains, dividends, and inheritance taxes, and the minimization of regressive taxes such as food tax and sales tax.

2. Social Morality y-Axis

a. Government authority (Up)

[3:103] The extreme up on the social moral axis emphasizes governmental authority with regard to social morality. This point of view maximizes governmental moral authority and minimizes the importance of personal moral autonomy (informed consent). Individuals in this type of society are not respected for making autonomous (informed consent) moral choices through a process of fair procedures, rather individuals are forced into compliance by coercive threats and punished for noncompliance. This paternalistic point of view has little respect for personal autonomy (informed consent).

b. Personal liberty (Down)

[3:104] The extreme down on the social moral axis emphasizes individual autonomy (informed consent). This point of view maximizes personal moral autonomy (informed consent) and minimizes paternalistic government authority such as the professional practice standard. Individuals in this type of society are not forced into compliance by coercive threats and punished for noncompliance, rather their personal moral autonomy (informed consent) is maximized through a process of fair procedures. This antipaternalistic (anti professional practice standard) point of view has very high respect for personal autonomy (informed consent).

3. Four Quadrants

a. Libertarian right (Bottom-Right)

[3:105] The libertarian right (bottom right quadrant) emphasizes both economic and moral autonomy (informed consent). The focus is on the minimization of governmental authority, (professional practice standard) and the maximization of personal autonomy (informed consent). This personal autonomy (informed consent) is maximized by the establishment of individual rights and liberties and is implemented through the process of fair procedures. From this point of view as economies are determined by the process of the free-market system, they naturally tend towards trickle-down capitalistic monopolies.

b. Authoritarian left (Top-Left)

[3:106] The authoritarian left (top left quadrant) emphasizes both economic and moral authority of the government, (professional practice standard) usually in the form of trickle-up economics, and moral legislation. The focus is on the minimization of individual rights and liberties (minimize informed consent) and the maximization of governmental authority (professional practice standard). The authoritarian left is usually manifested as being totalitarian or fascist. Fascism and totalitarianism is when there is a centralized government that controls both the economy and the morality of a country while suppressing opposition. From this point of view as economies are determined by a centralized government, they naturally tend towards a trickle-up egalitarian economy.

c. Authoritarian right (Top-Right)

[3:107] The authoritarian right (top right quadrant) emphasizes both economic and moral governmental authority, usually in the form of trickle-down economics, and moral legislation. The focus, like the authoritarian left, is on the minimization of individual rights and liberties as implemented through the process of fair procedures (informed consent), and the maximization of governmental authority (professional practice standard). The authoritarian right is also usually manifested as totalitarian or fascist to the extent that there is a centralized government that controls both the economy and the morality of a country while suppressing opposition. From this point of view as economies are determined by a centralized government, they naturally tend towards trickle-down capitalistic monopolies.

d. Libertarian left (Bottom-Left)

[3:108] The libertarian left (bottom left quadrant) emphasizes both economic and moral autonomy (informed consent). The focus is on the minimization of governmental authority (professional practice standard), and the maximization of personal autonomy (informed consent). This personal autonomy (informed consent) is maximized by the establishment of individual rights and liberties and is implemented through the process of fair procedures. From this point of view as economies are determined by the process of fair procedures they naturally tend towards a trickle-up egalitarian economy.

4. Diversity in the Compass

[3:109] On any given issue a person may end up in different quadrants. However, when asked a variety of questions on a variety of subjects that relate to the economy and to social morality an average or a tally can be done and individuals can be plotted on the political compass. Then if others answer the same questions, then a person can compare themselves with them as well. Historical persons can also be plotted on the political compass even if they haven't directly answered the questions by answering the questions for them based on historical text. Although there are no units on this Cartesian graph the historical comparisons are interesting. (For more information and for a personal plotting on this graph go to http://www.politicalcompass.org/test)

5. Application of Justice

[3:110] The principlistic application of justice (be fair) can be accomplished using a variety of social justice perspectives.

a. Libertarians (Bottom-Right & Left)

[3:111] Libertarians will emphasize individual rights and liberties often times independently of the determinations of the benefits and burdens of society as a whole. Political libertarians in the United States have a tendency to be at the bottom right quadrant. However, most religious traditions, and rational moral evaluations generally argue for the libertarian left position.

b. Utilitarians (Bottom-Right & Left)

[3:112] Utilitarians are similar to libertarians in emphasizing individual rights and liberties but unlike libertarians, utilitarians greatly emphasize the maximization of benefits and the minimization of burdens of both the individual citizens and society as a whole. As a result utilitarians have a tendency to be higher up and further to the left on the compass than the bottom-right libertarians.

c. Egalitarians (Top & Bottom Left)

[3:113] Egalitarians will emphasize equality both economically and with regard to social morality. This equality has a tendency to necessitate the empowering of authority for its implementation resulting in a tendency to be further up on the compass than the libertarian left.

d. Communitarians (Top & Bottom-Left)

[3:114] Communitarians will emphasize the importance of culture, traditions, relationships, and casuistry (professional practice standard) and deemphasize individual rights and liberties (informed consent). This deemphasization of rights and liberties has the tendency to move the communitarians further up on the political compass than the libertarian left.

6. Democracy

[3:115] What type or model of justice (be fair) is to be emphasized will be largely dependent on the conditions and environment that the community finds itself. Types of governments ought to be determined by the society's history, culture, diversity, economic and moral conditions along with the traits and abilities of its leaders and the citizens.

[3:116] Democracy would demand that its citizens be informed, competent, and tolerant of diverse points of views. To the degree that citizens lack those traits is the degree to which democracy ought not to be pursued as intolerant democratic societies end up being the tyranny of the majority. Constitutional checks and balances along with individual rights and liberties are usually associated with most forms of democracy in order to prevent the natural tendency towards the tyranny of the majority.

7. Communitarianism

[3:117] Communitarianism with its motto of "from each according to their ability and to each according to their need" may be the most ideal form of relationship based government but may also be one of the most practically unfulfillable with the current state of humanity and its tendency towards selfishness and being adversarial.

[3:118] However, morality has always been about the determining of ideal goals and objectives and striving towards that perfection along with the recognition and necessity of what does in fact practically work under the current environment that society finds itself.

[3:119] Interestingly, most American citizens, and most of the populations around the world, tend to be located in the bottom left quadrant of the political compass. Most American politicians tend to be located in the top right quadrant. Republican politicians push towards the very top right quadrant and Democrat politicians are a bit more moderate but are still also in the top right quadrant.

[3:120] On the one hand, this is a surprising conclusion considering that most voters believe that there democratic representatives share their views of the function and role of government when in fact it turns out that the citizen's representatives do not share the same views. On the other hand, perhaps this should be expected considering how corporate America demands the economic right position and many religious Americans demand an intolerant moral position towards diversity. The corporate and religious powers push or compel politicians to be in the top right quadrant.

8. Political Compass

[3:121] Answer the following propositions by circling option **A** for agree and option **D** for disagree and give no answer if you are neutral. There are no right or wrong answers. There are also no units to the Political Compass meaning that the only relevant data in the end is the comparison of one person's result with that of another person's result.

[3:122] After answering the propositions, go and circle the appropriate weighting in the box for each section. Add up the points. The maximum and minimum value is 16 and -16 respectively. Plot your x and y points and graph it. For example a -8 x axis and a -8 y axis will graph you in the center of the bottom left quadrant.

Political Compass

a. Economic X-Axis Propositions

A = Agree

D = Disagree

Neutral needs no response

[3:123] **Note:** If there is a (Left) at the end of a statement, then the statement will move you left on the political compass if you agree with it. If there is a (Right) at the end of a statement, then the statement will move you right on the political compass, if you agree with it. Lastly, for simplicity sake, the options available are "Agree" or "Disagree" even though it is recognized that the questions and responses are much more complex than just an agree or disagree.

[3:124]

1. AD From each according to his ability, to each according to his need. (Left)

2. AD The freer the market, the freer the people. (Right)

3. AD The rich are too highly taxed. (Right)

4. AD The poor are too highly taxed. (Left)

5. AD Controlling inflation is more important than controlling unemployment. (Right)

6. AD Controlling unemployment is more important than controlling inflation. (Left)

7. AD Tariffs or protectionism is sometimes necessary in international trade. (Left)

8. AD It is unjust that many personal fortunes are made by individuals that only manipulate money without contributing any labor towards production. (Left)

9. AD Tax payers ought not to fund museums or art, rather they ought to be able to provide for themselves solely on a commercial basis. (Right)

10. AD Those with the ability to pay should have the right towards better healthcare. (Right)

11. AD What is good for corporations is good for everyone. (Right)

12. AD Personal charity is better than social welfare. (Right)

13. AD Natural resources ought to belong to the community, not to individuals. (Left)

14. AD Workers ought to control the means of production, not individual "owners." (Left)

15. AD Aside from obeying civil laws, corporations have no other social responsibilities than to maximize profit to its shareholders. (Right)

16. AD Money flows from the working poor to the rich. (Left)

[3:125]

Circle the point value for each X-Axis proposition			
#	Agree	Neutral	Disagree
1	-1	0	1
2	1	0	-1
3	1	0	-1
4	-1	0	1
5	1	0	-1
6	-1	0	1
7	-1	0	1
8	-1	0	1
9	1	0	-1
10	1	0	-1
11	1	0	-1
12	1	0	-1
13	-1	0	1
14	-1	0	1
15	1	0	-1
16	-1	0	1
Total			
Sum Total: Agree + Disagree =			
Plot the sum on the X-axis [3:132]			

b. Governmental Authority Y-Axis Propositions

A = Agree

D = Disagree

Neutral needs no response

[3:126] **Note:** If there is an (Up) at the end of a statement, then the statement will move you up on the political compass if you agree with it. If there is a (Down) at the end of a statement, then the statement will move you down on the political compass, if you agree with it.

[3:127]

1. AD I'd always support my country, regardless of whether it was right or wrong. (Up)
2. AD Military action ought not to go against international law. (Down)
3. AD All governmental authority ought to be questioned. (Down)
4. AD Civil law ought to enforce an eye for an eye and a tooth for a tooth. (Up)
5. AD Government is to be limited to the assuring of rights and liberties. (Down)
6. AD The most important thing for children to learn is to accept authority. (Up)
7. AD Civil liberties are being excessively curbed in the name of counter-terrorism. (Down)
8. AD Government ought to be deeply involved in the public school curriculum. (Up)
9. AD An all-powerful government is better than a limited government. (Up)
10. AD The prediction of future events is not possible. (Down)
11. AD It is not the role of government to promote the majority's personal convictions. (Down)
12. AD You cannot be moral without being religious. (Up)

13. AD Government is to promote morality through the laws that it makes. (Up)

14. AD Public schools ought not to instill religious values. (Down)

15. AD It is important that our government leaders are religious. (Up)

16. AD Government is not to punish sexual activity that does not violate other's civil rights. (Down)

[3:128]

Circle the point value for each Y-Axis proposition			
#	Agree	Neutral	Disagree
1	1	0	-1
2	-1	0	1
3	-1	0	1
4	1	0	-1
5	-1	0	1
6	1	0	-1
7	-1	0	1
8	1	0	-1
9	1	0	-1
10	-1	0	1
11	-1	0	1
12	1	0	-1
13	1	0	-1
14	-1	0	1
15	1	0	-1
16	-1	0	1
Total			
Sum Total: Agree + Disagree =			
Plot the sum on the Y-axis [3:132]			

[3:129]

c. Political Compass Plot

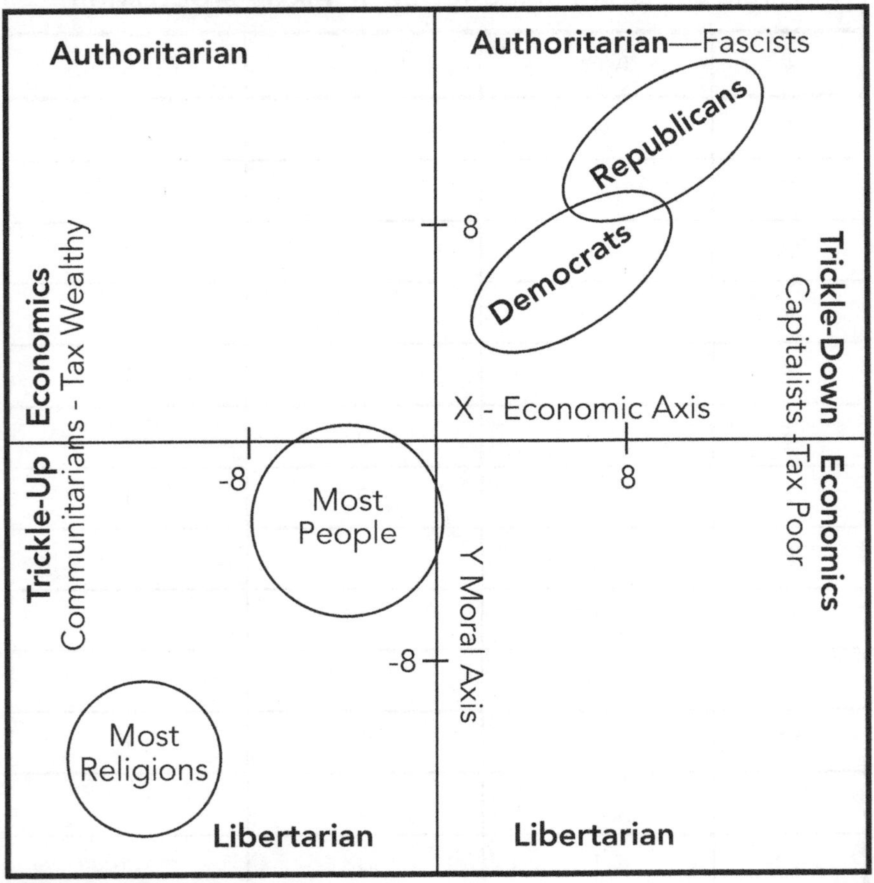

Conclusion

[3:130] The moral approach of Principlism has now been briefly presented. The discussion focused on the broad general principles of autonomy (informed consent), beneficence (do good), nonmaleficence (do no harm), and justice (be fair). Using this approach there will still be disagreements in the specification, balancing, and the coherent organization of these principles but through the process of inquiry, by multiple and diverse methods, there will be more agreement than disagreement on the resultant conclusions. Even though there are differences in epistemic justifications and beliefs between various individuals and groups within society, descriptively, there will still be wide intersubjective agreements on the general moral principles. Ideals, together with practicality, will help determine the specification and balancing of the principles of autonomy (informed consent), beneficence (do good), nonmaleficence (do no harm), and justice (be fair), and Principlism will ultimately result in a morally progressive society that respects the beauty and necessity of pluralism and diversity.

***

Va. INFORMED CONSENT

Utilitarian & Deontological Perspectives

Overview

[1:1]

The issue of informed consent and the proper amount of information disclosure has become a prominent issue regarding research on human subjects and patient care. In spite of the numerous discussions on the criteria to be used for obtaining informed consent there has been little agreement on the epistemic justifications of such criteria. This is because most discussions approach the issue of informed consent from reasonable and rational yet incompatible comprehensive worldviews. The position developed in this chapter will overcome this epistemic problem by using Rawls' "metaphysically neutral" political conception of justice.

[1:2] The first section of this chapter will present the historical elements of informed consent. Classical utilitarian and deontological arguments are used to show how these comprehensive worldviews can arrive at the same resulting viewpoint on consent.[1] However, even though the utilitarian and deontological positions can both come to the consensus that consent is the moral position both are still unable to come to an epistemic

---

[1] The consensus on the value of consent for both utilitarian and deontological positions will also be shown in §2 and §3 respectively.

agreement on the fundamental basis or argument(s) for each other's position on consent.[2]

[1:3] In the second half of this chapter, using the Rawlsian social-political position, which is significantly different from either classical utilitarianism or deontology,[3] it will be shown how Rawls' social-political philosophy is able to not only stay metaphysically independent of both the classical utilitarian and deontological moral positions, but is also able to absorb both of them even though they may be incompatible and/or even opposing positions.[4] Rawls' social-political process or arguments are fundamentally agreeable to both the classical utilitarian and deontological positions. This is possible not only because of the broad, general and noncomprehensive nature of Rawls' social-political philosophy but also because of the fundamental fairness of Rawls' hypothetical approach and because Rawls' political framework is metaphysically neutral in that his framework does not necessarily determine a specific comprehensive worldview such as utilitarianism or deontology. Rawls believes that this broad and general approach is a necessary and progressive step if we are going to live compatibly in a pluralistic democratic society composed of free and equal citizens.

---

2 Classical utilitarians argue from a consequential basis and classical deontologists or intuitionists argue from an intrinsic worth basis. However, there are individuals who disagree with this. In *Bioethics in a Liberal Society,* p. 113, Max Charlesworth argues that "Mill pretends that autonomy, liberty and individuality are based upon 'the principle of utility', but in fact the values of autonomy and personal liberty are for him as absolute as they are for Kant. They are intrinsic goods regardless of any consequences they may have and there is, for Mill, no envisageable set of circumstances in which the general recognition of autonomy and liberty might have such untoward consequences that their restriction would be justified." I do not accept this analysis as will be made clear in §2.

3 As we shall see this is not only because of its general and noncomprehensive nature but also because Rawls' theory is argued from a hypothetical "contractarian" political position.

4 The moral viewpoints are "absorbed" in the sense that both could successfully exist within the broad and general Rawlsian framework without being in "political" conflict with each other.

Introduction

[1:4] Informed consent addresses the issue as to what standard of information disclosure would be necessary for a proper informed consent in a pluralistic society comprised of free and equal citizens who hold to differing comprehensive worldviews. This political approach ends up being fundamentally liberal in that it does not judge whether reasonable and rational comprehensive worldviews are correct or incorrect regardless of whether they are considered to be liberal or conservative positions.

[1:5] Historically the principles of beneficence (do good), and nonmaleficence (do no harm), have dominated the medical culture and have been undergoing both internal and external pressure to reevaluate itself because of the contemporary focus and emphasis on autonomy (informed consent). The fundamental basis typically used in this reevaluation, of what amount or type of information disclosure is necessary in order to obtain a proper informed consent, has been classical consequentialism or deontological reasoning. However, consequentialism and deontology are appeals to specific comprehensive worldviews; they are not broad and general political conceptions that all citizens with differing comprehensive worldviews can hold to at the same time. Since our pluralistic society is composed of many differing incommensurable reasonable and rational comprehensive worldviews there is great resistance to any type of religious, philosophical or moral agreement that would put one group's reasoning, as correct and others as being wrong.

[1:6] To cross this impasse it is necessary to establish broad and general political conceptions that all or most reasonable and rational comprehensive worldviews can agree to. It is not necessary, for example, to present arguments for and against utilitarian or deontological reasoning as they are both reasonable and rational comprehensive worldviews consistent within themselves. Thus the task is to construct a political system in which incommensurable comprehensive worldviews can agree on based on a freestanding interrelated consensus, i.e. broad and general metaphysical claims that are not specific to a limited number of comprehensive worldviews.

[1:7] This is accomplished in the second half of this Chapter by presenting Rawls' political conception of justice (be fair), as expressed in *A Theory of Justice* and *Political Liberalism*. From this metaphysically neutral political conception of justice an ideal standard of information disclosure for a proper autonomous informed consent is extrapolated. This is possible because Rawls' metaphysical claims are so broad and general that his political framework is derivable from, consistent with, or at least not in contradiction with a majority of traditionally held comprehensive worldviews.

[1:8] Once the proper amount of information disclosure necessary for an autonomous informed consent has been determined for an ideal political society, argument as to how this ideal conception of disclosure needs to be modified in order to be justly applied to our nonideal political society is presented.

I. Informed Consent

A. Importance Of Informed Consent

1. Nuremberg Code

[1:10] Since the Nuremberg Trials the topic of informed consent has dominated the subject of research on human subjects. The world was shocked that in the German concentration camps horrible and brutal experiments were conducted on nonconsenting subjects.[5] The Nuremberg Code was articulated in a court opinion concerning the trial of twenty-three German physicians for "war crimes and crimes against humanity" during World War II.[6]

[1:11] In terms of consent the Nuremberg Code says:

> "The voluntary consent of the human subject is absolutely essential. This means that the person involved should have legal capacity to give consent; should be so situated as to be able to exercise free power of choice, without the intervention of any element of force, fraud, deceit, duress, overreaching, or other ulterior form of constraint or coercion; and should have sufficient knowledge and comprehension of the elements of the subject matter involved as to enable him to make an understanding and enlightened decision. This latter element requires that before the acceptance of an affirmative decision by the experimental subject there should be made known to him the nature, duration, and purpose of the experiment; the method and means by which it is to be conducted; all inconveniences and hazards reasonably to be expected; and the effects upon his health or person which may possibly come from his participation in the experiment. The duty and responsibility for ascertaining the quality of the consent rests upon each individual who initiates, directs or engages in

---

[5] Tom L. Beauchamp, James F. Childress, *Principles of Biomedical Ethics*, Second Edition (New York: Oxford University Press, 1983), p. 66.

[6] George J. Annas, Leonard H. Glantz, Barbara F. Katz, *Informed Consent to Human Experimentation: The Subject's Dilemma* (Cambridge: Ballinger Publishing Company, 1977), p. 6.

the experiment. It is a personal duty and responsibility that may not be delegated to another with impunity." [7]

2. Nuremberg Code's four elements of consent

[1:12] As a response to these Nazi experiments, in which the consent of the human subjects was not even considered, the Nuremberg Code established four characteristics of consent. Consent was to be 1. voluntary, 2. competent, 3. informed, and 4. with understanding.[8] However, the Nazi actions were crimes not merely because they violated consent rather, they were crimes mainly because their actions were not beneficent, or do good, and were not nonmaleficent, or do no harm.

B. History Of Beneficence And Nonmaleficence

[1:13] Historically,[9] what was considered important was beneficence, or do goo, and nonmaleficence (do no harm), not the consent of the patient. This is clearly expressed in the Hippocratic tradition of medicine[10] where the paternalistic injunction was "I

---

[7] *Trials of War Criminals before the Nuremberg Military Tribunals under Control Council Law No. 10,* vol. 2 (Washington, D.C.: U.S. Government Printing Office, 1949), pp. 181-82.

[8] Annas, Glantz, Katz, *Informed Consent to Human Experimentation: The Subject's Dilemma*, p. 7.

[9] For "A Brief Historical Overview" see T. M. Grunder, *Informed Consent: A Tutorial* (Owing Mills: National Health Publishing, 1986), pp. 1-9.

[10] Assumed traditionally to have been written by Hippocrates, the Oath exemplifies only the Pythagorean school rather than Greek thought in general. The Oath of Hippocrates is one of the earliest and most important statements on medical ethics. Estimates of its actual date of origin vary from the sixth century B.C. to the first century A.D. Not only has the Oath provided the foundation for many succeeding medical oaths (e.g. the Declaration of Geneva), but it is also still administered by many medical schools to graduating medical students either in its original form or in a slightly altered version. To see an example of a graduating oath that follows very closely the Hippocratic Oath see the *Solemn Oath of a Physician of Russia* which can be found in the *Kennedy Institute of Ethics Journal* Vol. 3, No. 4 (Baltimore: The Johns Hopkins University Press, 1993), p. 419. This Oath has been approved by the Minister of Health and the Minister of Higher Education of the Russian Federation and has been taken by the 1992 and 1993 graduating classes of Moscow Medical University.

will keep them [patients] from harm and injustice."[11] In contrast, it might be argued that today the healthcare maxim is "I will get the patient's informed consent."

C. Informed Consent As A Contemporary Myth

[1:14] Most of the recent medical codes have held that physicians must obtain the informed consent of patients before undertaking any healthcare procedures.[12] However, it is still questionable whether informed consent, in its true sense, has really arrived in clinical medicine.

> [1:15] "Katz's view [is] that informed consent in clinical medicine has more the quality of a fairy tale, myth, or mirage than reality.[13] As he sees it, informed consent has done nothing to change historical medical practice because informed consent has never really arrived in medicine, never really taken hold. … Katz seems right in his thesis that informed consent has not changed the fundamental character of the physician-patient relationship. … The beneficence model is overwhelmingly predominant. Patients routinely acquiesce to medical interventions rather than autonomously authorizing them. From this perspective all the changes are surface displays, while below the surface there are no more real "informed consents" than in the past." [14]

D. Immorality Of Being Submissive or Controlling

[1:16] Both classical utilitarian and deontological perspectives would argue that the patient who is competent and acquiescent,

---

[11] See Ludwig Edelstein, "The Hippocratic Oath: Text, Translation, and Interpretation," *Supplements to the Bulletin of the History of Medicine* 30, Supplement 1 (Baltimore: The Johns Hopkins University Press, 1943); reprinted in Owsei Temkin and C. Lillian Temkin, eds., *Ancient Medicine: Selected Papers of Ludwig Edelstein* (Baltimore: The Johns Hopkins University Press, 1967).

[12] Beauchamp and Childress, *Principles of Biomedical Ethics*, 2nd ed., pp. 67.

[13] Jay Katz, *The Silent World of Doctor and Patient* (New York: Free Press, Macmillan Inc., 1984), pp. 83-85.

[14] Ruth R. Faden, Tom L. Beauchamp, *A History and Theory of Informed Consent*, (New York: Oxford University Press, 1986), p. 100.

i.e., submissive, and the healthcare provider who is dominant, i.e., controlling, are both acting immorally.[15]

[1:17] Even though the utilitarian and deontological viewpoints are fundamentally different from each other[16] it is interesting how practically they will still arrive at the same conclusion: two competent individuals that are involved in a compromised consent situation, i.e. the submissive and dominant positions, would be violating, if not their own political liberties, the political liberties of others as citizens in a free and equal democratic society.[17]

[1:18] The ones who are submissive fail to have a proper regard for themselves and can in a very real sense cause or perpetuate the dominant party to have an improper view of the submissive party. The ones who are dominant fail to have a proper perspective on how they are to view others and can cause or perpetuate the submissive party to have an improper view of the dominant party.

[1:19] Therefore, on the one hand, if seeing oneself as submissive implies being less free and equal then that would be an improper view of oneself in a free and equal society. Also, if seeing oneself as submissive causes others to see themselves as dominant—in

---

[15] Immoral in the sense that to be either "acquiescent" or "dominant" would be inconsistent with the development of the person for the utilitarian and would be inconsistent with the dignity of persons for the deontologist. However, I am not saying that both are on the same "order" of immorality, e.g. it may be the case that in many or most situations that there is a greater degree of "immorality" on the part of the "dominant" person as they generally have greater control and responsibility. This might be especially true, for example in a doctor-patient relationship where the doctor takes the "dominant" position.

[16] Different at least to the extent that classical utilitarian and deontological positions appeal *fundamentally* to extrinsic and intrinsic values respectively. This does not mean that one would necessarily be involved in a contradiction if one were to believe consent/autonomy was both intrinsically and extrinsically valuable. However, as we shall see in §2 and §3 Mill's classical utilitarianism and Kant's classical deontology stresses extrinsic values and intrinsic worth respectively.

[17] If these arguments about consent are in fact sound, then we will have come to the same basic conclusion by using not only the two most dominant and classical ethical viewpoints but also by using a modern social-political philosophy that claims to be independent or freestanding from these classical moral positions.

the sense of perceiving others as less than free and equal, that also is an improper view of individuals in a free and equal society.

[1:20] Conversely, on the other hand, if seeing oneself as dominant implies seeing others as less free and equal than oneself then that would be an improper view of oneself and others in a free and equal society. Also, if seeing oneself as dominant causes others to see themselves as less than free and equal, in comparison to oneself, that also is an improper view of individuals in a free and equal society.

II. Informed Consent: Utilitarian Support

[1:22] Both historically and contemporarily, utilitarianism and deontology[18] have dominated the discussions about informed consent.[19] Classical utilitarianism supports informed consent insofar as informed consent involves autonomy. Classical deontology supports informed consent insofar as informed consent presents a duty to ourselves, and to others, to treat, and to be treated, as persons having intrinsic worth, i.e., having the ability and responsibility to conform to civil law for the purpose of peace and to self-legislate maxims of actions for the purpose of self-perfection and the happiness of others.

A. Utilitarianism As Maximizing Best Interest

[1:23] Utilitarians *could* argue that the purpose and justification for healthcare is to promote benefit, and to protect persons from various risks of harm. The autonomous choice, or informed consent of the patient, would then be a secondary issue, and beneficence, or the professional responsibility to do good, the primary issue. This type of paternalism[20] could be supported by the utili-

---

[18] "Theories of normative ethics fall into two main groups: *consequentialist* (or *utilitarian*) theories and *deontological* theories (from Greek *deon* = duty)" Henrik R. Wulff, Stig A. Pedersen, Raben Rosenberg, *Philosophy Of Medicine*, (London: Blackwell Scientific Publications, 1990), p. 179.

[19] "This study of the theoretical aspects in medical ethics is highly developed with an abundance of primary and secondary texts. ... Almost universally these topics are treated from the viewpoint of either utilitarian or deontological ethics. An essential grasp of the principles and complexities of these theories is mandatory for the practicing of medical ethics" William J. Ellos, *Ethical Practice In Clinical Medicine* (New York: Routledge, 1990), p. 2.

[20] For an excellent discussion on the nature of strong and weak paternalism see, Beauchamp and Childress, *Principles of Biomedical Ethics*, 2nd ed., pp. 168-79.

tarian as a form of consequential justification.[21] Here the utilitarian's *summum bonum* or the "ultimate good" does not include autonomous decision-making or informed consent but rather only the well being of the patient. Those who would subscribe to this reasoning with regard to beneficence (do good), and/or non-maleficence (do no harm), would be inclined to protect patients against unwise assumptions of risk(s) regardless of whether it was the patient's autonomous and/or informed choice.

B. Utilitarianism As Maximizing Autonomy

1. Autonomy usually outweighs other concerns

[1:24] Other classical utilitarians (in particular Mill) argued that liberty or autonomy[22] ought not to be interfered with unless it is to prevent harm to others.

[1:25] Mill in his book *On Liberty* says:

> "The interference of society to overrule his judgment and purposes in what only regards himself, must be grounded on general presumptions: which may be altogether wrong, and even if right, are as likely as not to be misapplied to individual cases. ... [H]e himself is the final judge. All errors which he is likely to commit against advice and warn-

[21] Max Charlesworth, *Bioethics in a Liberal Society,* (New York: Cambridge University Press, 1993), pp. 112-113, argues that "... for the utilitarian an efficient and effective health system is a good health system regardless of whether the health choices of individuals are diminished or not. (It might be argued that utilitarianism could accommodate itself to the goal of enlargement of choice in this area in that a good health strategy would be one which had the consequence or outcome of maximizing autonomy and choice ...But, ... it is not possible to quantify and measure and do sums about such a consequence or outcome [greater autonomy] in the way required by the theory of utilitarianism.)"

[22] The meaning of the term "autonomy", like many other words in our language, depends upon who is using the term and the context in which it is used. "Autonomy" or "self-rule" can be used to mean what Mill refers to as "liberty". "Liberty" for Mill implies the "internal" capacity to choose on one's behalf but primarily it means the lack of imposition from others when making a choice. This is important for Mill as this liberty or what I have called "autonomy" is the fundamental basis for the development of what Mill would call individuality, which is the "best thing" a human being can be. (John Stuart Mill, "On Liberty" in *Essential Works of John Stuart Mill,* ed. Max Lerner [New York: Bantam Books, 1961], p. 312.).

> ing, are far outweighed by the evil of allowing others to constrain him to what they deem his good." [23]

2. Protection of others from harm may override autonomy

> [1:26] "[T]he only purpose for which power can be rightfully exercised over any member of a civilized community, against his will, is to prevent harm to others. His own good, either physical or moral, is not a sufficient warrant. He cannot rightfully be compelled to do or forbear because it will be better for him to do so, because it will make him happier, because, in the opinions of others, to do so would be wise, or even right. ... In the part which merely concerns himself, his independence is, of right, absolute. Over himself, over his own body and mind, the individual is sovereign."[24]

3. Individual harmful actions may negatively effect others

[1:27] However, Mill also realized that no action in society can ever be totally individual or isolated. It is difficult to come up with actions or decisions that merely concern the individual. Mill argues that when a person does anything harmful to himself it will usually not only affect those who are close to him but will also affect the community at large. An individual's action that results in an injury to one's property, body or mental faculties will usually affect others. And even if it does no direct harm to others it could result in harm by that person's example.

> [1:28] "If he injures his property, he does harm to those who directly or indirectly derive support from it, and usually diminishes, by a greater or less amount, the general resources of the community. If he deteriorates his bodily or mental faculties, he not only brings evil upon all who depended on him for any portion of their happiness, but disqualifies himself for rendering the services which he owes to his fellow creatures generally; perhaps becomes a burden on their affection or benevolence; and if such conduct were very frequent, hardly any offense that is committed would detract more from the general sum of good. Finally, if by his vices or follies a person does no direct harm to

---

[23] *Ibid.*, p. 324.

[24] *Ibid.*, p. 263.

> others, he is nevertheless (it may be said) injurious by his example; and ought to be compelled to control himself, for the sake of those whom the sight or knowledge of his conduct might corrupt or mislead.
>
> And even (it will be added) if the consequences of misconduct could be confined to the vicious or thoughtless individual, ought society to abandon to their own guidance those who are manifestly unfit for it? If protection against themselves is confessedly due to children and persons under age, is not society equally bound to afford it to persons of mature years who are equally incapable of self-government?"[25]

[1:29] Mill argues that although it may be the case that a person's actions towards himself may possibly be a bad example to society he believes that on the whole that a person's hurtful actions towards himself will be a good example because of the painful or degrading consequences that will be a result of most of those bad actions.[26]

4. Tyranny of the majority must be avoided

a. Majority is usually wrong

[1:30] The strongest argument Mill gives against society having the power and ability to control other person's personal decisions is that more often than not the interference would be wrong. Whenever the public tries to determine categorically what is good or bad for other people the public will be wrong just as (or

---

[25] *Ibid.*, p. 327.

[26] "With respect to what is said of the necessity of protecting society from the bad example set to others by the vicious or the self-indulgent ... [W]e are now speaking of conduct which, while it does no wrong to others, is supposed to do great harm to the agent himself; and I do not see how those who believe this, can think otherwise than that the example, on the whole, must be more salutary than hurtful, since, if it displays the misconduct, it displays also the painful or degrading consequences which, if the conduct is justly censured, must be supposed to be in all or most cases attendant on it." *Ibid.*, p. 330.

more) likely as they are right.[27] And often times this social imposition results in the majority oppressing the minority[28] with the majority's preferences.[29]

b. Actions that do not violate other's rights should not be obstructed

[1:31] As a result, whenever a person's decision(s) affect others only contingently, not violating any specific duty to the public or causing any direct hurt to any assignable individual(s), society ought not to obstruct the person's liberty for making that decision. The resulting personal and social benefits of this liberty far outweigh any resulting social inconvenience or burden.

---

[27] "But the strongest of all the arguments against the interference of the public with purely personal conduct, is that when it does interfere, the odds are that it interferes wrongly, and in the wrong place. On questions of social morality, of duty to others, the opinion of the public, that is, of an overruling majority, though often wrong, is likely to be still oftener right; because on such questions they are only required to judge of their own interests; of the manner in which some mode of conduct, if allowed to be practiced, would affect themselves. But the opinion of a similar majority, imposed as a law on the minority, on questions of self-regarding conduct, is quite as likely to be wrong as right; for in these cases public opinion means, at the best, some people's opinion of what is good or bad for other people; while very often it does not even mean that; the public, with the most perfect indifference, passing over the pleasure or convenience of those whose conduct they censure, and considering only their own preference. There are many who consider as an injury to themselves any conduct which they have a distaste for, and resent it as an outrage to their feelings; as a religious bigot, when charged with disregarding the religious feeling of others, has been known to retort that they disregard his feelings, by persisting in their abominable worship or creed. But there is no parity between the feeling of a person for his own opinion, and the feeling of another who is offended at his holding it; no more than between the desire of a thief to take a purse, and the desire of the right owner to keep it. And a person's taste is as much his own peculiar concern as his opinion or his purse." *Ibid.*, p. 330-331.

[28] "When we compare the strange respect of mankind for liberty, with their strange want of respect for it, we might imagine that a man had an indispensable right to do harm to others, and no right at all to please himself without giving pain to any one." *Ibid.*, p. 354.

[29] "There is no reason that all human existences should be constructed on some one, or some small number of patterns. If a person possesses any tolerable amount of common sense and experience, his own mode of laying out his existence is best, not because it is the best in itself, but because it is his mode." *Ibid.*, p. 315.

[1:32] "But with regard to the merely contingent, or, as it may be called, constructive injury which a person causes to society, by conduct which neither violates any specific duty to the public, nor occasions perceptible hurt on any assignable individual except himself; the inconvenience is one which society can afford to bear, for the sake of the greater good of human freedom. ... If society lets any considerable number of its members grow up mere children incapable of being acted on by rational consideration of distant motive, society has itself to blame for the consequences."[30]

[1:33] "The maxims are, first, that the individual is not accountable to society for his actions, in so far as these concern the interests of no person but himself. Advice, instruction, persuasion, and avoidance by other people if thought necessary by them for their own good, are the only measures by which society can justifiably express its dislike or disapprobation of his conduct. Secondly, that for such actions as are prejudicial to the interests of others, the individual is accountable, and may be subjected either to social or to legal punishments, if society is of opinion that the one or the other is requisite for its protection."[31]

5. Autonomy promotes individuality which increases both personal and social happiness

[1:34] Thus the *summum bonum*—the ultimate good—in healthcare, for example, is not necessarily the healthy recovery of the patient; rather it is the broad and general classical utilitarian value of happiness.[32] Mill argues that it is through the exercise of our liberty that we as individuals develop our character and increase happiness.

---

[30] *Ibid.*, p. 329.

[31] *Ibid.*, p. 340.

[32] [Utilitarianism] "views morality as concerned with the production of desirable or valuable states of affairs or experiences—commonly human happiness, welfare, or desire satisfaction; their production is the goal of morality. Human actions are morally evaluated in terms of their tendency to promote these goals, and right action is that action which, among the alternatives open to an agent, maximizes these valuable consequences for any and all persons affected. The consequences for any one person count for no more than for any other" (Dan W. Brock, *Life and Death: Philosophical Essays In Biomedical Ethics*, [New York: Cambridge University Press, 1993], p. 96).

[1:35] "In proportion to the development of his individuality, each person becomes more valuable to himself, and is therefore capable of being more valuable to others. There is a greater fullness of life about his own existence, and when there is more life in units there is more in the mass which is composed of them." [33]

[1:36] Mill believed that if the perfecting of man is of first importance and if the human faculties of perception, judgment, discriminative feeling, mental activity, and even moral preferences are exercised only by the making of choices, then it is imperative that persons concern themselves with not only what moral agents do, but also with the manner in which moral agents perform those actions, i.e. by making autonomous choices.[34] Thus, regardless of whether a person's decisions are in truth or error, the greatest freedom for the competition of ideas will have the best result.[35] Since a well-developed human being can only be produced by the cultivation or development of individuality through decision-making, it follows that what Mill calls wrong is that which obstructs decision-making and that which is right is that

[33] Mill, "On Liberty", p. 311.

[34] "The human faculties of perception, judgment, discriminative feeling, mental activity, and even moral preference, are exercised only in making a choice. He who does anything because it is the custom, makes no choice. The mental and moral, like the muscular powers, are improved only by being used. … He who lets the world, or his own portion of it, choose his plan of life for him, has no need of any other faculty than the ape-like one of imitation. He who chooses his plan for himself, employs all his faculties. … It really is of importance, not only what men do, but also what manner of men they are that do it. Among the works of man, which human life is rightly employed in perfecting and beautifying, the first in importance surely is man himself." *Ibid.*, p. 307.

[35] "[Mill's] conception of the good society was a humane and generous one: the society in which there was the greatest freedom for the competition of ideas, whether in truth or error, and for diversity of personality and styles of life." (Max Lerner, Preface to "On Liberty" in *Essential Works of John Stuart Mill*, p. 252.).

which promotes the development of human beings, i.e. autonomous choices.[36]

> [1:37] "Actions are right in proportion as they tend to promote happiness, wrong as they tend to produce the reverse of happiness." [37]

[1:38] In other words:

UTILITY AND INFORMED CONSENT
1. If the principle of utility has as its *summum bonum* happiness, and
2. if autonomy is the surest route to this happiness, and
3. if autonomy involves informed consent, whenever two or more parties are involved
4. **then** utilitarians must defend informed consent.

[1:39] Therefore, in classical utilitarianism, or at least in the case of Mill, either autonomy (informed consent), is a supreme value, i.e. part of the ultimate good, or autonomous choice is at least the best means to maximize what is of supreme value.

[1:40] Utilitarians may argue that the authority to make decisions should rest with the agent because it will benefit them by enabling them to make the decision that best promotes their welfare. These arguments could range from the simple contention that making one's own decisions promotes one's psychological well-being to the more controversial claim that agents generally know themselves well enough to be the best judges ultimately of what is and what is not beneficial for them. It can also be argued

[36] "Having said that Individuality is the same thing with development, and that it is only the cultivation of individuality which produces, or can produce, well-developed human being, I might here close the argument: for what more or better can be said of any condition of human affairs, than that it brings human beings themselves nearer to the best thing they can be? or what worse can be said of any obstruction to good, than that it prevents this?" Mill, "On Liberty", p. 312.

[37] John Stuart Mill, *Utilitarianism* (Indianapolis: Hackett Publishing Company, 1979), p. 7.

that rules of consent will curb social fears about being used by others as a mere means, promoting a climate of trust.[38]

6. Utilitarianism defends informed consent by defending autonomy

[1:41] Thus the utility justification[39] for informed consent maintains that consent requirements will benefit all parties involved, society and its individual citizens. However, it is also clear that, insofar as a recognition of the value of autonomy forms a part of the justification for informed consent, this is perfectly compatible with the point of view that autonomy is not itself being regarded as an intrinsic good, rather it is being valued as an extrinsic good, i.e. for the sake of best interest.[40]

---

[38] Charles Fried describes the trust relationship in the following terms: "Although trust has to do with reliance on a disposition of another person, it is reliance on a disposition of a special sort: the disposition to act morally, to deal fairly with others, to live up to one's understandings, and so on. Thus to trust another is first of all to expect him to accept the principle of morality in his dealings with you, to respect your status as a person, your personality" ("Privacy", Hughes, ed. *Law, Reason and Justice*, 1969), p. 52.

[39] "Total" utilitarianism argues that "it is possible to conceive of a higher population with a lower quality of life that is compensated for by the increased numbers enjoying it. ... Average utilitarianism bids us take into account utilities to possible people only to the extent that they would affect the average utility per life lived" (R. M. Hare, *Essays On Bioethics* [Oxford: Clarendon Press, 1993], pp. 68-69). Classical utility justifications increases the 'average' utility of all involved when it comes to the issue of autonomy.

[40] Faden and Beauchamp, *A History and Theory of Informed Consent*, p. 14.

III. Informed Consent: Deontological Support

A. Informed Consent: Direct Duty Of Autonomy

1. Intrinsic value as a perfect duty

[1:45] The deontological position sees the requirement of informed consent as following from a direct duty[41] to respect each individual's autonomy.[42] Instead of assessing the moral worth of an action solely on the consequences of that action, there is a focus on other moral features of the action.[43] Kant and others who subscribe to the protection of individual autonomy, because of

---

[41] "A duty-based moral view posits a moral ideal for a person in the form of a set of moral commitments, constraints, or prohibitions of behavior that can be violated only at the cost of one's moral integrity ... This kind of moral position focuses directly on individual decision and action, and evaluates that decision and action not solely on the consequences it brings about. ... The moral categories of a duty-based view are all constraints on our action to which we must conform at the peril of our moral integrity. These constraints commonly derive from the general idea of relations between persons, and the moral requirement that what we do to others be justified by features of that specific other, and our relation to him. Duty-based views attempt to account for the intuition that a person has a special responsibility for what he deliberately and directly does to others, different from his responsibility for the actions of others. In this sense, duty-based views take the distinction between persons more seriously than do goal-based views, and focus on persons as agents whose own deliberate actions put them into morally significant relations with specific other persons." Dan W. Brock, *Life and Death: Philosophical Essays In Biomedical Ethics* (Cambridge University Press: New York, 1993), pp. 97-98.

[42] For Kant, "autonomy is the ground of dignity of human nature and of every rational nature" (436). "The principle of autonomy is this: Always choose in such a way that in the same volition the maxims of the choice are at the same time present as universal law" (440). "What else, then, can freedom of the will be but autonomy, i.e. the property that the will has of being a law to itself? The proposition that the will is in every action a law to itself expresses, however, nothing but the principle of acting according to no other maxim than that which can at the same time have itself as a universal law for its object. ... Thus a free will and a will subject to moral laws are one and the same" (447). "the will of a rational being can be a will of its own only under the idea of freedom, and that such a will must therefore, from a practical point of view, be attributed to all rational beings" (448). Immanuel Kant, *Grounding for the Metaphysics of Morals,* 1785, translated by James W. Ellington (Indianapolis: Hackett Publishing Company, 1981); page references are to the German *Akademie der Wissenschaften* edition of Kant's Morals included in the margins of Ellington's translation.

[43] Henrik R. Wulff, Stig A. Pedersen, Raben Rosenberg, *Philosophy Of Medicine* (London: Blackwell Scientific Publications, 1990), p. 181.

such duty, usually base their arguments on synthetic *a priori* statements about the intrinsic worth of rational persons.[44] Conceptually and logically, this concept of autonomy has been linked with the concept of rational beings—"persons"—as having intrinsic value, i.e. dignity, independent of special circumstances that confer value, i.e. utility justifications. Autonomous persons are ends in themselves—having intrinsic value—and thus all rational beings have a perfect duty[45] to others and to ourselves not to treat others or ourselves merely as means to an end. Kant's categorical imperative states:

---

[44] Categorical Imperative: Determines which maxims are acceptable moral principles by their ability to serve as practical norms of conduct for everyone, that is, as laws within a civil community. The first formulation, called the Formula of Universality is a purely formal standard and so is analytically true. "Act only on that maxim through which you can at the same time will that it should become a universal law." or, alternatively, if its maxim can "coexist with the freedom of everyone in accordance with a universal law" of freedom. The second formula adds the moral matter, the notion of persons as ends, i.e., intrinsically valuable, and is a synthetic claim. "Act in accordance with a maxim of *ends* that it can be a universal law for everyone." All other imperatives are conditional. The moral *imperative* makes this constraint known through the categorical nature of its pronouncement (the unconditional ought). Such constraint, therefore, does not apply to rational beings as such (there could also be *holy* ones) but rather to *human beings*, rational *natural* beings, who are unholy enough that pleasure can induce them to break the moral law.

[45] H. J. Paton in *The Categorical Imperative* (London: Hutchinson & CO., 1965), pp. 147-148, says "Kant attaches great importance to the distinction between perfect and imperfect duties, but he seems nowhere to define the distinction clearly ... Perfect duties ... admit of no exception in favour of inclination, and this would suggest that imperfect duties do admit of such exceptions. ... In the case of perfect duties we are obliged to perform a definite *act*—for example, to pay precisely the ... [money] which we owe. In the case of imperfect duties we are bound to act only on a *maxim*: ... it is left to our discretion to decide whom we ought to help, and to what extent we ought to help."

Therefore, I define perfect and imperfect duties as follows: perfect duties—that is duties that are determinate both with respect to the particular content of the duty on any particular occasion, and the identity of the person to whom the duty is owed. Whereas imperfect duties are duties which are indeterminate with respect to both the particular content of the duty on any particular occasion and to whom the duty is owed.

> [1:46] "Act in such a way that you treat humanity, whether in your own person or in the person of another, always at the same time as an end and never simply as a means."[46]

[1:47] Following the lead of Kant, deontologists are therefore not usually inclined to protect agents against the consequences of their choices, on grounds that such constraints would violate both society's or the professional's own duty not to treat persons merely as a means to an end and to respect the agent's own duty to act autonomously as a rational person.[47]

2. Deontological and utilitarian differences with regard to consent

[1:48] The justifications based on duty recognize consent as valid because the consenting party is an intrinsically valuable autonomous person. Utilitarian arguments proceed differently, namely, by considering the extent to which respect for a person's autonomy would maximize the benefits of personal and social welfare and minimize harm.[48] When informed consent is justified by the principle of duty, it is done so not primarily to facilitate social benefits, but rather as a check against social benefits as being the sole reasoning for the informed consent. In other words, the principle of duty focuses on the intrinsic dignity of the person

[46] Immanuel Kant, *Grounding for the Metaphysics of Morals,* p. 429.

[47] "For the Kantian, as Nozick sees him, the proper treatment of persons is not itself a goal of action, but rather a 'side constraint' on action in pursuit of any goal. It cannot be sacrificed for a greater good, not even for a greater incidence of proper treatment. ... Kantians do not actually deny that men may be used as means. They object only when men are treated merely as means. But this distinction is not on its face illuminating. They cannot mean that men should be valued both as ends and means much as, say, tennis is desirable both in itself and as a means to health. For, if tennis were bad as a means to health, its intrinsic value might be outweighed; but the value of a person cannot be balanced off in this way." Arthur Flemming, "Using a Man as a Means," *Ethics: An International Journal Of Social Political And Legal Philosophy, vol.* 88 (1978), pp. 283-98.

[48] "The utilitarian theory of distribution calls for realizing the greatest good for the greatest number. It involves a calculation of the consequences of an action, counting pleasures and benefits as positive factors and pains and losses as negative factors. These factors are summed up, and the state of affairs with the greatest total is the proper one" (Thomas M. Garrett, Harold W. Gaillie, Rosellen M. Garrett, *Healthcare Ethics: Principles And Problems,* 2nd ed. [Englewood Cliffs: Prentice Hall, 1993], p. 88.

rather than on social benefits. Therefore, deontologically, persons have a right to receive information that is necessary for making an informed consent, and to deny the agent the necessary information to make an informed consent is the same as denying the agent the right to make an informed consent, which is a violation of that person's dignity.

[1:49] A utilitarian might argue that autonomous decision-making is that which will maximally promote the agent's and society's greatest-happiness. By contrast, a deontologist might argue that there is a direct duty to honor autonomous decision-making, as that is how a person respects an agent's intrinsic worth as a person.

B. Competing Theoretical Approaches Result In Intractable dilemmas

[1:50] Although the principle of the respect for autonomy is believed by some to be the grounding principle in the obligation or duty to obtain informed consent, it is apparent that several issues will limit this obligation or duty. It is controversial, to say the least, whether this principle of autonomy, whether supported by utilitarian or deontological reasoning, is the exclusive or even the primary justification of consent requirements. Further, and more importantly, what demands does the principle of autonomy make with regard to the amount and type of information that is to be disclosed so that the individual can make an autonomous decision? To what extent does society have a duty or obligation to restrict autonomous decisions when they conflict with other societal values or principles? Some considerations might be that of endangering the public health—nonmaleficence (do no harm), the using up of scarce resources—justice (be fair), whether or not the treatment conforms to acceptable medical practice, etc. If there are restrictions to a person's autonomy, it must be because of some competing value(s)/duties or principles.[49] In turn, these competing value(s)/duties or principles might themselves be linked to either utilitarian or deontological principles. It is difficult to know, on either approach, where such competition from competing values is likely to come to an end.

> [1:51] "As long as the debate between Kantians and utilitarians continues, and as long as the Western political and philosophical tradition embraces both the principles of respect for persons and beneficence, there cannot be a resolution of dilemmas traceable to those competing theoretical approaches."[50]

[1:52] However, through a nontraditional approach, great progress can be made with regard to informed consent, by absorbing or bypassing those competing worldviews through the use of a metaphysically neutral political framework of justice.

---

[49] The President's Commission for the Study of Ethical Problems in Medicine and Biomedical and Behavioral Research argues that "The ethical foundations of informed consent can be traced to the promotion of two values: personal well-being and self-determination. To ensure that these values are respected and enhanced, the Commission finds that patients who have the capacity to make decisions about their care must be permitted to do so voluntarily and must have all relevant information. ... Nevertheless, patient choice is not absolute. a. Patients are not entitled to insist that healthcare practitioner furnish them services when to do so would violate either the bounds of acceptable practice or a professional's own deeply held moral beliefs or would draw on a limited resource on which the patient has no binding claim." (b, c, d, and e expresses how the patient choice is not absolute when decision-making capacity is lacking.) President's Commission for the Study of Ethical Problems in Medicine and Biomedical and Behavioral Research, *Making Healthcare Decisions: The Ethical And Legal Implications of Informed Consent in the Patient-Practitioner Relationship* (Washington, D.C.: U.S. Government Printing Office, 1982), pp. 2-6.

[50] Barry Hoffmaster, Benjamin Freedman, Gwen Fraser, *Clinical Ethics: Theory and Practice* (Clifton N.J.: Humana Press, 1989), p. 118.

IV. Informed Consent: Justice

[1:54] This nontraditional approach of addressing the subject of informed consent is through the use of the broader concept of justice instead of principles of utility[51] or duty.

[1:55] Because most literature that addresses the issue of informed consent by way of justice does not appeal to a distinctive principle of justice independent of other principles such as utility or duty, they end up presenting a confused picture. The term "just" is sometimes used in a broad and unspecified sense to refer to that which is "justified," or "morally right." Justice emerges more often than not when it is believed that someone's legal or moral rights have been infringed or violated. Complaints of injustice rarely arise in connection with informed consent. Autonomy or beneficence principles are usually cited instead.[52]

[1:56] Beauchamp and Faden argue that:

> "the major moral and conceptual problems about informed consent are not justice-based and do not directly confront issues of social justice." [53]

[1:57] What they say is true of the discussion to date on informed consent. However, what would reasonable and rational agents agree to under certain hypothetical conditions of justice, i.e. free and equal citizens living in a pluralistic constitutional

---

[51] "Utilitarianism is not a theory of justice or of distribution, but a theory of the public good in which justice plays a subordinate role. A just distribution in utilitarianism would involve no more than maximizing the benefits of goods and services within the society": Thomas M. Garrett, Harold W. Gaillie, Rosellen M. Garrett, *Healthcare Ethics: Principles And Problems*, p. 88.

[52] Faden and Beauchamp, *A History and Theory of Informed Consent*, p. 14.

[53] *Ibid.*, p. 16.

democratic society.[54] Once this just political framework is constructed, a standard of information disclosure will need to be determined that will be considered the most appropriate under this metaphysically neutral just system. If a standard of information disclosure can be chosen under ideal circumstances, then perhaps it will be possible to glean some insights into what type of information disclosure should be striven towards in less than perfect situations.

***

[54] "Some ethicians [categorize social contract theories] as part of deontological ethics in that the contract spells out the duties which we have to each other as a result of that contract. It might also or better be conceived as part of a utilitarian approach to ethics in that a good social contract would insure as much as possible the greatest happiness of the greatest number with the contract providing the best climate for this outcome" (William J. Ellos, *Ethical Practice In Clinical Medicine*, p. 154). Rawls, as we shall see in chapter 5b, develops a theory of justice that is not based on any type of deontological or utilitarian ethics. Rawls' theory of justice is free standing and independent of any of these "associational views".

Vb. INFORMED CONSENT

Overview - Rawlsian

[2:1]

Informed consent and other issues of ethics have usually been investigated through the use of various traditional ethical theories of utilitarianism, or consequentialist based theories, and deontology, or duty based theories. The justice approach differs by appealing to a broader political spectrum of hypothetical contractarianism. Because of the multicultural society people now find themselves living in, it is next to impossible for them to find broad social agreement on any type of associational or personal philosophical positions like consequentialism or deontology. Yet individuals still must get along socially and society must make policy decisions in spite of religious, philosophical and moral plurality. As a result, there is a need to deviate from the traditional methods of ethical inquiry. Concentration must instead be on the broad and general constitutional rights and liberties that all or most people can agree on, no matter what their personal, social or comprehensive doctrines might be. Rawls' hypothetical contractarian theory is such an approach as its metaphysical assumptions are neutral enough so that they are derivable from, consistent with or at least not in contradiction with a broad number of traditional comprehensive worldviews.

[2:2] Although the subject of informed consent could be presented using a variety of approaches, the following discussions will be based on the construction and application of Rawls' theory of justice. This process will determine what type of information disclosure would be politically *ideal* under a Rawlsian political framework. It may be the case that the perfect solution on the subject of information disclosure will never be determined but perhaps this will be one step in the right direction, at least for those who fit the criteria for a Rawlsian reasonable and rational competent citizen.

I. Social Contract: Justice

A. Justice: Independent Of Utility and Duty

[2:3] Rawls' guiding aim in his books, *A Theory Of Justice, Justice as Fairness* and *Political Liberalism,* is to work out a theory of justice that is a viable alternative to classical utilitarianism and deontological conceptions of justice that have long dominated our philosophical tradition.[55]

> [2:4] "[T]he features of a political conception of justice are, first, that it is a moral conception worked out for a specific subject, namely, the basic structure of a constitutional democratic regime; second, that accepting the political conception does not presuppose accepting any particular comprehensive religious, philosophical, or moral doctrine; rather, the political conception presents itself as a reasonable conception for the basic structure alone; and third, that it is not formulated in terms of any comprehensive doctrine but in terms of certain fundamental ideas viewed as latent in the public political culture of a democratic society." [56]

1. Informed Consent: Independent of Utility and Duty

[2:5] Since the derivation of a standard of informed consent will be through the application of Rawls' political framework that is independent of classical utilitarian and deontological conceptions, it follows that the derived political standard of informed consent will also be independent of classical utilitarian and deontological conceptions.

2. Political Liberalism: a misnomer

[2:6] In light of Rawls' pluralistic approach to justice it can be argued that the title of his book Political Liberalism is an unfortunate choice. This title unnecessarily alienates those who consider themselves to be conservative even though Rawls' political system is quite compatible with either political conservatism or

---

[55] John Rawls, *A Theory of Justice* (Cambridge: Belknap Press of Harvard University Press, 1971), p. 3.

[56] John Rawls, *Political Liberalism* (New York: Columbia University Press, 1993), pp. 174-5.

political liberalism as commonly understood. Rawls would have been more inclusive if he would have given his book a title more like Political Democracy: A Multicultural Foundation of Social Justice.

[2:7] Rawls' political conception of justice generalizes and carries to a higher order of abstraction the traditional social contract doctrines of Locke, Rousseau, and of course Kant,[57,58,59] and Political Liberalism accomplishes this task in a much different way.

3. Pluralistic societies: develop naturally when citizens are free and equal

a. Plurality of reasonable and rational comprehensive worldviews

[2:8] Rawls' conception is that in a democratic society in which all citizens are able to exercise their human reason freely and without coercion (within the constraints of social deterministic aspects) citizens will naturally end up with a plurality of reasonable and rational comprehensive[60] views or comprehensive worldviews.[61]

> [2:9] "Comprehensive doctrines of all kinds—religious, philosophical, and moral—belong to what we may call the "background culture" of civil society. This is the culture of the social, not of the political. It is the culture of daily life,

---

[57] *Ibid.*, p. xv.

[58] Rawls, *A Theory of Justice*, p. 11.

[59] John Locke's *Second Treatise of Government,* Jean-Jacques Rousseau's *The Social Contract*, and Immanuel Kant's ethical works beginning with *The Foundations of the Metaphysics of Morals* as definitive of the contract tradition.

[60] "A conception is said to be general when it applies to a wide range of subjects ...; it is comprehensive when it includes conceptions of what is of value in human life, as well as ideals of personal virtue and character, that are to inform much of our nonpolitical conduct ... ." Rawls, *Political Liberalism*, p. 175.

[61] "Comprehensive worldview" is a better descriptive term than what Rawls calls a "comprehensive doctrine". A worldview is the perspective of an agent and how she perceives and interprets the world around her including her concept of the good. Even though this is the same as what Rawls calls a comprehensive doctrine, the term "doctrine" usually is not used in this personal, broad and universal sense.

of its many associations: churches and universities, learned and scientific societies, and clubs and teams to mention a few." [62]

[2:10] "Political liberalism assumes that, for political purposes, a plurality of reasonable yet incompatible comprehensive doctrines is the normal result of the exercise of human reason within the framework of the free institutions of a constitutional democratic regime." [63]

b. Incompatible rational & reasonable comprehensive worldviews

[2:11] Not only will there be a plurality of comprehensive worldviews[64] but some of them will also be incompatible even in a well-ordered society[65] where citizens act fairly.

[2:12] A modern democratic society is characterized not simply by a pluralism of comprehensive religious, philosophical, and moral doctrines but by a pluralism of incompatible yet reasonable comprehensive doctrines.[66]

[2:13] This notion of plurality relates to informed consent in that many of the problems that are faced with the issue of information disclosure are the result of people having reasonable and rational worldviews that differ or are incompatible with each other. Al-

---

62 Rawls, *Political Liberalism*, p. 14.

63 *Ibid.*, p. xvi.

64 Mill in *On Liberty* says: "Individuals, classes, nations, have been extremely unlike one another: they have struck out a great variety of paths, each leading to something valuable; and although at every period those who traveled in different paths have been intolerant of one another, and each would have thought it an excellent thing if all the rest could have been compelled to travel his road, their attempts to thwart each other's development have rarely had any permanent success, and each has in time endured to receive the good which the others have offered." Mill, "On Liberty", p. 321.

65 To say that a society is well-ordered conveys three things:
1. It is a society in which everyone accepts, and knows that everyone else accepts, the very same principles of justice.
2. Its basic structure is publicly known, or with good reason believed, to satisfy these principles.
3. Its citizens have a normally effective sense of justice and so they generally comply with society's basic institutions, which they regard as just.
Rawls, *Political Liberalism*, p. 35.

66 *Ibid.*, p. xvi.

though it would be expected that most pluralistic decision-making would be focusing more on the concrete situation(s), rather than theoretical worldviews, it is still the worldviews that give interpretation and meaning to the concrete situation(s). For example, one party might view a situation as a test of their faithfulness to God whereas another might view a situation as an unfortunate fact of life that needs to be dealt with. The former party may as a result have a submissive or an acceptance type of attitude towards "God's test" whereas the latter party may have an aggressive or a take charge type of attitude. Rawls' hypothetical political system will help to shed some light on what up to now has proven to be an intractable problem.

B. Political Liberalism: Fair Cooperation

1. Liberalism vs. Conservatism: tolerance vs. intolerance

[2:14] The important question for Rawls is: can there be developed a political framework which will make it possible for people with differing reasonable and rational comprehensive worldviews to function socially, i.e. exercise fair cooperation, within a free and equal democratic society?[67] The political framework that Rawls develops is what he calls Political Liberalism. Why liberalism? Because liberalism, in contrast with conservatism, is that which is tolerant and accepting of other reasonable and rational comprehensive worldviews.[68] But if this is the reason why Rawls calls it liberalism then he has confused his own political conception of democracy with that of various incompatible comprehensive worldviews, as Rawls argues that his political framework is not a metaphysical position, or is at least metaphysically neutral, making his political framework acceptable for many if not most comprehensive worldviews.

---

[67] It is true that we are assuming that the society is composed of free and equal citizens in a democratic society. This assumption I believe is valid in working out a political system applicable, for example, to the United States. Whether this is itself a worldview will be discussed later.

[68] Rawls, *Political Liberalism*, p. 3.

2. Interrelated consensus: even with incompatible worldviews

[2:15] Political democracy builds itself on what Rawls calls an overlapping consensus or what might be better understood as interrelated consensus[69] not just on a liberal comprehensive worldview. It may be true that Rawls' political liberalism has *prima facie* more in common with the liberal than the conservative point of view. However, the purpose of this endeavor is to show how vastly differing comprehensive worldviews, i.e. conservative or liberal, can agree independently to this democratic political system designed for a pluralistic society without compromising their *basic* social values.[70] For Rawls, the realm of the political deals with those social values that are interrelated, primary and basic.

[2:16] Rather than looking for and finding capital "T" Truth in what could be called The Political System, we are looking to develop *A* Political System that will make it possible for people with differing comprehensive worldviews (a given if people are free and equal in a democratic society) to function socially within a society.

C. Free & Equal and Rational & Reasonable Citizens

[2:17] Political persons, i.e. citizens, are regarded as free and equal in virtue of their possession of the two moral powers, the rational and reasonable.[71]

---

69 The term "overlapping consensus" gives the false impression that what is being agreed to is something shared, like the union of several circles (overlapping each other). Rawls makes it clear that this is not what is meant. What is being agreed upon are principles that are/can be free-standing of various comprehensive worldviews. However, the principles are interrelated with the various comprehensive worldviews in that they *can* be viewed from the perspective of one's worldview as either derivable from, consistent with, or at least not in conflict with their other values. They are also interrelated in that the principles do have the added effect of constraining, guiding and maybe even determining to some extent, through the political structure, what worldviews are acceptable to have or pursue.

70 How this is possible shall be made clearer.

71 Rawls, *Political Liberalism*, p. 34.

[2:18] "Justice as fairness works from the fundamental ideas of society as a fair system of cooperation together with the conception of the person as free and equal. These ideas are taken as central to the democratic ideal." [72]

[2:19] "... the conception of citizens as free and equal persons ... is a political conception affirmed for the sake of establishing an effective public conception of justice." [73]

[2:20] "... since persons can be full participants in a fair system of social cooperation, we ascribe to them the two moral powers ... namely, a capacity for a sense of justice [reasonable] and a capacity for a conception of the good [rational]." [74,75]

D. Political Democracy Is Not A Comprehensive Worldview

[2:21] This system of political democracy is unique in that it is not a comprehensive worldview that imposes itself on others, rather political democracy is something that most if not all reasonable and rational comprehensive views would agree to—an interrelated consensus. Thus the goal is not to find "The" Political System rather the goal is to find *"A"* Political System that does a better job promoting and maintaining a stable society of free and equal citizens than the *classical* views of utilitarianism or deontology. The goal is to find a better alternative than what most other political philosophers have held on to or combined up to this point in time. If Rawls is successful, and if it is possible to

[72] *Ibid.*, p. 167.

[73] *Ibid.*, p. 367.

[74] *Ibid.*, p. 19.

[75] "These two powers are the capacity for a sense of right and justice (the capacity to honor fair terms of cooperation and thus to be reasonable), and the capacity for a conception of the good (and thus to be rational)."*Ibid.*, p. 302.

apply Rawls' political system, through extension,[76] to the concept of informed consent then it will be possible to determine which standard of information disclosure would be most appropriate for Rawls' political persons.

76 As we shall see in § 8 & 9 we will not be extrapolating the "Rawlsian" informed consent principle by philosophical argument tracing back to the basic liberties under the first principle, as it would be unlikely that those with differing philosophical arguments would ever be able to convince others that they are correct. Rather the basis of agreement will be in the public culture of a democratic society and its underlying conception of the person and that of social cooperation. Our appeal will be to the constitutional bases which account for our fundamental constitutional rights and liberties establishing the social conception of the person. Thus legislation of a type of informed consent will be constrained by the two principles of justice and constitutional law in hierarchical order.

II. Political Persons

[3:1]

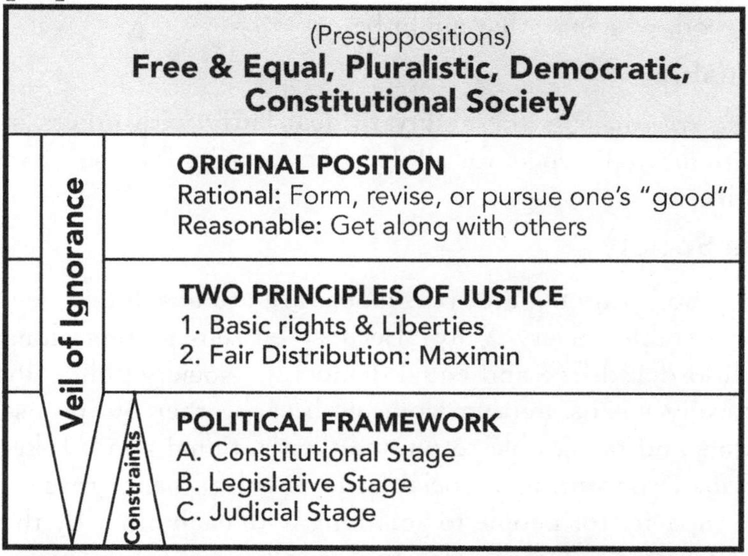

[3:2] In developing this system the logical place to start, other than the assumption of a free and equal democratic society, is with the subjects involved—political persons.

A. Two Moral Powers: Rational & Reasonable

[3:3] A political person is comprised of two indispensable parts Rawls calls the two moral powers the rational and the reasonable. Of course the political person *qua* person will be actually comprised of more than just the rational and the reasonable, but the rational and reasonable are essential for the political person. Rawls uses the terms rational and reasonable in a very broad and general sense that is absolutely necessary to understand if one is to understand his position. Likewise it may be the case that the terms rational and reasonable may have a fuller meaning but the broad and general meaning of the terms is as follows.[77]

[77] The political person needs to be defined as broadly and generally as possible in order not to be a metaphysical conception. A fuller discussion of this issue follows shortly.

1. Rational

[3:4] Being *rational* is the capacity to freely form, revise, and pursue one's good, whatever that might be.

2. Reasonable

[3:5] Being *reasonable* is the ability to deal fairly with others in society with mutual respect for all. It is the capacity for a sense of right and justice.

B. Stable Society

[3:6] Being both rational and reasonable are are absolutely necessary for a stable society. Why? Because citizens getting along in this well-ordered free and equal democratic society politically and practically means, getting along with each other by the use of fair terms and being able to pursue their rational good. Likewise informed consent, as a social issue, involves being reasonable—the capacity for people to get along with each other by the use of fair terms, i.e. a sense of justice—and as an autonomy issue informed consent involves being rational—the capacity for people to pursue their rational good, i.e. to freely form, revise, and pursue their own good. But caution as to what it practically means to be rational and reasonable needs to be addressed.

C. Just Political Construction / Process

[3:7] In Rawls' political democracy, a just political construction or process needs to be followed in all interpersonal transactions. In other words, it is not possible to entirely derive what informed consent would entail from knowing that citizens are rational and reasonable. A political process must be followed that in effect assumes a rational and reasonable political system that all must follow in order for them to function and flourish as a pluralistic society.

III. Original Position: Hypothetical & NonHistorical

A. Veil Of Ignorance: Fairness

[4:1] Using as a model this full conception of the political person as rational and reasonable, Rawls argues that it is also rational and reasonable to construct a hypothetical nonhistorical original position in which the representatives in the original position are purely rational representatives of citizens of a free and equal democratic well-ordered society, constrained by the reasonable or fair (i.e. thick) veil of ignorance.

> [4:2] "…in the fundamental case of social cooperation within the basic structure of society, the representatives of citizens as reasonable and rational agents must be situated reasonably, that is, fairly or symmetrically, with no one having superior bargaining advantages over the rest. This last is done by the veil of ignorance."[78]

[4:3] The result is a rational (i.e. able to freely form, revise, and pursue one's good) and reasonable (i.e. socially cooperation) political system compatible with a plurality of rational and reasonable worldviews that may have irreconcilable, incompatible, and incommensurable conceptions of the good (i.e. a pluralistic society which is a natural result of being free and equal).

B. Two Moral Powers Essentials: Principles of Justice

1. Political democracy: is but one workable system

[4:4] If the purpose of the original position is to represent political persons the question arises as to what are the essentials for the development of the two moral powers that is the development of the political person as reasonable and rational? Rawls' argues that what is essential for the development of the political person is a rational and reasonable political structure and process, of which political democracy is but one workable system.

[78] Rawls, *Political Liberalism*, p. 52.

2. Standard of disclosure: for inform consent

[4:5] As relating to the task of choosing an appropriate standard of information disclosure for an informed consent it will be shown that the basis of agreement for informed consent will be in the public culture of this democratic society, i.e. in its underlying conception of the political person and that of social cooperation.

[4:6] This means that the standard of information disclosure to be chosen as necessary for an informed consent will be the one that can be considered as being rational and reasonable. Rational, but not that the standard of information disclosure can form, revise or pursue its own good as a standard of information disclosure cannot have a good of its own. Reasonable, but not that the standard of information disclosure can personally deal fairly with others. The standard of information disclosure necessary for an informed consent will be rational and reasonable to the extent that the public culture, in its underlying conception of the political person—as rational and reasonable—and that of social cooperation, from which the standard is derived, is a result of Rawls' constructive political process.

3. Representatives: equal under the veil of ignorance

[4:7] The reasonable or fair terms of this structure and process starts out as the veil of ignorance ranging from being thick at the point of agreeing on the principles of justice and getting thinner as the constitutional, legislative and judicial stages are developed respectively. The purely rational autonomous representatives, subject to the restrictions of the original position, are to agree on principles of fundamental justice. The representatives are symmetrically situated with respect to one another, because of the veil of ignorance, and are in that sense equal. It is their task to agree on certain principles of justice from a list of alternatives given by the traditions of moral and political philosophy.

4. Conception of the person and the principles: tautological

a. Traditional alternatives of principles

[4:8] The agreement of the parties on certain definite principles establishes a tautological connection between the conception of the person represented and the principles. However, it is not necessary to show that the principles of justice that are agreed upon would be adopted from *any* enumeration of alternatives. The aim of justice as fairness is only to show that the principles of justice would be adopted over the other *traditional* alternatives. Once this is done further refinements may be made.

b. Reasonable constraints: preferences of principles

> [4:9] "While it should be granted that any list of alternatives may be to some extent arbitrary, the objection is mistaken if it is read as holding that all lists are equally so. A list that includes the leading traditional theories is less arbitrary than one which leaves out the more obvious candidates. Certainly the argument for the principles of justice would be strengthened by showing that they are still the best choice from a more comprehensive list more systematically evaluated. I do not know how far this can be done. I doubt, however, that the principles of justice (as I have defined them) will be the preferred conception on anything resembling a complete list.... Justifying grounds do not lie ready at hand: they need to be discovered and suitably expressed, sometimes by lucky guesses, sometimes by noting the requirements of theory. It is with this aim in mind that the various conditions on the choice of first principles are brought together in the notion of the original position. The idea is that by putting together enough reasonable constraints into a single conception, it will become obvious that one among the alternatives presented is to be preferred."[79]

---

[79] Rawls, *A Theory of Justice*, pp. 581-82.

IV. Two Principles of Justice

[5:1] The following are two principles of justice that meet the above criteria. The first principle representing the rational and the second principle the reasonable:[80]

[5:2] 1. Each person has an equal claim to a fully adequate scheme of equal basic rights and liberties, which scheme is compatible with the same scheme for all; and in this scheme the equal political liberties, and only those liberties, are to be guaranteed their fair value.

[5:3] 2. Social and economic inequalities are to satisfy two conditions:

i) they are to be attached to positions and offices open to all under conditions of fair equality of opportunity; and

ii) they are to be to the greatest benefit of the least advantaged members of society.

[5:4] The first principle that the representatives in the original position would agree to is a fully adequate set of the equal basic liberties that are necessary for the individuals they represent to develop as political persons or citizens. A political person, Rawls argues, requires:

[5:5] 1. The development and use of their rational moral powers, (i.e. their determinate conception of good). Even though the representatives in the original position still do not know the content of this good, they do know the general structure of the facts of psychology and social institutions. That is they know that those whom they represent do in fact form, revise and pursue comprehensive worldviews and that the principles of justice also influence the content of these comprehensive worldviews.

[5:6] 2. The development and use of their reasonable moral powers, (i.e. sense of justice or fairness).

[5:7] The principles of justice will determine what is deemed to be as a worthy good or end to pursue to the extent that the polit-

---

[80] Rawls, *Political Liberalism*, pp. 5, 291.

ical culture, rules and regulations influence the choice of values. However, this does not mean that the political culture, rules and regulations are made supreme and that all other associational values are subordinated to them. This is true at least to the extent that the political culture, rules and regulations are so broad and general that they do not dictate any particular religious, philosophical or moral associational value(s). If it is argued that the associational values are subordinated to the political culture, rules and regulations it would only be to the extent that the associational values are to be constrained within the broad and general political values deemed necessary for individuals to develop their moral powers as rational and reasonable agents. As Rawls says:

> [5:8] "[This] does not imply that the exercise of the moral powers on the part of the citizens in society is either the supreme or the sole form of good. Rather, the role and exercise of these powers (in the appropriate instances) is a condition of good." [81]

[5:9] As a result the representatives in the original position would agree that it would be "just" that the citizens they represent would have a fully adequate scheme of equal basic rights and liberties necessary for the development of the political person, so long as they do not interfere with the liberties of others.

A. Freestanding: Independent Of Metaphysical or Comprehensive Worldviews

[5:10] The support for the agreement on these equal basic rights and liberties can be derived from either utilitarian or deontological arguments. A utilitarian could argue from the position of the promotion of the greatest degree of the good through consequences and a deontologist could argue from the position of logical consistency with the definition of a political person and the categorical imperative. The point of this is that various comprehensive worldviews, which may even be incompatible and incommensurable, can agree on political principles by being inter-

[81] *Ibid.*, p. 334.

related with the primary principles. However, this agreement is not because of an overlap or similarity between various comprehensive worldviews but because the two principles and the ensuing primary goods are freestanding. Freestanding in that instead of deriving agreement from comprehensive worldviews, like utilitarianism and deontology, the agreement is derived from the broad and general notions of what would be necessary for free and equal persons to function in a pluralistic society. That is, what would be necessary for persons to pursue freely and equally a) a determinate conception of a good and b) social cooperation, i.e. a rational conception of a determinate good and a reasonable conception of social cooperation. The two principles of justice is one such solution that is independent of any comprehensive moral doctrine because the principles have not been derived from any comprehensive worldview(s). Rather, the two principles have been derived from the "limited" point of view of what a free and equal political person in a well-ordered democratic society would need in order to develop as reasonable and rational. Thus the two principles are freestanding and as a result may or may not be part of various comprehensive worldviews.[82]

[5:11] It could be argued that Rawls is depending on a metaphysical conception of a political person such that his political conception is metaphysical instead of political and thus part of a, or a number of, comprehensive worldviews.[83] But Rawls' position is that political democracy is to be a freestanding view, independent of any particular metaphysical or comprehensive worldview. He argues that what is implied in a political conception is that there be no specific metaphysical or epistemological doctrine. But doesn't the construction of this political system presuppose in the original position a particular metaphysical conception of the political person as rational and reasonable?

---

[82] This is not like saying, for example, that although two languages are not intertranslatable they both can be translated into a third language. That would be too comprehensive of a notion. Rather, it is more like saying that the two non-intertranslatable languages have the broad and general notion of communication for whatever reason(s).

[83] Rawls, *Political Liberalism*, p. 10.

B. Original Position: No Metaphysical Implications On The Nature Of The Self

[5:12] Rawls does not think that he is using any particular metaphysical conception because the original position is only a device of representation. The veil of ignorance, Rawls argues, does not have any metaphysical implications concerning the nature of the self.

> [5:13] "When we simulate being in the original position, our reasoning no more commits us to a particular metaphysical doctrine about the nature of the self than our acting a part in a play, say of Macbeth or Lady Macbeth, commits us to thinking that we are really a king or a queen engaged in a desperate struggle for political power. We must keep in mind that we are trying to show how the idea of society as a fair system of social cooperation can be unfolded so as to find principles specifying the basic rights and liberties and the forms of equality most appropriate to those cooperating, once they are regarded as citizens, as free and equal persons." [84]

[5:14] Rawls in a footnote continues to argue that:

> Part of the difficulty is that there is no accepted understanding of what a metaphysical doctrine is. ... [T]o develop a political conception of justice without presupposing, or explicitly using, a particular metaphysical doctrine, for example, some particular metaphysical conception of the person, is already to presuppose a metaphysical thesis: namely, that no metaphysical doctrine is required for this purpose. One might also say that our ordinary conception of persons as the basic unit of deliberation and responsibility presupposes, or in some way involves, certain metaphysical theses about the nature of persons as moral or political agents. ... If we look at the presentation of justice as fairness and note how it is set up, and note the ideas and conceptions it uses, no particular metaphysical doctrine about the nature of persons, distinctive and opposed to other metaphysical doctrines, appears among its premises, or seems required by its argument. If metaphysical presuppositions are involved, perhaps they are so general that they would not distinguish between the metaphysical views—Cartesian, Leibnizian, or Kantian; realist, idealist,

[84] *Ibid.*, p. 27.

or materialist—with which philosophy has traditionally been concerned. In this case they would not appear to be relevant for the structure and content of a political conception of justice one way or the other.[85]

C. Nonmetaphysical Foundation For Laws: Necessary For Pluralistic Societies

[5:15]. The original position is a nonmetaphysical foundational conception of the basis of political morality to which we appeal. Now it is true that comprehensive worldviews are adequate within themselves to provide a metaphysical foundation for the basis of laws and regulations, including informed consent. But there is a need for a nonmetaphysical foundation because individuals are living within a pluralistic society, which are comprised of incompatible worldviews, in which it is necessary that they all get along socially.[86]

D. Political Interrelated Consensus vs Comprehensive Associational Worldviews

[5:16] The original position, as rational and reasonable, is this nonmetaphysical foundation that needs to be substituted for at least that part of the individual's worldview that deals with the political realm. Rawls, in a sense, splits up worldviews into two pieces; the political and the associational. This is not so different from what Descartes did with his Cartesian or psychological dualism, giving the soul to the Church and the body to science.

---

[85] *Ibid.*, p. 29.

[86] It is important to note here that Rawls' concept of "reasonable" and that of the reasonable person standard are quite different since for Rawls "reasonable" means dealing fairly with others whereas the reasonable person standard has more of the idea of establishing a rational end or purpose. Rawls' concept of "rational" on the other hand, is the forming, pursuing and/or revising of one's end or purpose in life, *whatever* that might be. The reasonable person standard is therefore different than Rawls' "rational" in that for Rawls there is no preference given to any particular end or purpose whereas the reasonable person standard does have a preference or at least a consensus on what range qualifies as a "reasonable standard". Thus Rawlsian rational persons may pursue any end they wish within the societal constraints of, for example, the constitution. With these differences in mind it would appear that the reasonable person standard would be closer to Rawls' concept of "rational" than his concept of "reasonable".

Here Rawls creates a dualism giving one half—the comprehensive worldviews—to the associations, like churches and so forth, and giving the other half—the general interrelated consensus—to politics. However, Descartes thought that the soul could exist independently of the body whereas Rawls is not so naive as to think that political interrelated consensus could exist independent of associational worldviews or vice versa.

[5:17] The political part of our interrelated consensus demands a type of political democracy if individuals are going to live in a society comprised of people holding to differing comprehensive worldviews without violence. The principles of this political democracy thus must be comprised of a reasonable and rational nonmetaphysical freestanding conception that most reasonable and rational associational worldviews are able to accept, i.e. interrelated. The other part of an individual's worldview, the nonpolitical aspects, are freely determined by their comprehensive worldview and may be incompatible with others in society. But as long as these differences are not politically incompatible mandates of law, i.e. force, then they should be able to cooperate and function as a stable and well-ordered democratic society where citizens are free and equal.[87] It is the interrelated political principles that most reasonable and rational worldviews can agree on that will form the basis of their concept of precisely how much information disclosure would be necessary for an informed consent.

E. Political Democracy: A Symphony

[5:18] People function within this realm of political democracy much like people do when they play harmoniously in a symphony.

---

[87] "[T]here is a sphere of action in which society, as distinguished from the individual, has, if any, only an indirect interest; comprehending all that portion of a person's life and conduct which affects only himself, or if it also affects others, only with their free, voluntary, and undeceived consent and participation. When I say only himself, I mean directly, and in the first instance: for whatever affects himself, may affect others through himself." Mill, *On Liberty*, p. 265.

[5:19] Rawls mentions that an orchestra illustrates the idea of a social union in that each member is dependent on the other for the final outcome.[88] Although not presented by Rawls, the orchestra can also illustrate the original position and the basic institutions. The original position, with its primary principles and primary goods, is the theory or foundation behind the staff, and keys yet still does not determining the style or type of music. The basic institutions, with its constitution, legislative and judicial stages, are the sheet music of the orchestra. Freedom is represented in the fact that the orchestra is composed of musicians who freely choose to master their particular instruments. Equality is represented in the fact that all the instruments are equally needed to create the music. The orchestra proceeds through the composition being guided by broad key changes like the constitution guides the broad social structure. The musicians try to play the sheet music as written, like legislation, and play in harmony with each other through the guidance and flexibility of a conductor, representing the judicial stage. Each musician uses their own instruments, or different worldviews, some the same, like two trombones, having the same worldview, but playing different parts of first and second chair—different talents. Various musical instruments may be quite different from each other, like the woodwinds, brass, percussion and strings—different worldviews—some may even sound terrible together—incompatible worldviews—yet with the basic structure of key changes—constitution—and of the notes on the sheet-music—legislation—and the conductor—judicial stage—they can play together harmoniously as a symphony, like a stable and just society.

F. Primary Goods: Five Categories

[5:21] In order to construct Rawls' stable and just pluralistic society, it is imperative to start out with an independent nonmetaphysical foundation—the original position. Rawls' rational representatives under the constraints of reason agree to a basic primary goods list, i.e. things that every rational citizen is presumed to

---

[88] Rawls, *Political Liberalism*, p. 321.

want.[89] These primary goods are comprised of five categories, each of which is believed to be necessary for all rational and reasonable persons in a pluralistic democratic society to have in order for them to form, revise or pursue their good no matter what their worldview is. This list is not comprehensive and thus may be made either longer or shorter. However, the larger the list, the more weak will be the protection of the essential goods as there will be more competition or exceptions to deal with. Each category may clash with other categories and thus have to be limited. This limitation is the central range of application of each liberty. This list is developed by trial and error through the process of reflective equilibrium[90] and could be continued indefinitely. Rawls is not trying to develop The Political System, but only *a* political system that works better than what is presently the case in terms of a social contract theory with a group of people who are free and equal citizens of a democratic well-ordered society.

Rawls lists the five categories of primary goods as follows:[91]

[5:22] 1. The basic liberties … these liberties are the background institutional conditions necessary for the development and the full and informed exercise of the two moral powers …; these liberties are also indispensable for the protection of a wide range of determinate conceptions of the good (within the limits of justice).

a. Freedom of thought
b. Liberty of conscience
c. Political liberty
d. Freedom of association
e. Freedoms specified by the liberty and integrity of the person
f. Rights and liberties covered by rule of law

---

89 Rawls, *A Theory of Justice*, p. 62.

90 "There is no such thing as absolute certainty, but there is assurance sufficient for the purposes of human life. We may, and must, assume our opinion to be true for the guidance of our own conduct. … [T]he source of everything respectable in man either as an intellectual or as a moral being, namely, that his errors are corrigible. He is capable of rectifying his mistakes, by discussion and experience." Mill, *On Liberty*, p. 271-272.

91 Rawls, *Political Liberalism*, pp. 181, 291, 308, 332-335.

[5:23] 2. Freedom of movement and free choice of occupation against a background of diverse opportunities: these opportunities allow the pursuit of diverse final ends and give effect to a decision to revise and change them, if it is so desired.

[5:24] 3. Powers and prerogatives of offices and positions of responsibility: these give scope to various self-governing and social capacities of the self.

[5:25] 4. Income and wealth, understood broadly as all-purpose means (having an exchange value): income and wealth are needed to achieve directly or indirectly a wide range of ends, whatever they happen to be.

[5:26] 5. The social bases of self-respect: these bases are those aspects of basic institutions normally essential if citizens are to have a lively sense of their own worth as persons and to be able to develop and exercise their moral powers and to advance their aims and ends with self-confidence.

[5:27] This is not a comprehensive list by any means, but a list that seems to be an adequate starting place that most reasonable and rational comprehensive views could agree to in a hypothetical, nonhistorical, well-ordered democratic society in which the citizens' possession of these primary goods specifies the guaranteed status of free and equal citizens.[92,93]

G. Three Grounds: For Adopting The Two Principles Of Justice

[5:28] Rawls gives three main grounds, each related to the capacity for a sense of justice, for the representatives in the original position to adopt the two principles of justice, which guarantee the equal basic liberties and assign them priority. These grounds are important for our study in that the basic liberties will be the foundation for determining what our constitution will be comprised of and thus the basis for our construction of our principles

---

92 See §3.3 for a discussion of how the principles of justice are agreed upon in relation to other *traditional* alternatives. These principles include the primary goods. Because this list is to some extent arbitrary and the justifying grounds do not lie ready to hand, i.e. they are discovered by lucky guesses and reflective equilibrium, it is of little interest, at least at this point, to analyze or evaluate Rawls' list.

93 "This, then, is the appropriate region of human liberty. It comprises, first, the inward domain of consciousness; demanding liberty of conscience, in the most comprehensive sense; liberty of thought and feeling; absolute freedom of opinion and sentiment on all subject, practical or speculative, scientific, moral, or theological. The liberty of expressing and publishing opinions may seem to fall under a different principle, since it belongs to that part of the conduct of an individual which concerns other people; but, being almost of as much importance as the liberty of thought itself, and resting in great part on the same reasons, is practically inseparable from it. Secondly, the principle requires liberty of tastes and pursuits; of framing the plan of our life to suit our own character; of doing as we like, subject to such consequences as may follow: without impediment from our fellow-creatures, so long as what we do does not harm them, even though they should think our conduct foolish, perverse, or wrong. Thirdly, from this liberty of each individual, follows the liberty, within the same limits, of combination among individuals; freedom to unite, for any purpose not involving harm to others: the persons combining being supposed to be of full age, and not forced or deceived.

No society in which these liberties are not, on the whole, respected; is free, whatever may be its form of government; and none is completely free in which they do not exist absolute and unqualified. The only freedom which deserves the name, is that of pursuing our own good in our own way, so long as we do not attempt to deprive others of theirs, or impede their efforts to obtain it." Mill, *On Liberty*, pp. 265-266.

of consent. A quick sketch of these three justifying grounds[94] is as follows:

[5:29] 1. The two principles of justice give priority to the equal basic liberties;[95]

a. advantage to everyone's conception of the good and of a just and stable scheme of cooperation—public knowledge rather than penal sanctions and

b. most stable conception of justice is the two principles of justice—perspicuous and concerned with the good of those with whom they represent.

[5:30] 2. Fundamental importance of self-respect presupposes;[96]

a. the development and exercise of the two moral powers and

b. the accepting of various plans of life or comprehensive worldviews as worthwhile.

[5:31] 3. A democratic society well ordered by the two-principles of justice can be for each citizen a more comprehensive good than the determinate good of individuals[97]—a social union of social unions.[98]

a. Society depends on various talents.

b. Society depends on cooperative endeavors.

---

94 "... [How is] justice as fairness, and indeed any other political conception, ... to be assessed. Here the test is that of reflective equilibrium: how well the view as a whole articulates our more firm considered convictions of political justice, at all levels of generality, after due examination, once all adjustments and revisions that seem compelling have been made. A conception of justice that meets this criterion is the conception that, so far as we can now ascertain, is the one most reasonable for us. Rawls, *Political Liberalism*, p. 28.

95 Rawls, *Political Liberalism*, p. 316.

96 *Ibid.*, p. 318.

97 "[T]his more comprehensive good cannot be specified by a conception of the good alone but also needs a particular conception of justice, namely, justice as fairness. Thus this more comprehensive good presupposes this conception of justice and it can be attained provided the already given determinate conceptions of the good satisfy the general conditions. *Ibid.*, p. 323.

98 *Ibid.*, p. 320.

c. Societies' notions of reciprocity in the principles of justice.[99]

H. Three Reasons: For Priority Of Basic Liberties Over Distribution Principle

[5:32] There are three reasons for the principle which guarantees that these equal basic liberties have priority over the second principle of just distribution are derived from:

[5:33] 1. "the explanation of why a liberty is basic,"[100] i.e. built on the concept of the political person and what it takes to develop as rational and reasonable citizens in a democratic well-ordered society,

[5:34] 2. "the procedural role of certain liberties and their fundamental place in regulating the basic structure as a whole, as in the case of the equal political liberties,"[101] and

[5:35] 3. the fact that "certain liberties are indispensable institutional conditions once other basic liberties are guaranteed; thus freedom of thought and freedom of association are necessary to give effect to liberty of conscience and the political liberties."[102]

I. Basic Liberties: Not Maximized Nor Do They Maximize Anything

[5:36] Since the primary goods are necessary for the development of the political person, it is tempting to think that the representatives in the original position would try to maximize them,

---

99 "[P]ublic culture is always in large part the work of others; and therefore to support these attitudes of regard and appreciation citizens must affirm a notion of reciprocity appropriate to their conception of themselves and be able to recognize their shared public purpose and common allegiance. These attitudes are best secured by the two principles of justice precisely because of the recognized public purpose of giving justice to each citizen as a free and equal person on a basis of mutual respect. This purpose is manifest in the public affirmation of the equal basic liberties in the setting of the two principles of justice. The ties of reciprocity are extended over the whole of society and individual and group accomplishments are no longer seen as so many separate personal or associational goods." *Ibid.*, pp. 322-333.

100 *Ibid.*, p. 309.

101 *Ibid.*, p. 309.

102 *Ibid.*, p. 309.

giving first priority to the scheme of basic liberties.[103] But the basic liberties are not maximized and the basic liberties do not maximize anything, including the two moral powers of the rational and reasonable.

1. Basic Liberties Only Provides The Social Conditions For Developing The Two Moral Powers

[5:37] Rather the basic liberties function only to guarantee the social conditions needed for the development of the full and informed exercise of the two moral powers.

> [5:38] "But in fact, …the scheme of basic liberties is not drawn up so as to maximize anything, and, in particular, not the development and exercise of the moral powers. Rather, these liberties and their priority are to guarantee equally for all citizens the social conditions essential for the adequate development and the full and informed exercise of these powers …." [104]

2. Maximizing Basic Liberties Is Incoherent

[5:39] The idea of maximizing the basic liberties is incoherent for at least two reasons. The first being that there is no coherent notion of what would be maximized. The second being that the two moral powers is only a part of what it is to be a person.

a. No Coherent Notion Of What To Maximize

> [5:40] "Now there are two reasons why the idea of a maximum does not apply to specifying and adjusting the scheme of basic liberties. First, a coherent notion of what is to be maximized is lacking. We cannot maximize the de-

---

[103] The first principle of justice in *Political Liberalism* is different than the one stated in *Theory*. The former states: "Each person has an equal right to a fully adequate scheme of equal basic liberties which is compatible with a similar scheme of liberties for all. … [T]he words "a fully adequate scheme" replace the words "the most extensive total system" which were used in *Theory*. *Ibid.*, p. 291. "Now, in *Theory* one criterion suggested seems to be that the basic liberties are to be specified and adjusted so as to achieve the most extensive scheme of these liberties. This criterion is purely quantitative and does not distinguish some cases as more significant than others; moreover, it does not generally apply and is not consistently followed. As Hart noted, it is only in the simplest and least significant cases that the criterion of greatest extent is both applicable and satisfactory." *Ibid.*, p. 331.

[104] *Ibid.*, p. 332.

velopment and exercise of two moral powers at once. And how could we maximize the development and exercise of either power by itself? Do we maximize, other things equal, the number of deliberate affirmations of a conception of the good? That would be absurd. Moreover, we have no notion of a maximum development of these powers. What we do have is a conception of a well-ordered society with certain general features and certain basic institutions. Given this conception, we form the notion of the development and exercise of these powers, which is adequate and fully relative to the two fundamental cases."[105]

b. Persons Are More Than Just The Two Moral Powers

[5:41] "The other reason why the idea of a maximum does not apply is that the two moral powers do not exhaust the person, for persons also have a determinate conception of the good. Recall that such a conception includes an ordering of certain final ends and interests, attachments and loyalties to persons and associations, as well as a view of the world in the light of which these ends and attachments are understood. If citizens had no determinate conceptions of the good, which they sought to realize, the just social institutions of a well-ordered society would have no point. Of course, grounds for developing and exercising the moral powers strongly incline the parties in the original position to adopt the basic liberties and their priority. But the great weight of these grounds from the standpoint of the parties does not imply that the exercise of the moral powers on the part of the citizens in society is either the supreme or the sole form of good. Rather, the role and exercise of these powers (in the appropriate instances) is a condition of good. That is, citizens are to act justly and rationally, as circumstances require. In particular, their just and honorable (and fully autonomous) conduct renders them, as Kant would say, worthy of happiness; it makes their accomplishments wholly admirable and their pleasures completely good. But it would be madness to maximize just and rational actions by maximizing the occasions that require them."[106]

---

105 *Ibid.*, pp. 333-4.

106 *Ibid.*, pp. 333-4.

V. Second Principle of Justice: Difference Principle

A. Difference Principle Defined: The Reasonable

[6:1] The second principle of justice, sometimes referred to as the difference principle, states that:

[6:2] Social and economic inequalities are to satisfy two conditions:

1. they are to be attached to positions and offices open to all under conditions of fair equality of opportunity; and

2. they are to be to the greatest benefit of the least advantaged members of society.[107]

[6:3] The two primary principles of justice—like the political person, the original position,[108] and comprehensive worldviews—reflect the rational and the reasonable. The first principle of justice reflects the rational. The second principle reflects the reasonable. Together the two principles of justice correspond to the two powers of moral personality, i.e. the rational and reasonable, reflecting that which is necessary to be a political person in a hypothetical, nonhistorical, democratic well-ordered society of free and equal citizens.

B. The Second Principle of Distributive Justice Is Not Necessary: An Erroneous Argument

[6:4] However, it *might*[109] be argued that the primary principles of justice should not include the reasonable. Remember that the

---

107 *Ibid.*, pp. 5, 291.

108 "Two different parts of the original position must be carefully distinguished. These parts correspond to the two powers of moral personality, or to what I have called "the capacity to be reasonable" and "the capacity to be rational." While the original position as a whole represents both moral powers, and therefore represents the full conception of the person" *Ibid.*, pp. 305.

109 Although the following argument is not Rawls' position, (and will be refuted in the following section §5.4), I believe that it helps us come to an understanding of why Rawls' rational and reasonable concepts are not derivative ideas but rather complementary ideas.

representatives in the original position are purely rational autonomous representatives who are reasonably constrained externally by a thick veil of ignorance. As the basic social structure is developed, going from issues that are very general, i.e. the principles of justice, to those that are more specific, i.e. constitutional, legislative and judicial stages, the veil of ignorance is gradually lifted as more information is needed in order to allow this construction. As this veil is gradually lifted there should be a transference of the just or reasonable from being externally imposed to becoming internally part of the basic structure. Thus when the outward constraints of the veil are thick the inward principles of the reasonable are thin. As the outward constraints of the veil become thinner the inward basic structure of the reasonable, just laws and regulations, becomes thicker.

1. Second principle of distributive justice is redundant: distributive justice & veil of ignorance

[6:5] Thus it *could* be argued that Rawls is being redundant since his second principle is reasonable and the original position is already under the constraints of the reasonable—the veil of ignorance—the original position is not the place to introduce the second principle of distributive justice.

2. Distributive justice should be introduced at legislative stage instead of Original Position

[6:6] Distributive justice thus should be introduced at the legislative stage, which still has a veil of ignorance but is much thinner or partial. The original position should be internally purely rational with external constraints of the reasonable, i.e. veil of ignorance. Thus the content of the original position and the agreed-on principles should be that of the rational only. It is not yet necessary to agree on the principles of reasonableness until the thick veil of ignorance, the external constraint of the reasonable, becomes thinner. The reason why the reasonable is not introduced at the constitutional stage is because Rawls argues that the constitution is to incorporate only the first principle of justice, i.e. the rational.

[6:7] The first principle of justice is to be applied at the stage of the constitutional convention. ... Although delegates have a notion of just and effective legislation, the second principle of justice, which is part of the content of this notion, is not incorporated into the constitution itself. Indeed, the history of successful constitutions suggests that principles to regulate economic and social inequalities, and other distributive principles, are generally not suitable as constitutional restrictions. Rather, just legislation seems to be best achieved by assuring fairness in representation and by other constitutional devices.[110]

[6:8] So why is the difference principle necessary or even allowable as a primary principle especially if it is not even incorporated into the constitution? Why not have, in the original position, just the rational principle, with its rational list of basic primary goods, agreed upon by the representatives under the (reasonable) thick veil of ignorance? It would still be modeling the political rational person on the rational and reasonable as the rational and reasonable are both being utilized in the original position. Then at the legislative stage the reasonable difference principle could be derived from the rational constitution. Thus it would be possible to start out with the pure rational principle, agreed upon through a pure reasonable veil of ignorance. The Constitution would then likewise be made up of the purely rational principles, and its basic liberties, under a thinning reasonable veil of ignorance. Then as the reasonable veil is thinned even more, the reasonable would be translated into legislation. As the basic institutions are developed through legislation and the judicial process, the reasonable veil of ignorance would gradually be lifted transferring progressively the external reasonable into the internal structure, i.e. rules of law and legislation. This would also, as a

---

110 *Ibid.*, pp. 336-7.

result, give the lexical order effect of giving priority of the rational over the reasonable.[111]

C. The Second Principle of Distributive Justice Is Necessary

1. The reasonable is not derivable from the rational

[6:9] However, if there is this transfer of the external reasonable into the internal reasonable on what bases will it be possible to determine what the internal reasonable is comprised of or built on? Certainly the external reasonable, i.e. the veil of ignorance, is not appropriate as a building block or foundation for the internal reasonable as the veil gives no guidance except for a lack of knowledge even though this lack of knowledge is for the purpose of impartiality.[112] Thus the reasonable would have to be derived from the only other aspect left, the rational. That which is internally reasonable would have to be derived from that which is rational and thus the reasonable would be dependent on the rational.

[6:10] But this is not what Rawls wants or has in mind. The rational and the reasonable are two distinct but complementary basic ideas. In particular, the reasonable is not derivable from the rational. David Gauthier, in his book *Morals by Agreement,* tries to derive the reasonable from the rational, thinking that since the rational is more basic and sure, deriving the reasonable from the rational would at last give the reasonable, or just, a firm foundation.

---

111 Allen Buchanan explains Rawls' concept of lexical ordering as follows; "A principle 'P' is lexically prior to a principle 'Q' if and only if we are first to satisfy all the requirements of 'P' before going on to satisfy the requirements of 'Q'. Lexical priority allows no trade-offs between the demands of conflicting principles: the lexically prior principle takes absolute priority." Buchanan, *Justice: A Philosophical Review,* p. 6.

112 However, the veil of ignorance is defended on the basis of a concept of impartiality, which may be related to Rawls' category of the reasonable as a mechanism of representation.

2. The reasonable and rational are complementary: one cannot exist without the other

[6:11] Rawls rejects this idea of deriving the reasonable from the rational, arguing that they are complementary ideas. And as complementary ideas the reasonable and the rational are unable to exist without the other. This becomes clear when it is realized what would happen if the political person were to be split up. On the one hand, a political person that was solely a reasonable agent would have nothing to be reasonable about as there would be no rational good or end to pursue. On the other hand, a political person that was solely rational would lack the sense of justice that comes from being reasonable and thus would not be able to recognize the independent validity of the claims of others in a pluralistic democratic society.

[6:12] To see justice as fairness as trying to derive the reasonable from the rational misinterprets the original position.[113]

3. Foundation of reasonable laws necessitates the second principle of justice

[6:13] The constitution is the first of the basic institutions and it is developed using only the rational principle of justice behind the veil of ignorance. Thus, even in the development of the rational constitution, the reasonable and the rational are complementing each other. But at the legislative stage the veil of ignorance is thinner as there is a need for incorporating or transferring the external reasonable into internal reasonable. This is where the reasonable second principle is a necessary component in the original position. It gives us a foundation on which to build our reasonable rules and laws. Just as the constitutional stage is built on or derived from the rational principle in the original position so now the reasonable part of the legislative stage is derived from the reasonable principle in the original position keeping intact the lexical ordering of the rational preceding the reasonable. The reasonable second principle of justice is thus a necessary compo-

---

113 Rawls, *Political Liberalism*, p. 52.

nent to Rawls' original position if the reasonable is in fact not to be derived from the rational.

> [6:14] "It is, of course, impossible to prove that the reasonable cannot be derived from the rational as it is impossible to know and evaluate all past, present and future arguments for that conclusion. Thus negative statements like this are at best just conjectures. The most we can do is look at those arguments that seriously attempt to derive the reasonable from the rational and show how they fail in their attempt.[114] To the extent that the arguments are successful in deriving the reasonable from the rational we must show that they rely at some point on conditions expressing the reasonable itself." [115]

> [6:15] "The way to resolve the matter is to consider after due reflection which view, when fully worked out, offers the most coherent and convincing account. About this, of course, judgments may differ." [116]

[6:16] The important point is that for Rawls the rational and the reasonable are complementary and that they are the necessary political components for free and equal political citizens in this just, stable, nonhistorical, hypothetical, democratic, and well-ordered society.

D. Representatives Are Purely Rational

[6:18] But how then is it possible to justify the reasonable principle of justice in the original position when the representatives are acting as purely rational autonomous agents? It is important to see that the representatives are rationally autonomous in two respects.

> [6:19] "First, in their deliberations they are not required to apply, or to be guided by, any prior or antecedent principles of right and justice. Second, in arriving at an agreement on which principles of justice to adopt from the alternatives available, the parties are to be guided solely by

---

[114] Gauthier is an example of someone who attempts to derive the reasonable from the rational. See David Gauthier, *Morals By Agreement* (New York: Oxford University Press, 1986).

[115] Rawls, *Political Liberalism*, p. 53.

[116] *Ibid.*, p. 53.

what they think is for the determinate good of the persons they represent, so far as the limits on information allow them to determine this." [117]

1. Rational representative know the citizen's two moral powers

[6:20] These rationally autonomous representatives, although under the constraints of the veil of ignorance, know at least two things about the political persons they represent:

1. the persons are rational in that they have the capacity to form, revise and pursue a good and

2. the persons need to be able to deal fairly with others, i.e. to be reasonable, so as to be able to promote their good.

2. Two moral powers require two principles of justice especially if complementary

[6:21] Even from a purely rational perspective, with this knowledge in hand, it would be clear that there would be a need for at least two primary principles[118] if the rational and the reasonable are to be seen as complementary (one cannot exist without the other) and not derivable from each other, that is:

1. a primary principle that would provide the foundation for freedom and equality to pursue, develop or exercise their good—the rational, and

2. a primary principle that would provide the freedom and equality to deal fairly with others—the reasonable.

[6:22] Thus, the reasonable is not being derived from the rational rather the rational just sees the reasonable as a complementary part of our two-faceted political person—the reasonable and rational—both being necessary for the promotion of the good. Thus the reasonable is not derived from the rational nor is the

---

[117] *Ibid.*, p. 307.

[118] A single principle could also represent the reasonable and the rational if it were comprised of both aspects. However, as we saw above, Rawls holds that the two principles are to be in lexical order. If we were to have only one principle the lexical ordering would not be as straight forward.

rational derived from the reasonable. Rather the reasonable and rational are complementary to each other.

E. Difference Principle: Maximin

[6:23] As mentioned at the outset of this section the second principle of justice is often times referred to as the difference principle and states that:

Social and economic inequalities are to satisfy two conditions:

1) they are to be attached to positions and offices open to all under conditions of fair equality of opportunity; and

2) they are to be to the greatest benefit of the least advantaged members of society.[119]

[6:24] The second principle of justice—the difference principle—is justified using maximin reasoning.

[6:25] "The term maximin means the maximum minimorum; and the rule directs our attention to the worst that can happen under any proposed course of action, and to decide in the light of that." [120]

1. Maximin is for background justice, not for specific morality

[6:26] The maximin principle has the limited role of being used only as a criterion of background justice. Rawls is constructing a general political structure or framework, not a specific comprehensive worldview. As a result, Rawls' makes clear that the maximin principle and the two principles of justice are all to be confined to the basic structure or framework and not to be used as a basis for specific morality. To do otherwise would be to shortcut the political construction process and the basic institutions, which are inevitable in a pluralistic democratic society, whose structures were systematically designed to insure that all citizens, with their same or different comprehensive worldviews, are dealt with, politically speaking, reasonably and rationally.

---

[119] *Ibid.*, pp. 5, 291.

[120] Rawls, *A Theory of Justice*, p. 154.

[6:27] The political maximin principle maximizes the minimum position with the hope of guaranteeing the best social conditions for the least advantaged. This Rawls feels is what the rational representatives would agree to as the conditions necessary for ensuring that those whom they represent would be guaranteed the best social conditions possible for their development as political persons.

2. Maximin & two principles of justice are to be confined to the basic structure

[6:28] Even though the maximin theory and the two principles of justice, in our political construction, are to be confined to the basic structure and not used as a basis for specific morality, i.e., a comprehensive worldview, people still have built elaborate "Rawlsian" informed consent arguments failing to understand this fundamental point. The following argument is an example of such a mistake.[121]

F. Cust's Misuse Of Maximin Results In Erroneous Conclusions

[6:29] Cust expresses correctly that Rawls, in his book *A Theory Of Justice,* presents what has been described as hypothetical contractarianism. In this hypothetical situation, there are people in the original position (Pops),[122] behind a veil of ignorance, who decide what principles of justice would be fair.[123] The veil of ignorance is characterized by Rawls as follows:

> [6:30] "Among the essential features of this situation is that no one knows his place in society, his class position or social status, nor does anyone know his fortune in the distribution of natural assets and abilities, his intelligence,

---

[121] Cust, "Hypothetical Contractarianism and the Disclosure Requirement Problem in Informed Consent", pp. 125-128.

[122] This is an acronym Cust uses. Cust, "Hypothetical Contractarianism and the Disclosure Requirement Problem in Informed Consent", p. 125.

[123] This, of course, is different from the description in *Political Liberalism*. In *Theory* Rawls has people in the original position choosing for themselves the principles of justice. In *Political Liberalism* Rawls has rational representatives choosing the principles for those whom they represent.

strength, and the like. I shall even assume that the parties do not know their conceptions of the good or their special psychological propensities." [124]

[6:31] Under the constraints of the veil of ignorance, Pops would still be rational, free, equal, and disinterested agents. The principles of justice chosen under these condition would establish not only what would be considered as primary social goods (PSG's)[125] but also how those PSG's should be distributed.

[6:32] Rawls states in *Theory* that the two principles of justice[126] could be justified in a number of ways.[127] One way of justification is to show, for example, how consequentialists could come to the same agreement of principles of justice through the use of actual and predictive consequences. But another way of defending the choice of the principles of justice is by showing how the principles are compatible with the risk aversiveness of Pops, i.e. the maximin solution.[128]

> [6:33] "[I]t is useful as a heuristic device to think of the two principles as the maximin solution to the problem of social justice. There is an analogy between the two principles and the maximin rule for choice under uncertainty. This is evident from the fact that the two principles are those a person would choose for the design of a society in which his enemy is to assign him his place. The maximin rule tells us to rank alternatives by their worst possible outcomes: we are to adopt the alternative the worst outcome of which is superior to the worst outcomes of others. The persons in the original position do not, of course, assume that their initial place in society is decided by a malevolent opponent." [129]

---

[124] Rawls, *A Theory of Justice*, p. 12. also see pp. 136-150.

[125] This is an acronym Cust uses. Cust, "Hypothetical Contractarianism and the Disclosure Requirement Problem in Informed Consent", p. 126. Primary social goods, or PSG's for short, are defined as those "things that it is supposed a rational man wants whatever else he wants." Rawls, *A Theory of Justice*, p. 92. also see pp. 90-95.

[126] For a formulation of the two principles of justice see *Ibid.*, pp. 302-303.

[127] *Ibid.*, p. 152.

[128] *Ibid.*, p. 152.

[129] *Ibid.*, p. 152-153.

[6:34] In employing the "maximin rule," in the determination of the "principles of justice," Pops would be trying to choose the best "worst outcome."

[6:35] Cust strikes off on his own by thinking that it would be consistent with Rawls' theory to use this maximin principle in the determination of what would be a just standard of information disclosure necessary for the making of an informed consent. Cust argues that if Pops were to choose a standard of information disclosure instead of the two principles of justice, Pops would choose the professional practice standard.[130] Cust believes this decision would be governed by these three considerations.[131]

> [6:36] "First, they [Pops] do not know, at least until the veil is lifted, whether they are the doctor or the patient, that is they have to make a choice on the assumption that they stand an equal chance of being either the doctor or the patient.
>
> Second, the choice they make has to be based on the minimax[132] rule, which, it will be recalled, tells them to maximize their minimum expected utility.
>
> Third, they are mutually disinterested, which is to say that once they are behind the veil of ignorance they are completely unconcerned with each other's interest." [133]

[6:37] Cust argues that Pops would reason as follows:

"[T]he maximin rule tells them [Pops] to minimize the worst possible outcome and assuming that the worst possible outcome

---

[130] See §8. Deciding On A Standard Of Disclosure.

[131] Cust, "Hypothetical Contractarianism and the Disclosure Requirement Problem in Informed Consent", p. 127.

[132] Cust refers here to the maximin rule as the minimax rule. Cust gives the minimax rule the same definition as the maximin rule: "the minimax rule, which, it will be recalled, tells them to maximize their minimum expected utility". *Ibid.*, p. 127.

[133] *Ibid.*, p. 127.

is one's death,[134] one would want to minimize the likelihood of that outcome. The best possible way to minimize that outcome, *ceteris paribus*, would be to allow the doctor to choose on behalf of the patient the nature and amount of information to disclose such that the likelihood of the worst possible outcome was minimized. Why the doctor? Because she is better informed both with respect to knowledge and expertise. Hence, insofar as disclosure requirements are concerned in decision making this is an argument in favor of the professional standard of disclosure." [135]

[6:38] However, if Cust were to truly follow his own maximin reasoning it might lead him to dispense with the requirement for patient informed consent altogether. If the doctor is always or usually in the best position to make medical decisions, and if in doctor/patient relationships the sole concern is the maximization of the patient's worst off condition, then the patient's informed consent may have little relevance in securing the maximin.

[6:39] Cust has misunderstood Rawls' intention for the use of the maximin theory. In *Political Liberalism* Rawls clearly states that:

> "The maximin principle was never [i.e., not in *Theory* either] proposed as a basis for morality; in the form of the difference principle it is one principle constrained by others that applies to the basic structure; and when this principle is seen in this limited role as a criterion of background justice, its implications in normal cases are not, I believe, implausible. Finally, confining the application of the principles of justice to the basic structure does not imply that only the number of persons involved determines which principles hold for a given case." [136]

[6:40] The important point is that the political maximin principle maximizes the minimum amount of primary goods and nothing

---

[134] Cust in a footnote says "Death may not be the worst possible outcome for, as some would surely argue, there are cases where being alive and in extreme pain is far worse than being dead. Nevertheless, even if death is not the worst possible outcome the argument goes through for whatever is the worse possible outcome is the outcome that the hypothetical contractors would want to minimize the likelihood of." Ibid., p. 128.

[135] *Ibid.*, p. 128.

[136] Rawls, *Political Liberalism*, p. 261.

else and the primary goods do not necessarily maximize anything. Rather the primary goods function only to guarantee the social conditions necessary for the development of the full and informed exercise of the two moral powers. The maximin theory was not meant to be used for deriving what type of information disclosure would be necessary for a reasonable and rational informed consent.

VI. Basic Institutions: Foundations

A. Political Person: Foundation Of The Constitution, Laws, And Justice

[7:1] The foundation of the constitution, legislative stage, and judicial stage is the conception of the political person as rational and reasonable.

1. Reasonable: always constrains the rational

[7:2] In the process of building the framework of the basic institutions, the reasonable always constrains the rational.

2. As the veil gets thinner the accumulated restrictions get greater

[7:3] "As you proceed from stage to stage, from the conception of a person to the two principles and then to the establishment of a constitution and next to legislation and finally to the judicial stage, what varies is the task of the rational agents of deliberation, i.e. going from general to specific and thus requiring a progressively "thinner" veil, and the constraints, that is the reasonable, to which they are subject, i.e. going from weak to strong as a result of accumulated restrictions of justice."[137]

> [7:4] "The autonomous representatives in the original position are under the constraints of the thick veil of ignorance and have the general task of determining the primary principles of justice necessary for the development of the political person. In the constitution stage although those selecting a constitution are under a thinning veil of ignorance[138] they are also under the constraints of the primary principles adopted in the original position. Legislators are constrained even more, despite the fact that they are under a thinner veil of ignorance, as any laws they enact must be in accord with all of the previous constraints,

[137] *Ibid.*, p. 340.

[138] The veil must thin as decisions become more specific. As decisions become more particular and situational there is a proportional need for particular and situational information. Conversely, in proportion to the extent that the decisions being made in the original position are broad and general so it was deemed just to restrict specific information, i.e. "thick" veil of ignorance.

> i.e. laws chosen must be in accord with not only the two primary principles but now also with the constitution. Thus the exercise of both the rational and the reasonable changes as the representatives proceed from stage to stage."[139]

[7:5]

1. Changes in the tasks of the rational;
   a. their tasks become less general and
   b. their tasks become more specific.
2. Changes in the constraints of the reasonable;
   a. the constraints of the reasonable becomes stronger or more complex because of previous agreements and
   b. the veil of ignorance becomes thinner, a necessary feature if the rational tasks are to be more specific.

[7:6] Thus the constraints on the rational from the reasonable changes at each stage as the task of the rational changes.

> [7:7] "While the constraints of the reasonable are weakest and the veil of ignorance thickest in the original position, at the judicial stage these constraints are strongest and the veil of ignorance thinnest. The whole sequence is a schema for working out a conception of justice and guiding the application of its principles to the right subject in the right order. This schema is not, of course, a description of any actual political process, and much less of how any constitutional regime may be expected to work. It belongs to a conception of justice, and although it is related to an account of how democracy works, it is not such an account." [140]

B. Constitutional Democratic Regime: Modern Reality

[7:8] After the reasonable and rational principles have been chosen by the rationally autonomous representatives in the original position they then must be applied to the basic structure which Rawls takes to be a modern constitutional democratic regime. The basic structures of society are:

---

[139] Rawls, *Political Liberalism*, p. 340.

[140] *Ibid.*, p. 340.

> [7:9] "the main political, social, and economic institutions, and how they fit together into one unified system of social cooperation, from one generation to the next." [141]

[7:10] The framework of the basic institutions consists of the constitutional branch, the legislative branch and the judicial branch.

1. Constitutional Branch

[7:11] The constitution is composed of two primary essentials:

a. General structure and process of government: variable

> [7:12] "The fundamental principles that specify the general structure of government and the political process: the powers of the legislature, executive and the judiciary; the scope of majority rule."[142]

[7:13] The constitutional essentials of the first kind could be illustrated by the difference between presidential and cabinet government. But once the structure of government is agreed on it should be changed only as a result of political justice or the general good and not because of some political advantage of some group or party. [143]

b. Basic rights and liberties: not variable

> [7:14] "Equal basic rights and liberties of citizenship that legislative majorities are to respect: such as the right to vote and to participate in politics, liberty of conscience, freedom of thought and of association, as well as the protections of the rule of law." [144]

1) Equal basic rights and liberties:

Simple to agree on and to realize.

> [7:15] "In contrast with the general structure and process of government, the second essential of the constitution,

[141] *Ibid.*, p. 11.

[142] *Ibid.*, p. 227.

[143] *Ibid.*, p. 228.

[144] *Ibid.*, p. 227.

which deals with equal basic rights and liberties, can only be specified within small variations."[145]

[7:16] "The distinction between the principles covering the basic freedoms and those covering social and economic inequalities is not that the first expresses political values while the second does not. Both express political values. ... In the first role that structure specifies and secures citizens' equal basic rights and liberties and institutes just political procedures. In the second it sets up the background institutions of social and economic justice appropriate to citizens as free and equal. The first role concerns how political power is acquired and the limits of its exercise." [146]

[7:17] "Unlike the essentials covering social and economic inequalities, it is fairly clear to see whether the constitutional essentials covering basic freedoms are satisfied. Social and economic inequalities are always subjected to wide differences of reasonable and rational opinions, inferences and intuitive judgments. This is because the subject, of social and economic inequalities, is complex, not very predictable and poorly understood." [147]

[7:18] "Thus, ... we can expect more agreement about whether the principles for the basic rights and liberties are realized than about whether the principles for social and economic justice are realized." [148]

[7:19] "Because a democratic constitution, as an expression of higher law, is to be widely supported "it is best not to burden it with many details and qualifications." It is also because of this fact that the basic institutions should be able to reflect and make visible the essential constitutional principles." [149]

[7:20] To conclude: there are four grounds for distinguishing the constitutional essentials specified by the basic freedoms from the principles governing social and economic inequalities.

[7:21]

---

[145] *Ibid.*, p. 228.

[146] *Ibid.*, p. 229.

[147] *Ibid.*, p. 229.

[148] *Ibid.*, p. 229.

[149] *Ibid.*, p. 232.

"a. The two kinds of principles specify different roles for the basic structure.

b. It is more urgent to settle the essentials dealing with the basic freedoms.

c. It is far easier to tell whether those essentials are realized.

d. It is much easier to gain agreement about what the basic rights and liberties should be, not in every detail of course, but about the main outlines."[150]

2) Distribution principle:

Little agreement, difficult to realize

[7:22] These considerations explain why basic liberties "count as constitutional essentials while the principles of fair opportunity and the difference principle do not."[151] This is an important point for our enterprise as it is the constitution that will establish the foundation for the principles of consent requirements.

> [7:23] "[I]f a political conception of justice covers the constitutional essentials and matters of basic justice—for the present this is all we aim for—it is already of enormous importance even if it has little to say about many economic and social issues that legislative bodies must regularly consider. To resolve these more particular and detailed issues it is often more reasonable to go beyond the political conception and the values its principles express, and to invoke nonpolitical values that such a view does not include. But so long as there is firm agreement on the constitutional essentials and established political procedures are reasonably regarded as fair, willing political and social cooperation between free and equal citizens can normally be maintained." [152]

c. Political Power: co-dependently held by the three branches of government

[7:24] The basic generality of this constitution to guarantee basic rights explains why political "power cannot be left to the legisla-

---

[150] *Ibid.*, p. 230.

[151] *Ibid.*, p. 230.

[152] *Ibid.*, p. 230.

ture or even the supreme court, which is only the highest judicial interpreter of the constitution." The legislature is to be constrained by the constitution. The supreme court may be the "highest judicial interpreter of the constitution" but it also is constrained by the constitution. Political power is held co-dependently by the three branches, i.e. the constitutional branch, the legislative branch, and the judicial branch, "in a duly specified relation with one another with each responsible to the people."

1) Electorate: can mold the interpretation of the constitution

[7:25] It is true that in a democratic society "a strong majority of the electorate can eventually make the constitution conform to its political will."[153] This comes about because:

> [7:26] "The constitution is not what the Court says it is. Rather, it is what the people acting constitutionally through the other branches eventually allow the Court to say it is. A particular understanding of the constitution may be mandated to the Court by amendments, or by a wide and continuing political majority ..." [154]

2) Abuse of institutional procedures:

Can result in laws that are inconsistent with the constitution

> [7:27] "No institutional procedure exists that cannot be abused or distorted to enact statutes violating basic constitutional democratic principles." [155]

2. Legislative Branch

a. Protects distribution principle

[7:28] Since the constitution protects mainly the equal basic rights and liberties of citizenship the legislative stage is needed to protect all the other legal rights and liberties specified by the two principles of justice.

b. Distribution is contextual

---

[153] *Ibid.*, pp. 232-233.

[154] *Ibid.*, pp. 237-238.

[155] *Ibid.*, p. 233.

[7:29] "This implies, for example, that the question of private property and the means of production or their social ownership and similar questions are not settled at the level of the first principles of justice, but depend upon the traditions and social institutions of a country and its particular problems and historical circumstances." [156]

[7:30] "Even if it were possible to construct a philosophical argument tracing legislation back to the first principle of justice, i.e. basic rights and liberties, there is good reason for working out a conception of justice that does not do this. For one thing, in a pluralistic society you probably will not find philosophical agreement. Secondly, the legislative stage is to be defined and arranged by both the conception of the person and social cooperation. Since the principles of justice account for our fundamental constitutional rights and liberties, the remaining questions of justice are to be settled at the legislative stage with the two principles of justice functioning as a possible common court of appeal." [157]

3. Summary of Constitutional and Legislative Stages

[7:31] "In sum, then, the constitution specifies a just political procedure and incorporates restrictions which both protect the basic liberties and secure their priority. The rest is left to the legislative stage. Such a constitution conforms to the traditional idea of democratic government while at the same time it allows a place for the institution of judicial review.[158] This conception of the constitution does not found it, in the first instance, on principles of justice, or on basic (or natural) rights. Rather, its foundation is in the conceptions of the person and of social cooperation most likely to be congenial to the public culture of a modern democratic society." [159]

[7:32] "Once a constitutional consensus is in place, political groups must enter the public forum of political discussion and appeal to other groups who do not share their

---

[156] *Ibid.*, p. 338.

[157] *Ibid.*, p. 338-339.

[158] For a valuable discussion of judicial review in the context of the conception of justice as fairness, see Frank I. Michelman, "In Pursuit of Constitutional Welfare Rights: one View of Rawls' *Theory Of Justice*," *University of Pennsylvania Law Review* 121(5) (May 1973), pp. 991-1019.

[159] Rawls, *Political Liberalism*, p. 339.

> comprehensive doctrine. … Political conceptions of justice provide the common currency of discussion and a deeper basis for explaining the meaning and implications of the principles and policies each group endorses." [160]

a. Political discussions

1) Framework of justice: directs the discussions

[7:33] The point here is that citizens are to conduct their fundamental political discussions within the Rawlsian political framework of justice. "Each person must be able to explain their political position not by appealing to their associational point of view but rather by principles and guidelines they think other citizens may reasonably be expected to endorse as free and equal citizens in a pluralistic society."[161]

2) Social cooperation: disciplines the discussions

> [7:34] "Although it may be the case that others may fail to endorse their political position the fact that their public discussions are based on the common public conception of the political person and social cooperation imposes considerable discipline." [162]

b. Orderly contest of political conceptions

> [7:35] "It is inevitable and often desirable that citizens have different views as to the most appropriate political conception; for the public political culture is bound to contain different fundamental ideas that can be developed in different ways. An orderly contest between them over time is a reliable way to find which one, if any, is most reasonable." [163]

> [7:36] "In a constitutional system with judicial review, or review conducted by some other body, it will be necessary for judges, or the officers in question, to develop a political conception of justice in the light of which the constitution, in their view, is to be interpreted and important cases decided. Only so can the enactments of the legislature be de-

---

[160] *Ibid.*, p. 165.

[161] *Ibid.*, p. 226.

[162] *Ibid.*, p. 227.

[163] *Ibid.*, p. 227.

clared constitutional or unconstitutional; and only so have they a reasonable basis for their interpretation of the values and standards the constitution ostensibly incorporates. Plainly these conceptions will have an important role in the politics of constitutional debates." [164]

[164] *Ibid.*, p. 165.

VII. Public Political Culture vs Social Culture

[8:1] If there is a civil and just democratic pluralistic well-ordered society that is comprised of citizens who hold to vastly differing worldviews, a natural result of being free and equal persons, these worldviews, if we use Rawls' political construction, could be characterized as comprised of two parts: the public political part and the background or social culture part.

A. Public Culture: Interrelated Political Conception

[8:2] The political part is the interrelated conception of justice that is reflected in terms of the fundamental ideas seen as implicit in the public political culture of a democratic society.

[8:3] It is the public culture that is comprised of the interrelated public political institutions.[165]

B. Social Culture: Comprehensive Doctrines

> [8:4] "The social part or background culture of a civil society is not necessarily composed of anything that is interrelated with other comprehensive worldviews *per se* but rather of various comprehensive doctrines, i.e. religious, philosophical and moral doctrines that manifest themselves in many associations: churches, universities, learned and scientific societies, and clubs and teams to mention a few. The background culture is the culture of the social or associational, not of the political.
>
> [8:5] A conception of justice fulfills its social role provided that persons equally conscientious and sharing roughly the same beliefs find that, by affirming the framework of deliberation set up by it, they are normally led to a sufficient convergence of judgment necessary to achieve effective and fair social cooperation. My discussion of the basic liberties and their priority should be seen in this light. … Thus justice as fairness is addressed not so much to constitutional jurists as to citizens in a constitutional regime. It presents a way for them to conceive of their common and

165 "In justice as fairness the priority of right means that the principles of political justice impose limits on permissible ways of life; and hence the claims citizens make to pursue ends that transgress those limits have no weight." *Ibid.*, p. 174. "The priority of right gives the principles of justice a strict precedence in citizens' deliberations and limits their freedom to advance certain ways of life." *Ibid.*, p. 209.

guaranteed status as equal citizens and attempts to connect a particular understanding of freedom and equality with a particular conception of the person thought to be congenial to the shared notions and essential convictions implicit in the public culture of a democratic society. Perhaps in this way the impasse concerning the understanding of freedom and equality can at least be intellectually clarified if not resolved. It is particularly important to keep in mind that the conception of the person is part of a conception of political and social justice. That is, it characterizes how citizens are to think of themselves and of one another in their political and social relationships, and, therefore, as having the basic liberties appropriate to free and equal persons capable of being fully cooperating members of society over a complete life. The role of a conception of the person in a conception of political justice is distinct from its role in a personal or associational ideal, or in a religious or moral way of life. The basis of toleration and of social cooperation on a footing of mutual respect in a democratic regime is put in jeopardy when these distinctions are not recognized; for when this happens and such ideals and ways of life take a political form, the fair terms of cooperation are narrowly drawn, and free and willing cooperation between persons with different conceptions of the good may become impossible."[166]

C. Politically And Socially: Incompatible Worldviews Can Coexist Peacefully

[8:6] Thus it has been shown how Rawls' rational and reasonable conception of justice, with its primary principles and basic institutions and stages, i.e. political person, two principles, constitution, legislative stage and judicial stage, can in fact be interrelated with other reasonable and rational comprehensive worldviews that may even be incompatible with each other. Because of the broad and general abstractness of this political construction most rational and reasonable worldviews will see this political conception of justice as fairness as either derivable from, consistent with, or at least not in conflict with their *fundamental* values in their worldview. Rawls has tried to show how this political conception or structure is a just and stable structure that is exercis-

---

166 *Ibid.*, pp. 368-69.

able in a well-ordered fair and equal pluralistic democratic society giving, as a result, a sense of fair representation and stability to all. Rawls believes that this political system theoretically makes it possible for people with different comprehensive worldviews to function politically and socially within a pluralistic society.

VIII. Deciding On A Standard Of Disclosure

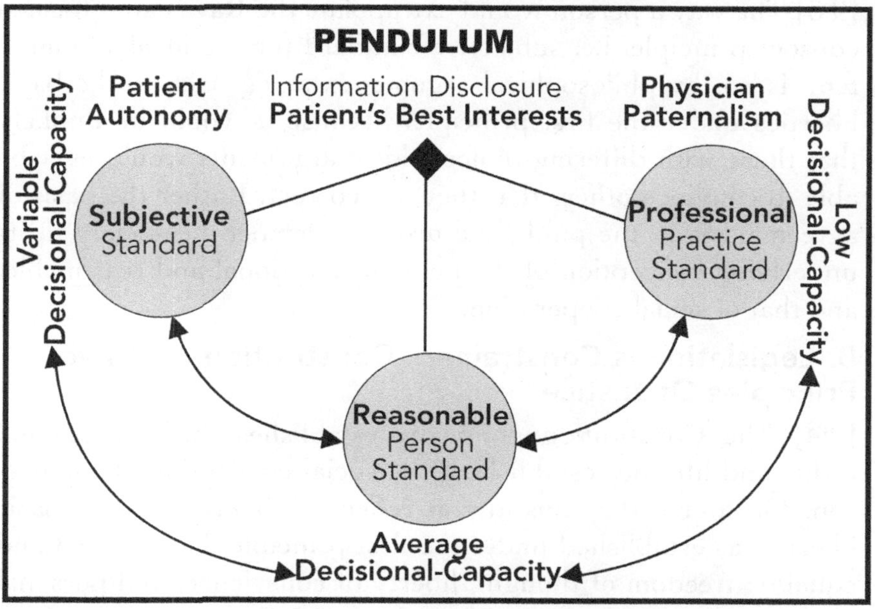

A. Rawls' Ideal Political Framework

[9:1] Using Rawls' just political framework to derive a public policy of information disclosure for an appropriate informed consent will result in the subjective standard.

1. Persons in Original Position: ideally competent

[9:2] In coming to this conclusion that the Rawlsian standard of information disclosure would be the subjective standard, it must be kept in mind that Rawls is dealing with a well-ordered society in which citizens would be ideally competent. In the real world there are people who are less than competent and thus the subjective standard might not be appropriate for them. As will be argued later, as the pendulum of competency swings towards ideal competency the subjective standard becomes more and more appropriate. As the pendulum of competency swings towards non-ideal competency you will likewise swing through the reasonable person standard toward the professional practice standard.

2. Persons in Original Position: two moral powers

[9:3] The way a person would extrapolate the Rawlsian informed consent principle, i.e. subjective standard for the ideally competent, is not by philosophical argument tracing back to the basic liberties under the first principle, because it would be unlikely that those with differing philosophical arguments would ever be able to convince others that they are correct. Rather the basis of agreement is in the public culture of a democratic society in its underlying conception of the person, as rational and reasonable, and that of social cooperation.[167]

B. Legislation Is Constrained: Constitution And Two Principles Of Justice

[9:4] The Constitution politically establishes the fundamental rights and liberties establishing the social conception of the person. Of course the constitution reflects and protects our basic liberties as established under the first principle, i.e. freedom and equality, freedom of thought, liberty of conscience, and personal liberty to mention a few. Thus the legislation of a type of informed consent that would be regarded as just would, of course, have to be constrained by constitutional law[168] and the two principles of justice.

1. Constitutional: rights and liberties

[9:5] In a well-ordered society of competent individuals the professional practice standard and the reasonable person standard fail to conform to the constitution because of the violations that would occur against some of the basic liberties the constitution would uphold. The professional practice standard, as held histor-

---

[167] The notions of the basic structure, of the veil of ignorance, of a lexical order, … as well as of pure procedural justice … [can not be expected] to work by themselves, but properly put together they may serve well enough. It is too much to suppose that there exists for all or even most moral problems a reasonable solution. Rawls, *Political Liberalism*, p. 89.

[168] Edmund Pellegrino says that constitutional liberties do apply to doctor patient relationships. "In a democratic society, people expect the widest protection of their rights of self-determination. Hence, the contemporary patient has a right to know the decisions involved in managing his case." Edmund D. Pellegrino, "The Hippocratic Ethic Revisited," in *Humanism And The Physician* (Knoxville: University of Tennessee Press, 1979), p. 98.

ically, violates at least freedom and equality, freedom of thought, liberty of conscience and personal liberty. This is a result of the conviction that the proper and moral role of the professional is to act in the agent's best interest as determined by the professional community rather than as determined by the agent.

2. Persons: free & equal

[9:6] However, in a Rawlsian system, persons are free and equal with basic rights and liberties—this includes, of course, professionals and agents. Competent agents and professionals are empowered to be free and equal with their constitutionally protected rights. Agents have the choice and the responsibility to take part in their determination of their good. Persons are in control of their lives to the extent that the constitution as a rational and reasonable social and democratic position empowers them with basic rights and liberties. Therefore, choices would fall under the umbrella of being free and equal along with freedom of thought and conscience.

3. Incommensurable beliefs: reasonable pluralism

[9:7] The reasonable person standard not only violates the constitutional rights and liberties such as freedom and equality, freedom of thought, liberty of conscience and personal liberty but it also does not take into consideration pluralistic standards of reasonable. It works on the presupposition that it is possible to come up with a reasonable protocol or standard that would be applied to all or most agents because that protocol or standard is believed to be universally reasonable. In a Rawlsian well-ordered society in which all are fully competent, the objection is not so much that the agents would not agree with the decisions, rather, it is the idea of taking away the decision making process from the autonomous agent who, incidentally, may have quite different beliefs than that of the standard agent, especially in a pluralistic society. Arguably, unreasonable choices are not autonomous or competent—as they would not promote the Rawlsian *reasonable* and *rational* person, however, the issue here is not that of unreasonable choices, rather, it is the fact that what is unreasonable for one group of individuals might be quite reasonable for another group who as autonomous persons share different beliefs. An example of this is the person who refuses to have a porcine heart valve put in because of the belief that pork is unclean, whereas another person accepts the porcine heart valve because they believe animals are here for their benefit and a third person who thinks that any use of a sentient animal for purposes that are not in the animal's best interests is immoral and wrong.

C. Subjective Standard

1. Respects: reasonable and rational agents

[9:8] The subjective standard of information disclosure appears to be the only reasonable and rational position under the constraints of a constitution, that upholds the basic liberties as derived under the first principle of justice, and also respects incommensurable worldviews.

2. Agent: may relinquish rights and liberties

[9:9] Now it may be the case that people may in fact relieve or relinquish their rights because of some associational beliefs or worldview. That is fine as long as people know that they do in fact have those political social rights. People must know that they have the constitutional right to relinquish not only their constitutional rights but also even more importantly to relinquish their associational constraints and to claim their constitutional rights and liberties as free and equal citizens.

3. Subjective standard: coherent

[9:10] Although it may be argued that none of the three standards of information disclosures is perfect, it seems clear that the subjective standard would be more coherent with free and equal competent citizens' constitutional rights and liberties. Certainly, since the subjective standard is inherently individual and private, people should have the freedom to receive less information but it would seem that from the options presented the subjective standard should be the social common standard for competent individuals, unless otherwise specified, as only this standard affirms competent persons as rational and reasonable.

[9:11] The conceptual, moral, and practical difficulties that were presented earlier in response to the subjective standard disappear in a Rawlsian well-ordered society in which all citizens are also ideally competent.

4. Joint responsibilities: professionals & agents

[9:12] The main objection to the subjective standard was that it unrealistically demanded too much from the professional. But in this Rawlsian society both the professional and the agent will not only have the proper conception of what it is to be a rational and reasonable person, both with respect towards themselves and towards others, but they will also have the capacity to be rational and reasonable. Thus, even though there is a demand on the professional to disclose relevant information there is also a joint responsibility on the part of the agent to participate in the determination of what informational needs are important.

5. Agents: ideally rational and reasonable

[9:13] The second and third objections dealt with not being able to make the right decisions and how decisions are in large part made prior to information disclosure. But once again these objections fall mute in a Rawlsian political framework as this well-ordered society is comprised of individuals who are rational and reasonable and who do in fact act and make decisions accordingly.

6. Nonideal circumstances: nonideal standard

[9:14] If this is indeed true, that the subjective standard would apply only towards those who are ideally rational, reasonable and thus ideally competent, then in the imperfect nonideal world some other disclosure may, and most probably is, more appropriate. However, even if this is the case, at least a standard of disclosure has been determined for those who fit the criteria for a Rawlsian rational and reasonable competent citizen.

***

VIa. CASE ANALYSIS PARADIGM

I. Principlism: Basic Paradigm

A. Principlism: Internationally Recognized

[1:1]

Writing a case study is not a difficult task if you have a basic paradigm. Principlism with its four basic principles of autonomy (informed consent), nonmaleficence (do no harm), beneficence (do good), and justice (be fair), provides such a paradigm and also benefits in being recognized nationally by U.S. Federal Law 45CFR46, and internationally by universally recognized human rights and liberties and by a wide variety of codes of ethics.

B. Principlism: Unified System

[1:2] Principlism is a unified approach in that each moral principle seems to converge into each of the other three principles. For example, it can be argued that Principlism, as a comprehensive moral approach, is just another term for justice. To the extent that justice is socially valued because of how it effectively establishes autonomy, nonmaleficence, and beneficence, both personally and socially, it can be argued that Principlism only needs its fourth principle—justice, in order to fulfill its moral function. However, this argument can also be made with regard to each of the four principles as each principle seems to be able to include each of the other three principles. Personal autonomy results in the maximization of personal benefits—beneficence and the minimization of personal burdens—nonmaleficence within a legitimate social structure—justice. Likewise, nonmaleficence is maximized, by maximizing autonomy, beneficence, and justice and beneficence is maximized, by maximizing autonomy, nonmaleficence, and justice.

[1:3] The fact that each of the four principles can be argued to be the supreme moral principle further validates the Principlistic approach towards moral decision-making. In other words, Principlism is a unified moral approach in which the addition of each principle strengthens the legitimacy of each of the other principles to the extent that each principle is specified and balanced using independent criteria and yet each principle still supports each of the other principles.[1]

C. Science: Unified System

1:4] Science illustrates the importance and necessity of such unification. For example, if several academically distinct fields converge on a unified position that would generally give more credence towards that position. On the other hand, if one academic discipline has a hypothesis that contradicts several or all of the other academic disciplines, then that would be reason either to reject that hypothesis or at least to give it some pause. One example of such unification would be the comparison of evolution vs. creationism. Evolution converges in several academic fields such as Biology, Microbiology, Astronomy, Cosmology, Geology, Paleontology, Oceanography, Pathology, Medicine, Anthropology, and more. Creationism, on the other hand, is based on the non-academic discipline of religious faith and is not supported by any of the empirical academic disciplines. As a result, creationism does not have the same academic stature as evolution and is therefore not considered as a plausible option by any of the empirical or rational academic disciplines.[2] Therefore, other than creationism being a curious sociological, anthropological, or psychological phenomena of culture, religion, and/or belief, creation-

[1] Chapter 1, page 6, [i:28] The fourth distinction, synthetic *a priori,* Kant held to be not only logically consistent but also one of the most important experiential and rational relationships. Synthetic meaning the predicate is not directly contained in the subject, and *a priori* because the synthetic statement can be verified independently of empirical sense experience.
[i:29] Immanuel Kant thought that mathematics and morality were synthetic *a priori* statements. For example, 5+7=12 is interesting in that 12, the predicate, is not directly contained in the subject of 5+7, and is therefore a synthetic statement. The relationship between "5", "7", and "+", i.e. axioms, cannot be determined by empirical sense experience, rather the relationship is determined *a priori* meaning independent of empirical sense experience.

[2] pp14-18, [1:13-25]

ism has no place in academic empirical rational discourse. Of course academic sciences are by definition limited to empirical and rational discourses and some knowledge is clearly not of that category[3]. For example, intersubjective experiences of sense data such as: sight, taste, smell, touch, hearing, and emotional states such as: love, and faith, are real and true experiences yet they elude rational and/or empirical quantification. However, since creationism claims to be an academic empirical conclusion, then it is legitimate to hold creationism to academic standards of universal academic consistency.

[1:5] Principlism validates itself with its universally recognized moral principles of autonomy (informed consent), nonmaleficence (do no harm), beneficence (do good), and justice (be fair). These principles are distinct moral attributes that converge and unifies moral decision-making even within pluralistic environments.

D. Moral Decision-Making Goal: Specify & Balance Principles

[1:6] The goal in moral decision-making is ultimately to specify and balance each of the four principles recognizing that there is no set hierarchical order of the principles in that one or more moral principle(s) may override one or more other moral principle(s) depending on the circumstances.

1. Specifying

[1:7] Specifying: the narrowing down or making the broad moral principles relevant for a particular situation.

2. Balancing

[1:8] Balancing: the attempt to maximize, as much as possible, all of the contributing or competing moral principles. However, situations do occur when one or more principles may be more relevant for a particular situation than one or more other principles.

---

[3] page 15, [1:15] Since academics uses empirical and rational evidence for establishing the nature of reality, and since this is an academic text, it follows that the study of the nature and origins of the principles of morality will also have to be presented using the empirical and rational scientific method, not those that are based on faith or some other nonscientific method.

3. Ten considerations when specifying and balancing

[1:9] Some considerations to take into account when specifying and balancing in no particular order:

1. **Rational:** Agent should have rational reasons for evaluating that one or more principles are more relevant than one or more other principle(s).
2. **Coherent:** Agent should choose an option that will maximize coherency between the principles.
3. **Universalizable:** Agent should make a decision in which it would be rational to universalize such a decision to others if they were to be in the same circumstances.
4. **Respect:** Agent should respect the beliefs of other individuals and the community at large.
5. **Minimization:** Agent should consider alternative actions that will minimize any "infringement" of one or more other principle(s) and or negative effects.
6. **Maximization:** Agent should consider alternative actions that will better maximize one or more relevant principles.
7. **Practical:** Agent should have pragmatic and/or empirical reasons for determining that one or more principles will be more practical than one or more other principle(s).
8. **Probable:** The agent should make a decision that has a reasonable chance of attaining the desired end.
9. **Simplicity:** Agent should choose a simple option over a more complex option if there is no relevant differences between the options.
10. **Influence:** Agent should not be influenced by morally irrelevant information about any party.

II. Case Study Paradigm

The following is an outline approach that can be used towards applying Principlism to a particular case.

[2:1]

A. Determine The Relevant Parties

1. Specifying The Relevant Parties

a. Positive rights

Obligation of others to provide something

1) Subject, guardian, or social institutions
2) Relatives
3) Community
4) State government
5) Federal government
6) International government
7) Other

b. Negative rights

Obligation of others to not interfere

1) Subject, guardian, or social institutions
2) Relatives
3) Community
4) State government
5) Federal government
6) International government
7) Other

2. Balancing the Relevant Parties:

If appropriate put the relevant parties in hierarchical order, and/or indicate if one or more parties has more compelling interests over one or more of the others.

[2:1]

B. Autonomy

1. Specifying Autonomy

Relate to negative and positive rights if relevant

a. Personal authorization

1) Intention
Usually communicated by Express, Implied, or Tacit Consent

a) **Negative Right**
Obligation of others to not interfere in the making of a choice.

b) **Positive Right**
Obligation of others to provide realistic options of choice.

1) **Substantial knowledge**
Usually provided using the Professional Practice Standard, Reasonable Person Standard, or Subjective Standard

a) **Negative Right**
Obligation of others not to interfere in the acquisition of knowledge

b) **Positive Right**
Obligation of others to provide information

3) **Substantial freedom**
Usually effected by such aspects as Persuasion, Coercion, and Manipulation

a) **Negative Right**
Obligation of others not to limit an agents freedom

b) **Positive Right**
Obligation of others to promote an agent's freedom

b. Institutional authorization

1) Intention
Usually implemented by a signed document

2) **Substantial knowledge**
Usually provided by a written document based on the Professional Practice Standard and/or the Reasonable Person Standard

3) **Substantial freedom**
If the document is not signed then the services are usually not provided

2. Balancing Autonomy

Balance the above by putting the obligations in hierarchical order, and/or by indicating if one has a more compelling interest over the other.

[2:2]

C. Nonmaleficence

1. Specifying Nonmaleficence

a. Burdens
What are the burdens of the various options for the subject and/or relevant parties?

b. Rights
What personal and social rights need to be considered?

1) **Positive Rights**
Obligations of others for providing potential or actual benefits

2) **Negative Rights**
Obligation(s) of others to not interfere in potential or actual benefits

2. Balancing Nonmaleficence

Balance the above by putting the obligations in hierarchical order, and/or by indicating if one has a more compelling interest over the other.

[2:3]

D. Beneficence

1. Specifying Beneficence

a. Benefits
What are the benefits of the various options for the subject and/or relevant parties?

b. Rights
What personal and social rights need to be considered?

1) Positive rights
Obligations of others for providing potential or actual benefits

2) Negative rights
Obligations of others to not interfere in potential or actual benefits

2. Balancing Beneficence

Balance the above by putting the obligations in hierarchical order, and/or by indicating if one has a more compelling interest over the other.

[2:4]

E. Justice

1. Specifying Justice:

a. Legal and/or social issues
What are the legal or social issues with regard to the subject and/or relevant parties?

b. Rights
How do the above issues relate to positive rights (obligations of others to provide) and negative rights (obligations of others to not interfere)?

1) Personal rights and liberties
Personal rights and liberties as provided by the state, federal, or international social structures

2) Social rights and liberties
Social rights and liberties as provided by the state, federal, or international social structures

3) Political rights and liberties
Political rights and liberties as provided by the state, federal, or international social structures

2. Balancing Justice

Balance the above by putting them in hierarchical order, and/or by indicating if one has a more compelling interest over the other.

[2:5]

F. Balance The Four Principles

1. Relevance
How many of the four principles are relevant for this case?

2. Importance
In this particular case, which principles are most influential and why?

3. Maximize or Override
Is it possible to maximize most or all of the four principles or do one or more of them have a stronger ground of obligation than one or more of the others and why?

[2:6]

Conclusion

Summarize the specification and balancing within each of the four principles and then summarize the reasoning behind the balancing of the four principles and present the reasons why the chosen moral decision would have a higher probability of accomplishing the desired end rather than some other decision.

***

VIb. Dr.Ethics™ Informed Consent

Introduction

[1:1]

This section will be evaluating the informed consent protocol of **DR. ETHICS™** an expert system developed for determining whether a valid informed consent has been given or not. However, the informed consent protocol in DR. ETHICS™ is a computer expert-system that is not easily put on paper in any type of coherent fashion. Ultimately the decision tree that would result in a judgment that would be deemed Ethical to Treat will be followed through in detail. However, responses that clearly would go outside of those constraints will also be evaluated.

[1:2] In the beginning of each major section a flow chart will be presented that will represent, as accurately as possible, the decision tree process used in DR. ETHICS™. The flow charts consist of boxes abbreviated for the full questions that will be shown in the text or on your computer. The arrows tell where DR. ETHICS™ is or could go depending on how the questions are answered.

[1:3] Certainly, nobody should be so naive as to think that DR. ETHICS™ should, or even could be used to determine real life situations on an individual case-by-case basis. DR. ETHICS™ is designed as a teaching tool to help explicate a rational and reasonable thinking process and criteria that are usually essential in making these types of considerations. However, it must be kept in mind that even though DR. ETHICS™ is compatible with Rawlsian political justice, DR. ETHICS™ still is only one of many ways in which these issues could be organized and/or addressed. Practically, if DR. ETHICS™ helps to formulate, clarify or reinforce a protocol already formulated for doing this type of work then DR. ETHICS™ will have achieved its aim. DR. ETHICS™ is and never was designed to take the person out of moral decision-making. Each individual agent needs to be considered on a case-by-case basis. Justice cannot be found neatly in a rule-book, legislation, or in an algorithm, rather, it is often times, if not most of the time, a practice of exceptions, i.e. a practice of judicial review.[1]

[1:4] Rawls would agree with this position especially since our society is becoming more and more pluralistic with fundamentally different and often times incommensurable worldviews. It is also a fact that society is not composed of anything like the Rawlsian notion of an ideal well-ordered society, rather society is not ideal or well-ordered and there exists various levels or degrees of competency and/or decisional-capacity.

[1] "Judicial review" is being used here in a broad and general sense meaning not only a mechanism like a court but also as something one could do in the process of decision making.

I. Dr. Ethics™: Ethical Perspective

[1:5] Dr. Ethics™ is a computer program that can analyze the ethical implications of case studies, particularly in clinical medicine. The Informed Consent Protocol is capable of interactively working through a variety of case studies, will help to expose the ethical dimensions related to the case, will ask for responses and/or decisions and then it will present its recommended resolution. This resolution can then be accepted or challenged and used as an advanced starting point and catalyst in ethical dialogue.

[1:6] Following the theme of the previous chapters, Dr. Ethics™ consists of a systematic approach not in a particular type of applied ethics or associational view, but rather an approach that is structured on principles of justice that a pluralistic society could agree on in order to establish and/or affirm the social conception of a rational and reasonable person. In trying to accomplish this task it is not necessary to take an eclectic approach in which one tries to combine all types of ethical approaches, as you would only end up with intractable reasonable and rational conflicts and contradictions. Dr. Ethics™ is an approach that is compatible with the Rawlsian social contract, i.e. upholding the primary basic liberties that a pluralistic society would hold of value. Dr. Ethics™ is not meant to be an approach establishing what an individual's values and goals should be, rather, it is an approach establishing what a pluralistic society as a whole should strive towards so that all individuals within that society can establish and or live according to their own personal worldview. In other words, it is an approach that tries to support those values and or rights that would provide free and equal individuals within a democratic pluralistic society the opportunity or environment to develop as rational and reasonable persons. As quoted in an earlier chapter on Rawls:

> [1:7] A conception of justice fulfills its social role provided that persons equally conscientious and sharing roughly the same beliefs find that, by affirming the framework of deliberation set up by it, they are normally led to a sufficient convergence of judgment necessary to achieve effective and fair social cooperation. My discussion of the basic lib-

> erties and their priority should be seen in this light. … Thus justice as fairness is addressed not so much to constitutional jurists as to citizens in a constitutional regime. It presents a way for them to conceive of their common and guaranteed status as equal citizens and attempts to connect a particular understanding of freedom and equality with a particular conception of the person thought to be congenial to the shared notions and essential convictions implicit in the public culture of a democratic society. Perhaps in this way the impasse concerning the understanding of freedom and equality can at least be intellectually clarified if not resolved. It is particularly important to keep in mind that the conception of the person is part of a conception of political and social justice. That is, it characterizes how citizens are to think of themselves and of one another in their political and social relationships, and, therefore, as having the basic liberties appropriate to free and equal persons capable of being fully cooperating members of society over a complete life. The role of a conception of the person in a conception of political justice is distinct from its role in a personal or associational ideal, or in a religious or moral way of life. The basis of toleration and of social cooperation on a footing of mutual respect in a democratic regime is put in jeopardy when these distinctions are not recognized; for when this happens and such ideals and ways of life take a political form, the fair terms of cooperation are narrowly drawn, and free and willing cooperation between persons with different conceptions of the good may become impossible.[2]

[1:8] It is with this in mind that DR. ETHICS™ approaches the issue of informed consent.

[1:9] DR. ETHICS™ and its informed consent protocol is meant to be a teaching tool and an example of what issues need to be addressed in dealing with informed consent. It is not an algorithmic program that is capable of replacing the judicial judgment of healthcare providers and patients. DR. ETHICS™ is only a starting point or a beginning, if you wish, at establishing a minimum standard which a democratic pluralistic society could all agree upon even though some would be satisfied with less strin-

---

2 Rawls, *Political Liberalism*, pp. 368-69.

gent requirements and others would prefer more stringent requirements.

[1:10] Where there is great dissent, e.g. abortion, euthanasia etc., public legislation should be minimized. Public debate and judicial review will be the means to change the broad social/personal beliefs and conceptions until general agreement can be reached and legislation passed. On issues of great disagreement legislation ought to be limited based on the idea that this lack of legislation would stimulate public debate benefiting the growth and development of the reasonable and rational political person, i.e. the ability to deal fairly with others in society with mutual respect for all and the capacity to freely form, revise, and pursue one's good, whatever that might be.

[1:11] In order to help orient users with DR. ETHICS™ and how it works through this informed consent protocol a visual guide of its decision-making processes will be provided through the use of flow charts.

II. Flow Chart One

[2:1] The following is the first of the four flow charts to be considered. Depending on how the user answers the questions presented will determine what direction the program will flow.

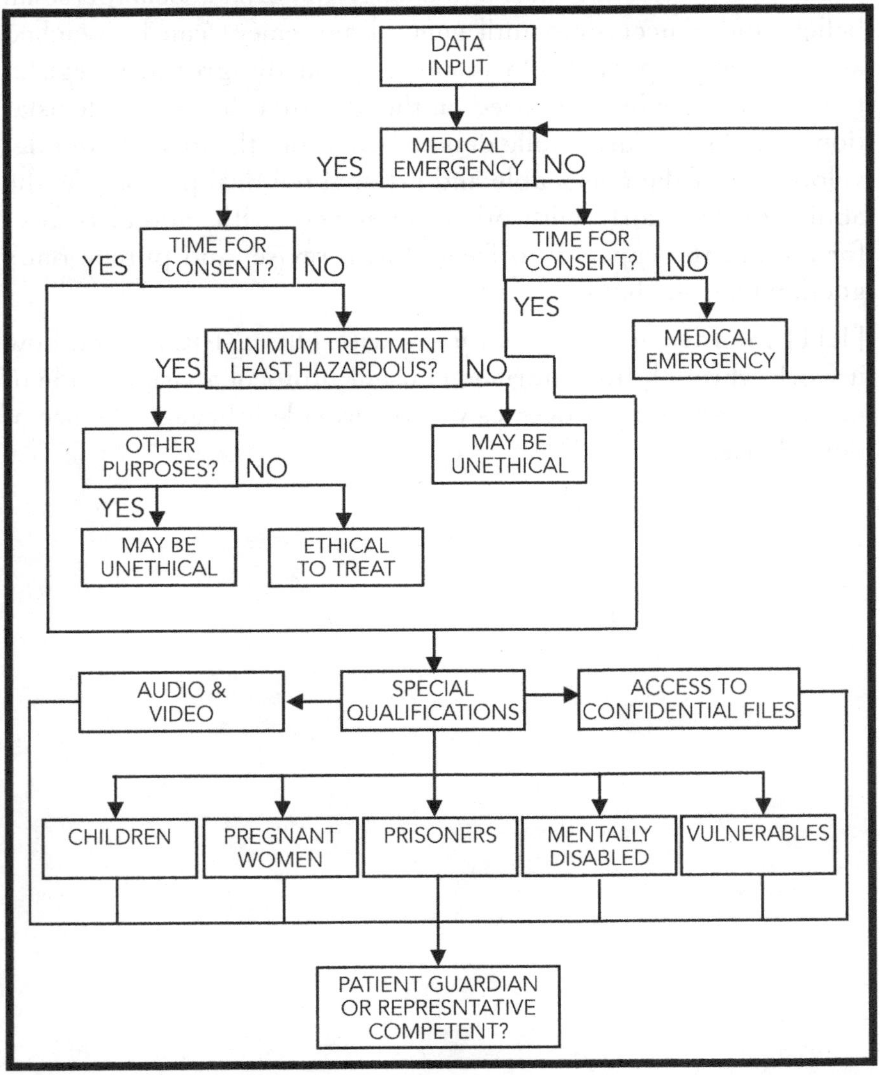

A. Preliminary Data

[2:2]

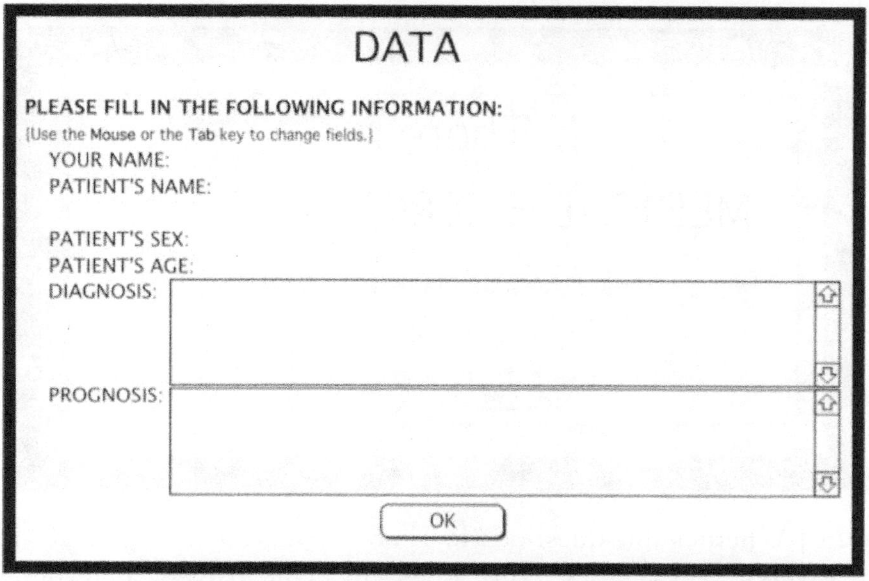

[2:3] The first couple of questions DR. ETHICS™ asks are for the purpose of acquiring preliminary data. These questions identify the background information about the patient and their prognosis and diagnosis. Although DR. ETHICS™ does not request a patient history, that information might later be important especially when trying to determine the prevalence rate with regard to the disease or state in question. More will be said on this later.

[2:4] Other questions that might be of importance in decision-making, are questions with regard to the patient's and healthcare provider's associational or personal worldviews—including religious views. These questions are not asked because DR. ETHICS™ is concerned with the pluralistic social-political values and not the more specific associational values. However, these associational or personal values and beliefs will be brought into the decision making process by the patient. DR. ETHICS™ wants to establish extensive liberties for a pluralistic democratic society.

B. Medical Emergency

[2:5]

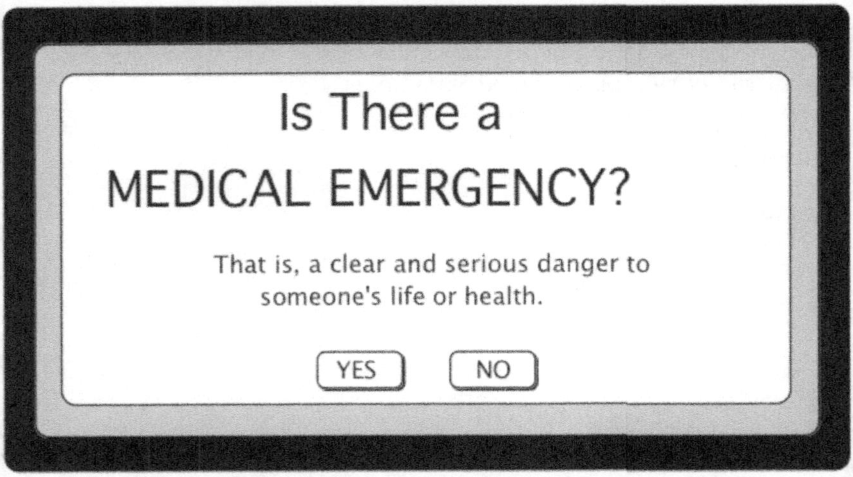

[2:6] Whether this question "Is There a Medical Emergency?" is answered "YES" or "NO" does not conclusively determine whether or not there is time to obtain the patient's, guardian's or representative's consent. Thus no matter how the user answers this question the user will next be asked, "Is there time to obtain the patient's, guardian's or representative's consent to treatment?" However, if a person were to select "NO," that this is not a medical emergency, and then answer the following question with regard to there not being time to obtain the patient's, guardian's or representative's consent to treatment the program would recognize the logical inconsistency and would promptly kick the user back to the previous question of whether or not it is a medical emergency.

[2:7] The rationale behind this is that if there is insufficient time to obtain consent before serious danger to the patient's life or health then perhaps the situation that the user thought was not a medical emergency is in DR. ETHICS™ terms a medical emergency. In this context it is not possible to have a non-emergency situation in which there is no time to get any type of consent, e.g. informed, proxy etc. In other words, if there is no time for any type of consent and there is a clear and serious danger to the patient, then by definition that is a medical emergency. This is not a justification for ignoring consent, rather it is a recognition of a situation in which getting consent is just not possible because of time constraints. Consent must be by-passed in those situations in order to prevent serious harm to the patient.

C. Time For Consent

[2:8]

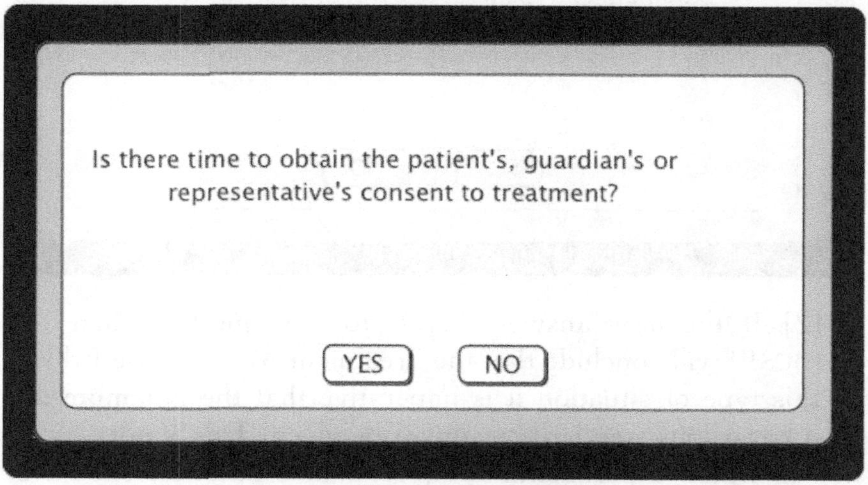

[2:9] Whether or not the case is a "medical emergency" if you answer "YES" to this question then DR. ETHICS™ will go to a section called Special Qualifications for Treatment/Research. The Special Qualifications section gives some additional precautions and guidelines that are necessary in obtaining consent from special individuals.

[2:10] If the situation is such that it is a medical emergency in which there is no time for consent, i.e. the user answers "NO" to this question, then DR. ETHICS™ will ask some additional questions. Two questions that follow from the fact that it is not possible to obtain consent in a medical emergency are the following:

D. Least Hazardous Treatment

[2:11]

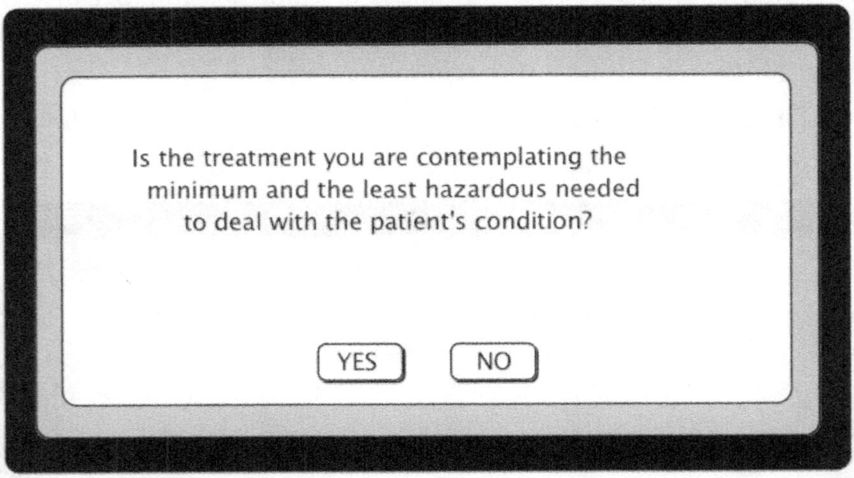

[2:12] If the user answers "NO" to this question then DR. ETHICS™ will conclude that the Treatment May Not Be Ethical. In this type of situation it is imperative that the minimum and least hazardous standard treatment be given. This is not a situation in which experimental or questionable practices should be used. The reasoning behind this is that since the patient is not at this time a competent reasonable and rational person with decisional-capacity, and since decisions concerning the patient's welfare must be made for them, then it follows that it would be best to err on the side of caution and towards those procedures that have been proven to be the minimum and the least hazardous. Thus in this particular situation, in which a consent is not possible, the minimum and least hazardous treatment, should be applied.

[2:13] This criterion does not violate the essential nature of the primary basic good of personal liberty that is necessary for someone to develop as rational and reasonable political persons as defined earlier. The situation is now nonideal in which the patient is not able to function rationally and reasonably.

[2:14] On the one hand, as competency for consent decreases the pendulum of informed consent swings towards the professional practice standard of consent. On the other hand, as competency for consent increases the pendulum of informed consent swings towards the subjective standard. The more a treatment deviates from the standard practice the more stringent the consent requirements become.

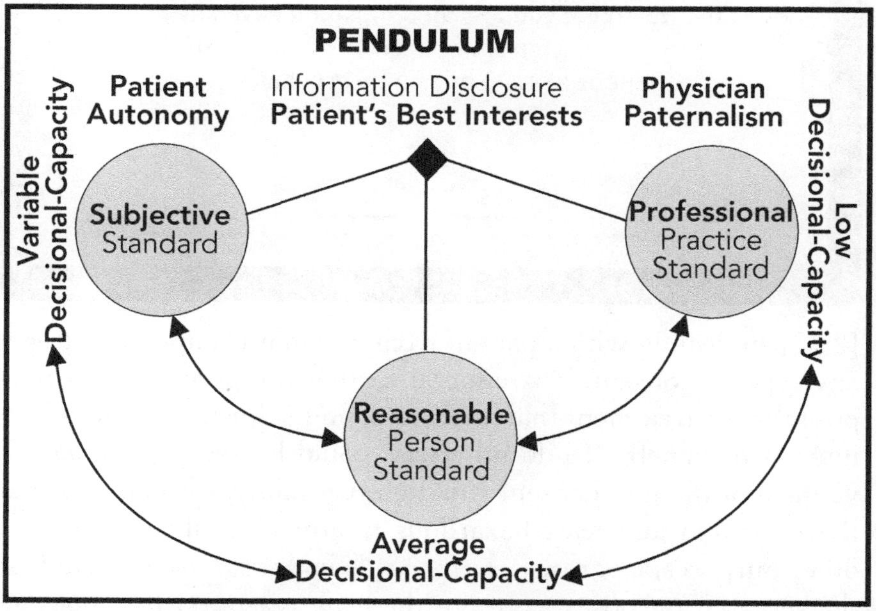

[2:15] Answering "YES" to the question of the treatment being the minimum and least hazardous necessary for treating this patient will generate the following question.

E. Other Purposes Than Patient Best Interest

[2:16]

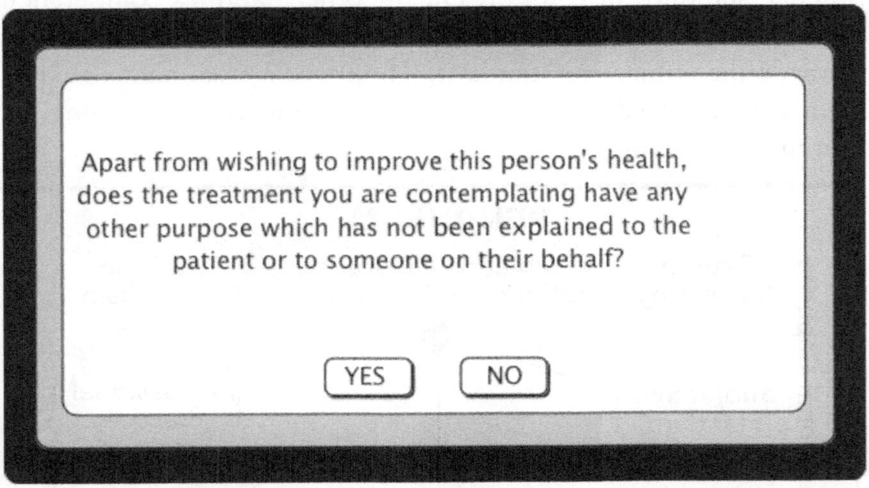

[2:17] In dealing with a patient from whom it is impossible to get any type of consent, it is imperative that the only or main purpose for the treatment that is being giving is for the patient's best interest or benefit. To do otherwise could be seen as taking advantage of the non-consent situation. Certainly if it happens that the minimum and least hazardous treatment could be used for other purposes, e.g. research, then it is important to indicate that the research purposes were not the *main* reason(s) for choosing the particular treatment. Again, because of this non-consent situation there is an emphasis towards the professional practice standard of treatment when the treatment is the minimum and least hazardous for a non-consenting patient.

F. Special Qualifications 45CFR46

[2:18] Going back to the case in which there is time to obtain the patient's, guardian's or representative's consent to treatment, the following Special Qualifications and Precautions section comes up. These Special Qualifications come directly from the Code of Federal Regulations Title 45: Public Welfare, Part 46: Protections of Human Subjects—45CFR46. Every Institutional Review Board—IRB is mandated to consider these Special Qualifications for Research on Human Subjects. (look at "flow chart one" to see what has been covered and to see what will be covered next.)

[2:19]

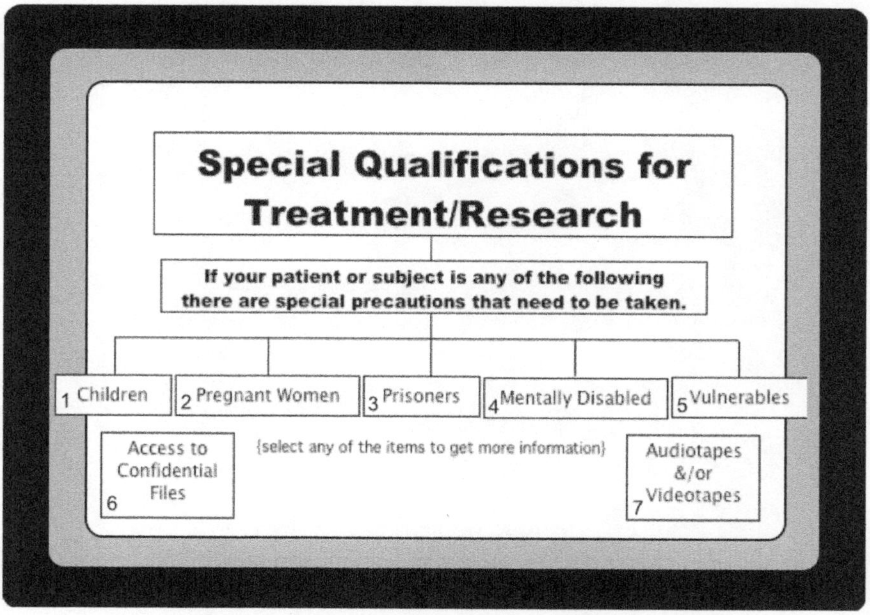

[2:20] As important as the details of this material is it will presently be by-pass at this point in order to provide the big picture and continuity as to how DR. ETHICS™ works. The goal is to devise a standard of practice that would be considered just in an ideal pluralistic democratic society of free and equal persons. The current approach is to concentrate not on the exceptions or special cases but on standard or normal circumstances first. Then once progress has been made then perhaps those normal procedures can be applied or modified in order to accommodate the special nonideal cases.[3] Therefore the focus is to delineate a basic standard of consent practice.

[3] A sketch of the basic issues are:

1) There are groups that present special problems for consent.
2) Their special status has been recognized by commissions drawing up research guidelines.
3) Similar issues arise for consent for treatment.

III. Flow Chart Two

[3:1] The second major "flow chart" to be considered is as follows:

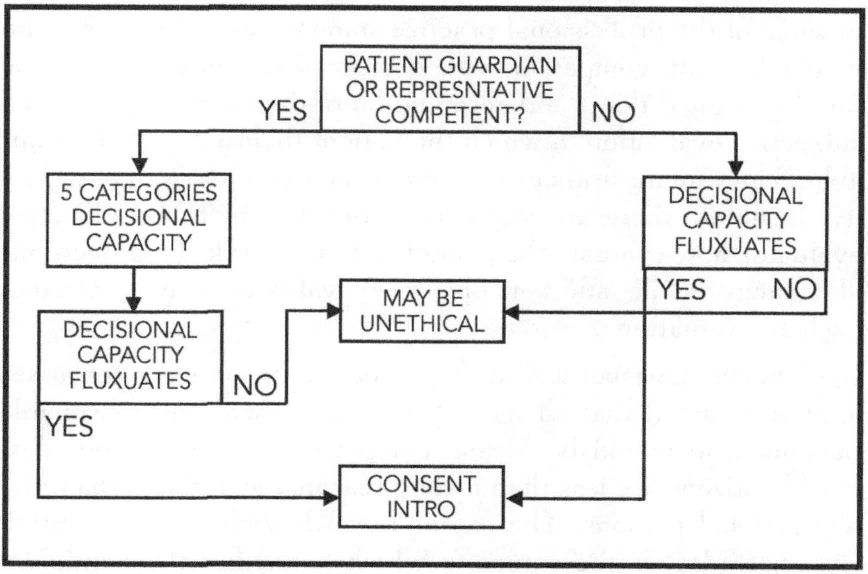

A. Competence

[3:2]

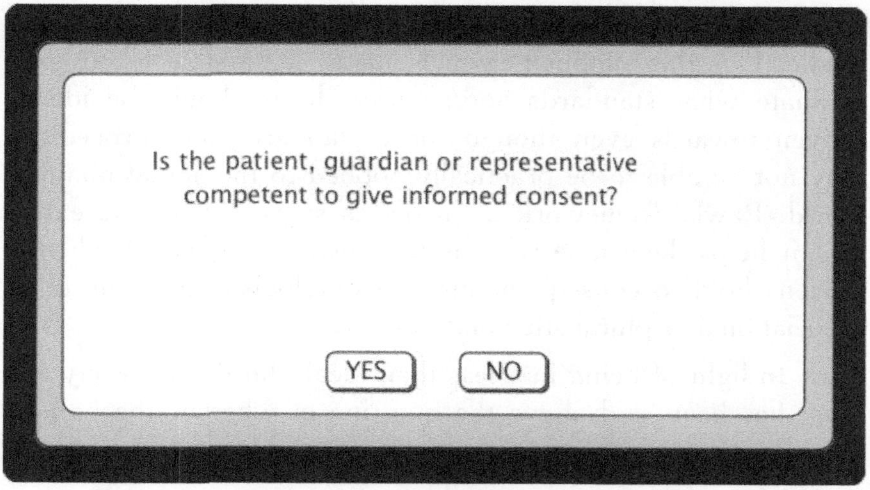

[3:3] Before explaining what happens when the user answers this question, "Is the patient, guardian or representative competent to give an informed consent," "YES" or "NO" it is necessary to address the implications of allowing the practitioner to make this judgment. The question here is whether or not this smuggles in some of the professional practice standard even for those who would be fully competent with decisional-capacity. It could be forcibly argued that the determination of decisional-capacity is a subjective evaluation in which the patient themselves is often unable to give an accurate evaluation of their own decisional-capacity. Certainly there are many situations in which one objective evaluator may evaluate the patient as having or lacking decisional-capacity while another objective evaluator may contradict such an evaluation.

[3:4] For a Rawlsian well-ordered society this issue never arises as it is assumed that all its citizens are rational and reasonable persons who would be ideally competent. But in the nonideal world, citizens are less than ideally reasonable and less than ideally rational persons. The extent towards which our society is less than ideal is the extent to which it justifies the pendulum swing towards the professional practice standard. Even though this is a less than ideal approach it is nonetheless a necessary practical approach.

[3:5] Rawls' well-ordered society is intentionally artificially simplistic. It is this simplicity which makes it possible to ethically evaluate what standards and/or procedures should be ideally striven towards even though those standards and procedures may not be able to be practically applied to the actual nonideal world. Rawls' framework of justice is successful to the extent that it helps determine what is the ideal regardless of whether citizens hold to consequentialism, deontologism, or some other associational or pluralistic point of view.

[3:6] In light of being in a less than ideal pluralistic society and what has been said above the question of whether the patient, guardian or representative is competent to give informed consent can now be discussed. If the response is "YES" to this question then DR. ETHICS™ will go to:

a. the question of defining the type of competency, then to

b. the section explaining how competency may fluctuate.

[3:7] If the response is "NO," then it will go to the section explaining how competency may fluctuate and the user is given the opportunity to change their mind. If the user thinks that the patient, guardian or representative is still lacking decisional-capacity and there is time to get consent, then it Might be Unethical to Treat the Patient. If user changes their mind and therefore thinks the patient, guardian, or representative has decisional-capacity then DR. ETHICS™ will move on to select one of the five types of competencies.

B. Competency Categories

[3:8]

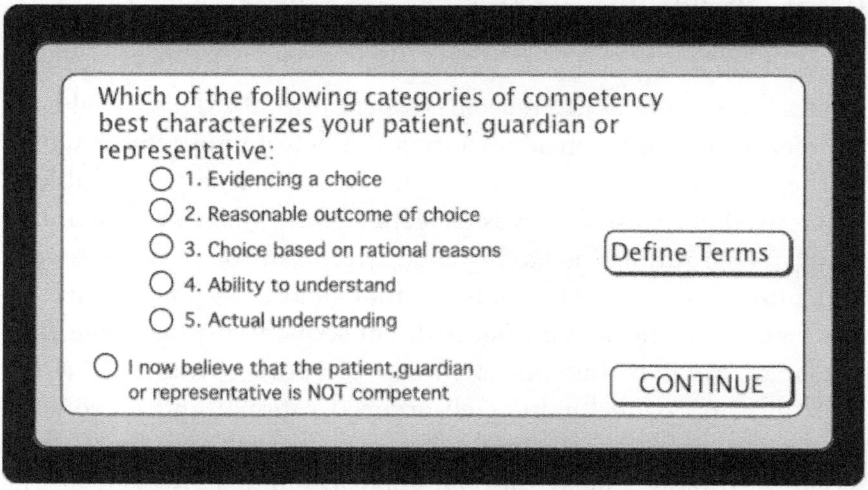

Five types of competency:

1. Evidencing a choice

[3:9] Evidencing a choice does not focus on the quality of the patient's decision but instead only on the presence or absence of a decision.

[3:10] Such a low level of function is usually not enough to establish decisional-capacity. Just because an individual shows evidence of choice it is not good enough to be defined as competent. An infant or an impaired adult may choose to play with something dangerous like a razor blade. Certainly it would be inappropriate to consider them competent and to let them do as they wish just because they show evidence of choice. However if the evidencing a choice is compatible with the best interests of the patient or in line with the professional practice then there will be a tendency to accept it as being sufficient evidence of decisional- capacity.

2. Reasonable outcome of choice

[3:11] Reasonable outcome of choice emphasizes the outcome of the decision—consequentialism—rather than on the mere fact of a decision or how it was reached.

[3:12] The way the term reasonable is being used here is somewhat different from the way Rawls uses the term reasonable. For Rawls being reasonable is having the ability to deal fairly with others in society with mutual respect for all. This would, of course, be a strong consideration in the determining the outcome of the decision being made. But the way the term reasonable is being used here also involves aspects of Rawls' term rational. For Rawls being rational is having the capacity to freely form, revise, and pursue one's good, whatever that might be. The pursuit of one's good has here been defined, consequentially, as some particular or range of outcomes. Rawls, of course, would not agree with this approach for his well-ordered rational and reasonable citizens as competency would be presupposed and the patient would also have a clear rational good in mind. However, in this situation it is not a well-ordered society of competent individuals. Thus the practical approach of emphasizing the outcome of the decision is used quite often by physicians and courts premised on the following syllogism: the patient needs treatment; the patient has not obtained treatment on his or her own initiative; The patient would in fact make a decision that would be in line with their best interests, therefore, the patient's decision is incorrect, which means that the patient does not have decisional-capacity with regard to this decision, thus justifying the involuntary imposition of treatment. Implicit in this reasoning is the belief that as the decisional-capacity for a particular decision diminishes so increases the power or need of others, who are competent, to make the decision for the patient.

3. Choice based on rational reasons

[3:13] Choice based on rational reasons emphasizes the quality of the patient's thinking, not the resultant outcome. This would be more of a deontological approach accentuating the perfect duty to oneself to act as an autonomous agent and the imperfect duty of others to respect the rational autonomous choices of rational agents.

[3:14] The way in which rational is being used here, like the reasonable outcome of choice, also encompasses both components of the terms rational and reasonable. Like Rawls' use of the word rational, there is an emphasis on the cognitive ability of the patient being able to freely form, revise, and pursue one's good, whatever that might be. Like Rawls' use of the word reasonable, there is also an emphasis on the ability to deal fairly with others in society with mutual respect for all.

[3:15] Choice based on rational reasons argues that as long as the reasoning is rational the patient has decisional-capacity. The problem here is distinguishing rational from irrational. In Rawls' well-ordered society this would not be a problem as all his citizens are by definition rational. In our case this becomes problematic as there is no clear way to absolutely determine the rationality of another person as it is to some extent subjective. This becomes even more difficult as our society becomes more pluralistic and other people's conception of the good are significantly different than the healthcare provider(s). Once again, implicit in this reasoning is the belief that as the decisional-capacity for a particular decision diminishes so increases the power or need of others, who are competent, to make that decision for the patient.

4. Ability to understand

[3:16] Ability to understand is the ability of the patient to comprehend or understand the risks, benefits, and alternatives to treatment, including no treatment, that is important, not how the patient weighs these elements, values them, or puts them together to reach a decision.

5. Actual understanding

[3:17] Depending on how sophisticated a level of understanding is to be required, this test delineates a potentially high level of evidence for decisional-capacity, one that may be difficult to achieve.

If you choose either 2, 3, 4, or 5, you will proceed to the following screen.

C. Competency Fluctuates Depending On Context

[3:18]

Competency Fluctuates Depending on Context

Patient's Decision	Risk/Benefit Ratio of Treatment	
	Favorable	Unfavorable or Questionable
Consent	Low Test of Competency	High Test of Competency
Refusal	High Test of Competency	Low test of Competency

The diagram above illustrates how the determination of a patient's competency tends to vary from one context to another depending on whether the patient refuses or consents to treatment in relation to the Risk/Benefit ratio determined by the health care providers.

It is impossible to evaluate another person's competency totally devoid from your own presuppositions and worldview(s). Although being aware of this influence can help to minimize the influence as much as possible.

The goal of the health care provider should be to evaluate the patient's competency from the patient's worldview and not your own.

After scrolling through the "Explain Table" and reading the above explanation do you still think the patient, guardian, or representative is competent?

D. Explanation Of Competency Table

[3:19]

EXPLANATION OF COMPETENCY TABLE

Patient's Decision	Risk/Benefit Ratio of Treatment	
	Favorable	Unfavorable or Questionable
Consent	Low Test of Competency (Cell A)	High Test of Competency (Cell C)
Refusal	High Test of Competency (Cell B)	Low test of Competency (Cell D)

1. Cell A

[3:20] If the risk/benefit ratio of the treatment is favorable and consent is given, Cell A, then a low test of decisional-capacity will be followed. If there is a refusal of consent, Cell B, then a high test of decisional-capacity will be followed.

[3:21] In Cell A the patient consents to have what the health professional(s) thinks to be a favorable risk/benefit ratio. Under these circumstances a test employing a low threshold of decisional-capacity may be applied to find even a marginal patient as having decisional-capacity so that the patient's decision may be honored and the doctor can do what they think is best for the patient—beneficence. This is what happens when uncomprehending patients are permitted to sign themselves into the hospital. For example, a patient may come in with a broken arm and be delusional because of the pain and shock. However, since it is an acceptable practice to reset broken arms the patient is considered competent enough for assent to the procedure even though they may be uncomprehending of the procedure as this will maximize what is considered to be the patient's best interests.

2. Cell B

[3:22] If the risk/benefit ratio of the treatment is unfavorable or questionable and consent is given, Cell C, then a high test of decisional-capacity will follow. If a refusal of consent is given, Cell D, then a low test of decisional-capacity is followed.

[3:23] In Cell B the patient does not consent to what the health professional(s) thinks to be a favorable risk/benefit ratio. Under these circumstances a test employing a higher threshold of decisional-capacity may be applied. Under such a test even a somewhat knowledgeable patient may be found to lack decisional-capacity so that consent may be sought from a substitute decision maker and treatment administered despite the patient's refusal under the belief that doing so would be to the patient's best interest.

[3:24] In both of these cases, Cell A & B, in which the risk/benefit ratio is favorable, health professionals and judges usually argue for providing treatment. Therefore, a test of decisional-capacity is applied that will permit the treatment to be administered irrespective of the patient's actual or potential understanding in order to maximize the patient's best interests.

3. Cell C

[3:25] In Cell C the patient consents to what the health professional(s) thinks is to be an unfavorable risk/benefit ratio. Under these circumstances a test employing a high threshold of decisional-capacity may be applied preventing even some fairly knowledgeable patients from undergoing treatment in order to maximize what is considered to be the best interest of the patient.

4. Cell D

[3:26] In Cell D the patient refuses to consent to what the health professional(s) thinks to be an unfavorable risk/benefit ratio. Under these circumstances a low threshold of decisional-capacity may be selected so that the patient will be found competent and the patient's refusal honored maximizing what is considered to be in the best interest of the patient.

[3:27] In both of these cases, Cells C & D, in which the risk/benefit ratio is unfavorable, health professionals and judges usually argue towards not providing the treatment based on best interests for the patient.

IV. Flow Chart Three

[4:1] Once decisional-capacity is determined (including the shifting standard) then there is the need to determine consent.

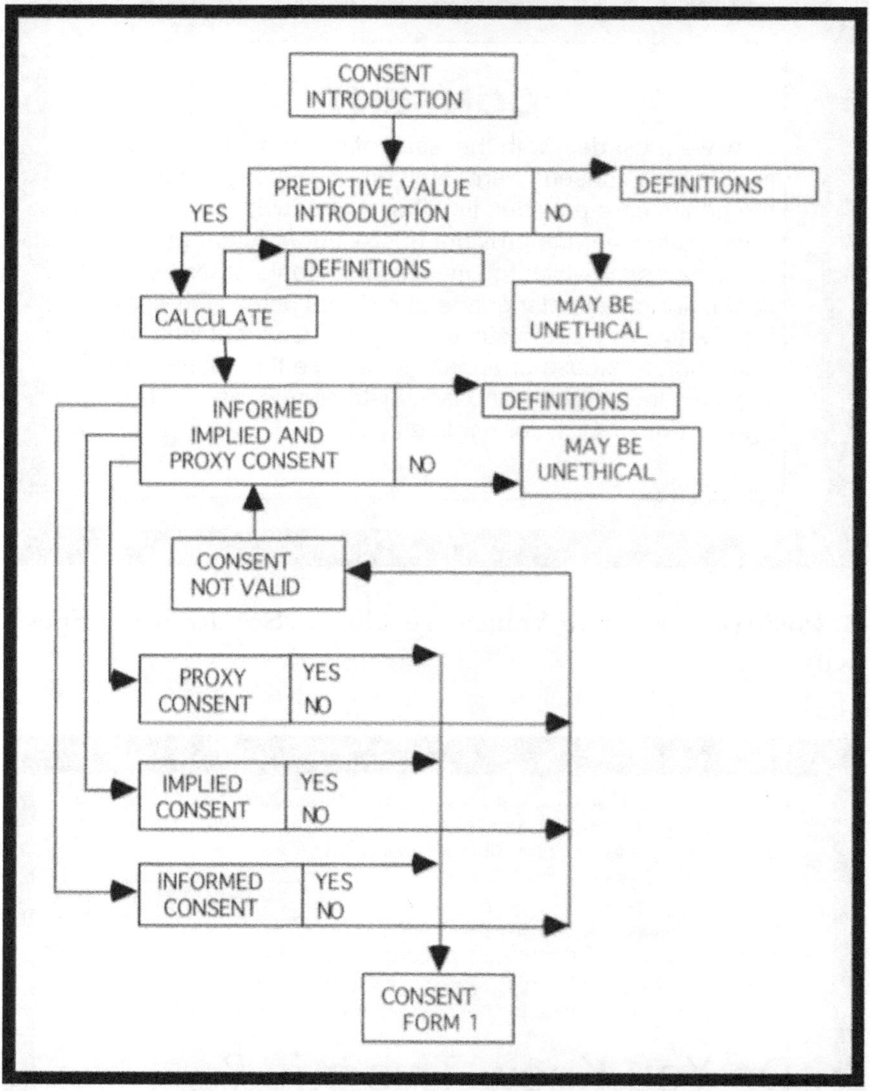

A. Consent: No Exculpatory Language

[4:2]

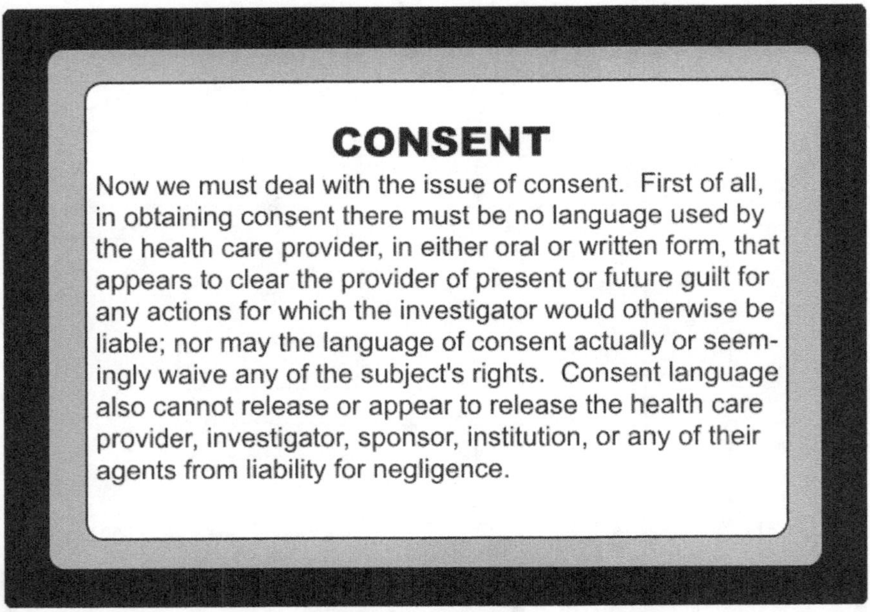

B. Positive Predictive Value: Prevalence, Sensitivity & Specificity

[4:3]

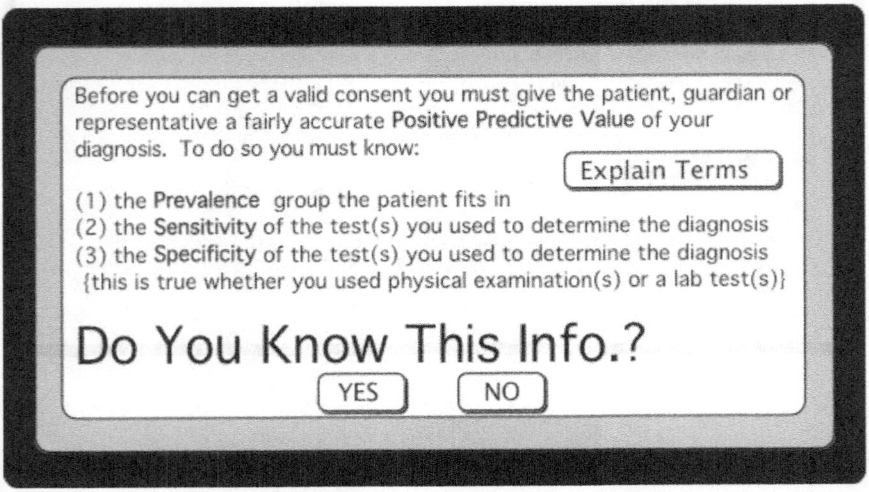

[4:4] If you select the button "Explain Terms," in the previous screen display, it will explain the terms Sensitivity, Specificity, Prevalence, Positive and Negative Predictive Values, Series and Parallel Sequential Testing and some of the ethical issues involved with diagnostic testing.

[4:5] This information is necessary in order for the patient to know to what extent the diagnostic test or evaluation of their condition is accurate. Many times a patient's diagnostic test is no more accurate than chance, i.e. no better than the patient's prevalence group. Therefore, in order to make a truly informed decision the positive and negative predictive values are imperative. However, it may be the case that since this is not an ideal society, it should be recognize that an acceptable consent may lack this qualification if it is not possible to acquire the positive and negative predictive values. Therefore, an option is given to bypass this requirement.

[4:6]

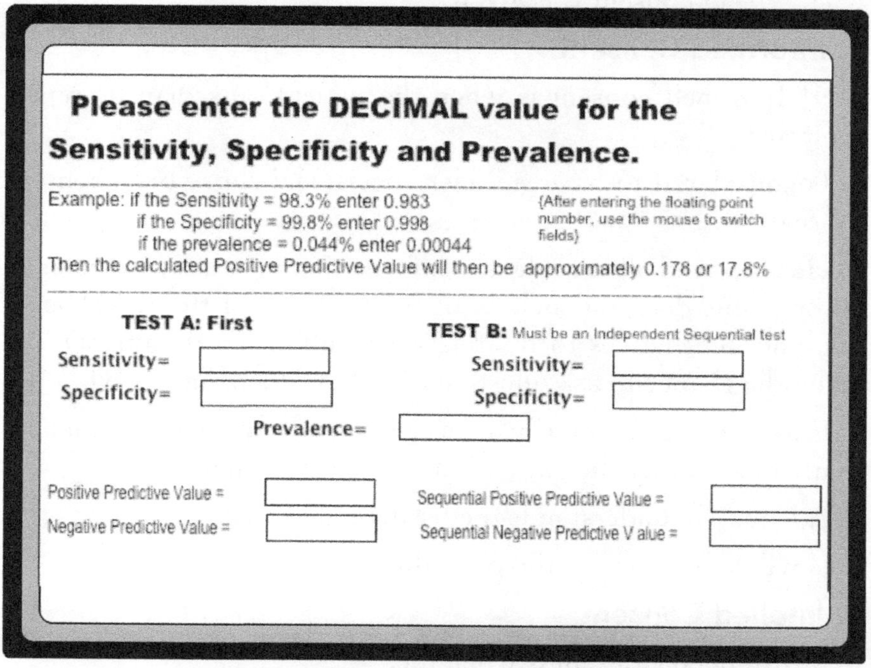

C. Types Of Consent

[4:7]

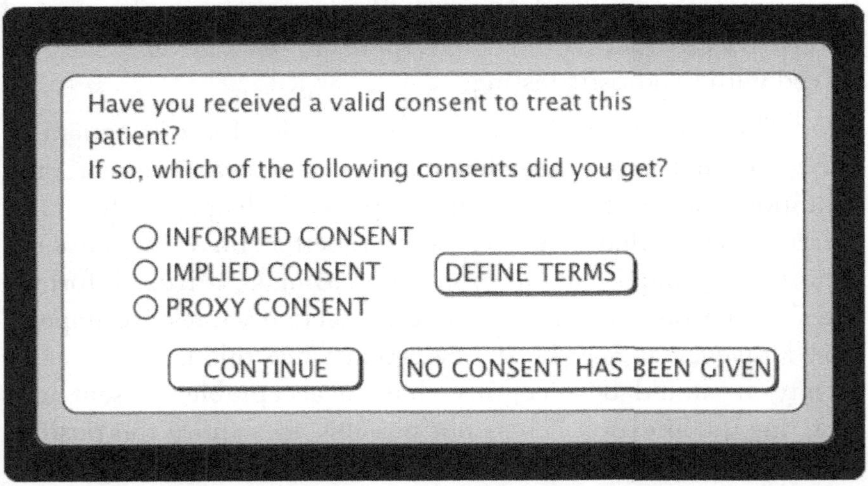

[4:8] Once the positive and negative predictive values have been disclosed DR. ETHICS™ will ask if consent has been attained and what type of consent was given.

1. Informed Consent:

[4:9] Informed consent is when the patient, guardian or representative:

a. Is considered to have sufficient decisional-capacity to consent to treatment.

b. Has received all the relevant information necessary to make an autonomous decision such as being informed of the risks, benefits, and alternatives to treatment (including no treatment) and given the chance to ask questions and have them answered.

c. Is able to act voluntarily, i.e. is sufficiently free from influences that would render the patient's decision involuntary.

d. Adequately understands the treatment.

e. Is willing to agree to the procedure.

2. Implied Consent:

[4:10] Implied Consent is when the:

a. Patient is in an emergency situation where it is not possible to get a voluntary informed or proxy consent and their life or health is threatened, or

b. Patient, guardian or representative initiated the contact for standard routine care.

3. Proxy Consent:

[4:11] Proxy consent is when another person, the guardian, makes a decision for another. Proxy consent usually takes place when the patient is not competent or lack the requisite decisional-capacity to consent to treatment or the patient is too young to make a legal informed consent decision.

The requirements are:

[4:12]

1. Guardian has the authority to make decisions for the patient.
2. Guardian is considered to have decisional-capacity.
3. Guardian is able to act voluntarily, i.e. is sufficiently free from influences that would render the guardian's decision involuntary.
4. Guardian has received all the relevant information necessary to make an autonomous decision such as being informed of the risks, benefits, and alternatives to treatment (including no treatment) and given the chance to ask questions and have them answered.
5. Guardian adequately understands the treatment.
6. Guardian represents the patient's point of view, if possible.
7. Guardian has made a decision regarding medical treatment.

V. Flow Chart Four

[5:1] The following is the fourth flow chart to be considered.

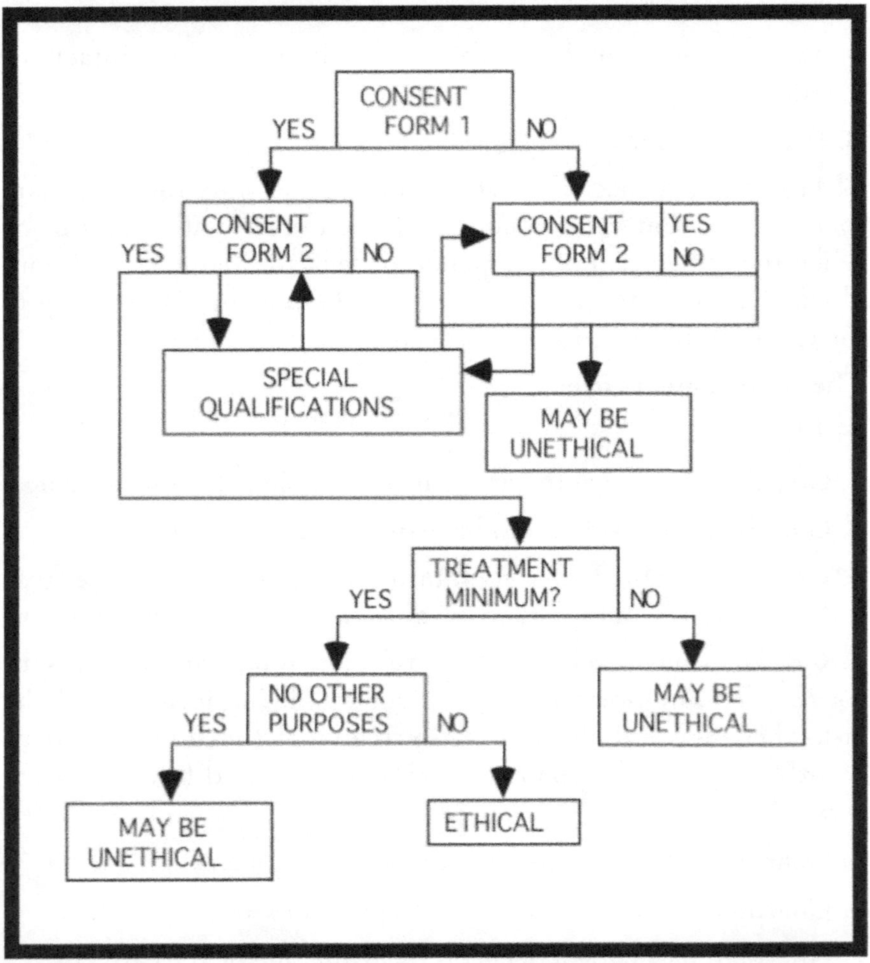

A. Consent Form 1

[5:2]

CONSENT FORM I

Does the consent form include each of the following basic elements?

YES	NO	
☐	☐	a. An explanation of the purposes of the procedure, and the expected duration of the patient's treatment?
☐	☐	b. A description of the procedures to be followed and identification of any procedures that are experimental?
☐	☐	c. A description of benefits to the patient or to others?
☐	☐	d. A description of any foreseeable risks or discomforts to the subject, or—if applicable—a statement that risks are minimal?
☐	☐	e. A disclosure of alternative procedures that may be advantageous to the subject (where research is combined with treatment or service)?
☐	☐	f. A statement describing the extent to which confidentiality of records identifying the subject will be maintained, along with the precise means of maintaining confidentiality?
☐	☐	g. For research involving more than minimal risk, the appropriate compensation and treatment availability statement?
☐	☐	h. An explanation of whom to contact for answers to pertinent questions about the research, including names, addresses, and phone numbers?
☐	☐	i. A statement that treatment is voluntary, refusal to participate will involve no penalty or loss of benefits, and the subject may withdraw or discontinue treatment at any time without penalty or loss of benefits?

Any "NO" answers will call for revision of the consent form or justification for the variance from normal form. A copy of the consent form must be left with the patient, guardian or representative.

B. Consent Form 2

[5:3]

CONSENT FORM 2

Does the consent form include each of the following basic elements?

YES	NO	
☐	☐	1. Is the consent form written in ordinary language, free of excess technicality, and styled to the nature of the subject (e.g., child, adult)?
☐	☐	2. Is the consent form free of exculpatory language through which the subject is made to waive or appear to waive any legal rights, including release of the investigator, sponsor institution, or agents from liability for negligence?
☐	☐	3. If young children are included as subjects, is provision made for securing the assent of the child as well as the consent of the parent or guardian?
☐	☐	4. If special subjects are used, such as pregnant women, prisoners, the mentally disabled, children, vulnerables or video/audio tapes or confidential data, are the required safeguards included?

Any "NO" answers will call for revision of the consent form or justification for the variance from normal form. A copy of the consent form must be left with the patient, guardian or representative.

[5:4] The next three screen displays were presented earlier when it was determined that there was no time for consent. Now it has been determined that there has been a valid informed consent.

C. Least Hazardous Treatment

[5:5]

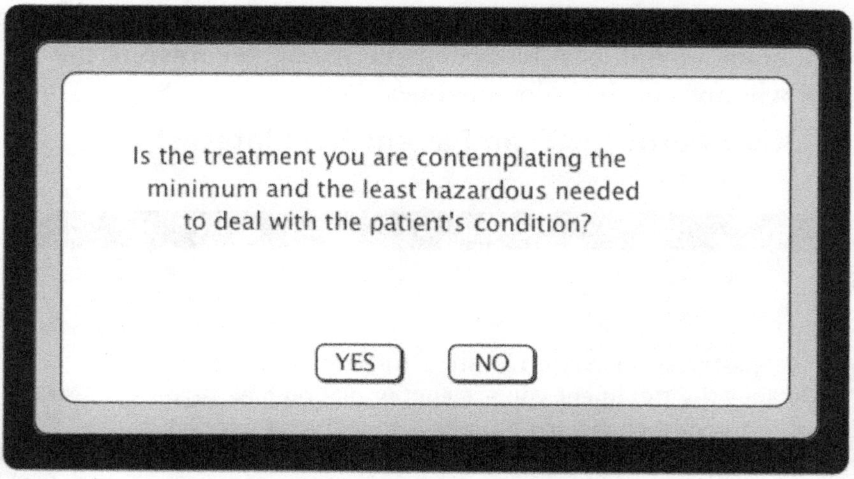

[5:6] If you answer "NO" to this question then DR. ETHICS™ will conclude that the Treatment May Not Be Ethical. The reasoning for this judgment is that even if all of the consent requirements have been given, if the healthcare professional deviates from the minimum and least hazardous standard treatment then it increases the risk for being not ethical as the treatment may not maximize the patient's best interest. However this judgment does not mean that it is in fact not ethical only that there is a greater probability that it could be.

[5:7] As mentioned before, as competency for consent decreases the more the pendulum swings towards the professional practice standard. On the other hand, as competency for consent increases the more the pendulum swings towards the subjective standard. The more a treatment deviates from the standard practice the more stringent the consent requirements become. The more stringent the consent requirements become the greater chance there is that the consent requirements could be violated.[4]

[5:8] Answering "YES" to the question of the treatment being the minimum and least hazardous necessary for treating this patient will present the following question.

D. Other Purposes Than Patient Best Interest

[5:9]

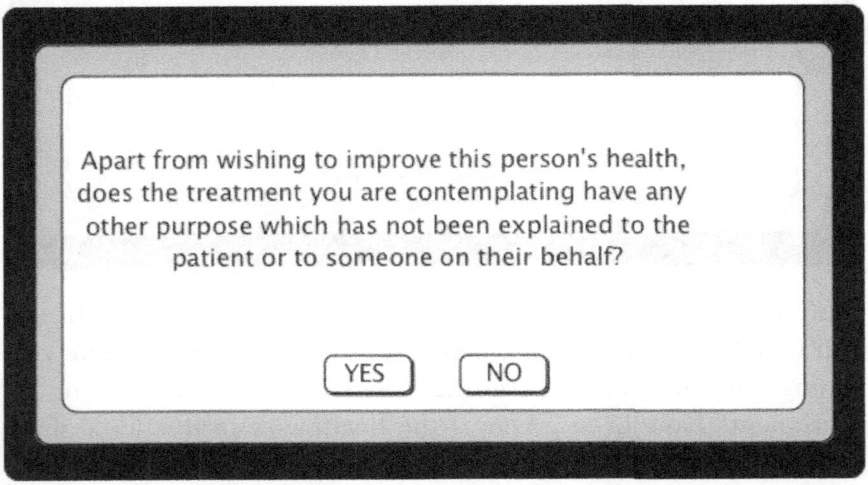

[5:10] Even though it is true that in order to get this far this requirement would have had to have already been met, it is repeated here in order to emphasize that the main purpose for the treatment being provided is for the patient's benefit. To do otherwise could be seen as taking advantage of the patient.

[5:11] If all of the above requirements have been met then DR. ETHICS™ will provide the following ethical analysis:

---

[4] At this point it should be clear that I am not defending the subjective standard over the professional practice or reasonable person standards. Rather, I am arguing that there is no one particular standard to appeal to in a nonideal society in which decisional-capacity varies. In other words, information disclosure varies along a spectrum—it is dependent on the level of decisional-capacity.

E. Ethical To Treat

[5:12]

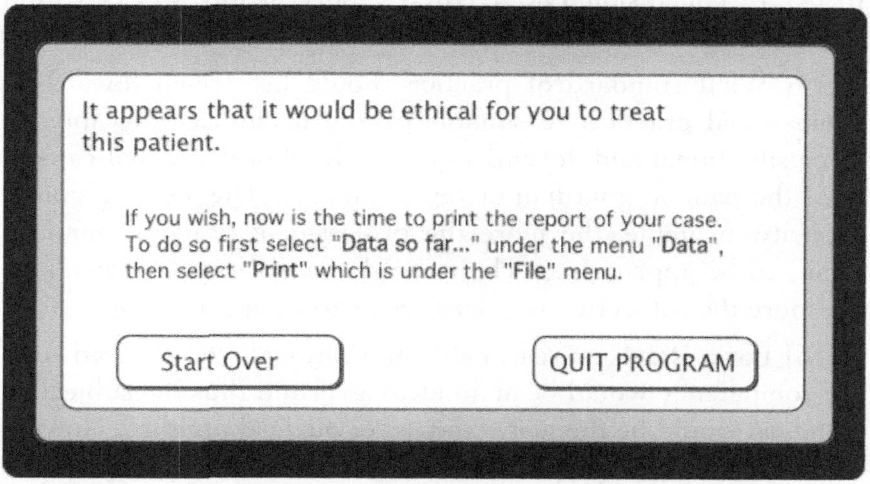

F. Thank You For Using Dr. Ethics™

[5:13]

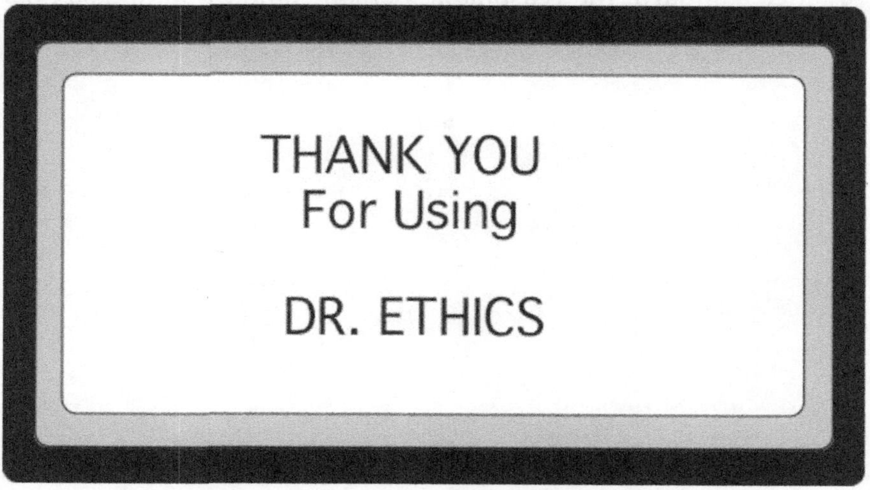

Conclusion

[5:14] In conclusion DR. ETHICS™ successfully works within the constraints presented in Rawls' *Political Liberalism.*

[5:15] What standard of practice should be striven towards—professional practice, reasonable person or subjective—appears to be situational and dependent on the level of decisional-capacity of the patient, guardian or representative. The less decisional-capacity available, the more the professional practice standard seems to be appropriate. The more decisional-capacity available the more the subjective standard seems to be appropriate.

[5:16] For a Rawlsian reasonable and rational well-ordered society competency would be at an ideal level and thus the subjective standard would be the just standard of medical practice. However, in a nonideal pluralistic society decisional-capacity varies from lacking decisional-capacity to full decisional-capacity and thus our standards of disclosure will vary from the professional practice standard, the reasonable person standard and, as a goal to be strived towards, the subjective standard.

VII. SEVEN READINGS

1. MORAL DEVELOPMENT

Why Researchers and IRBs Address 45CFR46 At the Expense Of Moral Principlism As Found In The Belmont Report

Abstract

[1:1]

Institutional Review Board's—IRB prime directive is the protection of human subjects. However, this federal mandate is flawed in its implementation because the Code of Federal Regulations Title 45 Part 46–45CFR46: Protection of Human Subjects and The Belmont Report (Principlism) attempt to protect human subjects independently of each other. 45CFR46 does not refer to the principles of autonomy (informed consent), beneficence (do good), and justice (be fair), as stated in the Belmont Report and the moral principles in the Belmont Report do not refer to the bureaucratic rules and regulations found in 45CFR46.

[1:2] Why is it that most researchers and IRBs focus primarily on the codified bureaucratic rules and regulations and rarely ever address specification and balancing of the moral principles as found in The Belmont Report?

[1:3] This pattern of focusing on codified rules and regulations at the expense of moral Principlism is what would be expected if Kohlberg's six stages of moral development are in fact descriptive true.

[1:4] However, Kohlberg failed to recognize the uniqueness of Principlism in that Principlism does offer the practical hope of being adopted by those in the lower stages of moral development if it is presented to them as derivable from, consistent with, or at least not in conflict with their personal, social or theoretical moral framework(s).

I. Moral Development

[1:5] Kohlberg's six stages of moral development can be broadly categorized as A. Self, B. Community, and C. Abstract.

A. Self

Stage One: Egoism Based On Punishment and Obedience (Authoritarian)

[1:6] In stage one, the researcher and/or IRB committee comply with 45CFR46 in order to promote their own self-interests and to avoid "physical punishment" based on federal noncompliance.

[1:6] (Note: although noncompliance would rarely result in corporal punishment, such as a good spanking, economic consequences can be considered to be a type of "physical punishment".) The more punishment associated with noncompliance the more "bad" the act is perceived to be by both the researcher and/or the IRB. Moral assessment is attributed to the unquestioned authority of federal law and the subsequent consequences for noncompliance with the perspective that there is only one right view.

[1:8] Stage 1 is the "might makes right" mentality. Avoidance of punishment, and/or forcing your will on others, is what it means to promote self-interests.

Stage Two: Egoism Based On Instrumental Exchange (Social)

[2:1] In stage two, the researcher and/or IRB committee comply with 45CFR46 to the degree that it might further their own interests as based on instrumental exchange. Concessions are made only if it is considered to be in their self-interests.

[2:2] Stage 2 reasoning recognizes that there are differing viewpoints but that the researcher and/or IRB is still pre-conventional in that there is still no identification with community values and the focus is still on what will maximize their personal needs, not the community needs. Justice is: "Do unto others as they have done unto you." Vengeance is a moral duty, and others are valued in terms of their utility.

[2:3] Stage 2 is the "what's in it for me" mentality. "Don't bite the hand that feeds you," "you scratch my back and I will scratch your back" and "an eye for an eye tooth for a tooth" is the basis of moral assessment.

B. Community

Stage Three: Social Conformity By Means Of Peer Pressure (Social)

[3:1] In stage three, the researcher and/or IRB committee comply with 45CFR46 because that is what it means to conform to the value expectations of their society and/or peers. Good behavior is that which pleases others in the group and self-sacrifice to the group's expectations is expected.

[3:2] Peer pressure is paramount and failure of the group to punish the individual nonconformist is considered to be "unfair." Individual vengeance is not allowed and individual forgiveness is promoted. This is the stage that most people never progress beyond.

[3:3] Stage 3 is the "good old boy" mentality.

Stage Four: Social Conformity By Means Of Law and Order (Authoritarian)

[4:1] In stage four, the researcher and/or IRB committee comply with 45CFR46 because the authority figure of federal law is considered to be right. Obedience is a matter of transcending personal needs and adopting a political ideology as based on the social contract. In this stage there is an obligation or duty to uphold the law because if everyone were to do otherwise society would not be able to maintain its social function.

[4:2] In stage one an individual must conform to the law and respect authority in order to avoid punishment. In stage four an individual must conform to the law and respect authority as a matter of social duty for the maintenance of social order. This is the highest moral stage of development for a majority of adults that progress beyond stage 3.

[4:3] Stage 4 is the "what if everyone did that" mentality.

Stage Four and a half: Disrespect of the Social Structure (The Cynic)

[4:4] In stage four and a half, the researcher and/or IRB becomes cynical as to the conventional morality. Kohlberg found that even though these individuals recognize the deficiencies of conventional morality as being say: socially constructed and/or relative and arbitrary, they still are unable to leave conventional morality behind because they have not discovered anything else to replace it with such as Principlism.

[4:5] As a result, much to the distress of Stage four individuals, these individuals often end up disrespecting community authority and indulging themselves in egoistic hedonistic pleasures. Such individuals also exercise uncritical cynicism such as "all lawyers are crooks," "all politicians are liars," or more specifically "all IRB members are against student and faculty academic freedoms" or "all researchers are out to take advantage of human subjects." Disillusionment and alienation is prevalent.

[4:6] Stage 4 1/2 is the "I might as well live my life any way I please as nothing will change anyway" mentality.

C. Abstract

Stage 5: Social Contract Theory (Theoretical)

[5:1] In stage five, the researcher and/or IRB committee start asking the question, "What ideally makes a good research protocol evaluation," "What ideally makes a good society?" Stage five participants step back from the conventional IRB protocols which are composed of a checklist of bureaucratic rules and regulations, and they start thinking theoretically as to what would be "ideal".

[5:2] For example, what rights and liberties ought to be recognized for human subjects and researchers. One such theoretical framework is the Rawlsian social contract theory of justice.

[5:3]

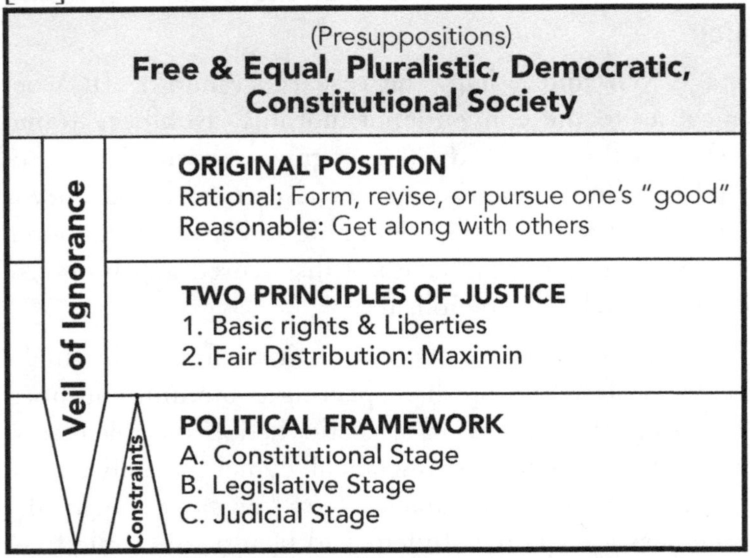

[5:4] Rawls' theoretical framework puts forth a hypothetical scenario in which he presupposes that there are individuals who live within a pluralistic, free and equal, democratic, constitutional society. He further presupposes that all the individuals in this hypothetical society are persons, that are rational and reasonable, (*rational* meaning the ability to form, revise, or pursue one's "good," i.e., one's "purpose and meaning of life," and *reasonable* meaning having the ability to get along with others). Rawls then presents us with the task of determining what principles of justice should be adopted for the citizens of this society if we were to be their representatives. To make sure that we do this fairly, Rawls puts us, or the representatives, behind a "veil of ignorance," called the "original position", in which all that is known is that the individual(s) that are represented are rational and reasonable as above defined. The task is to make sure that the citizen(s) have the "basic goods" that would be necessary for the continuation or development of their rational and reasonable states.

[5:5] Rawls argues that from this original position, it would be logically consistent to construct principles of justice that would ensure those necessary "basic goods." Rawls comes up with the following *Two Principles of Justice,* which are in hierarchical order. (Hierarchical order meaning; 1. that the first principle of justice must be established before establishing the second principle of justice and 2. that the first principle of justice can never be violated or infringed upon by the second principle of justice, or anything else lower in hierarchy). The *Two Principles of Justice* are summarily given as follows: 1. The establishment of basic rights and liberties, and 2. If there is going to be any unequal distribution it must benefit all, or at minimum the least well off, i.e., maximization of the minimal condition—maximin.

[5:6] The first principle of justice comes about by a) looking at what rights and liberties have historically worked well for democracy, b) lucky guesses/intuitions, and c) trial and error. These rights and liberties are then justified through a process of reflective-equilibrium—a back and forth process. Through this process of reflective-equilibrium, the specific rights and liberties become established and they mutually constrain each other.

[5:7] The second principle of justice is the distributive principle that utilizes the maximin principle, i.e., maximizes or improves the worse-off condition. In doing this, Rawls is not a "pure" egalitarian in that he does allow unequal distributions of "social goods" as long as it benefits all, especially the least well off. However, because of the hierarchical order, the distribution cannot violate any of the basic rights or liberties under the first principle of justice when implementing the distributive principles of the second principle of justice.

[5:8] Once the two primary principles of justice are established, Rawls believes that it is then logical to construct a just political framework that would be composed of the *Constitutional Stage, the Legislative Stage,* and the *Judicial Stage*. The *Constitutional Stage* would consist of the responsibility for the specifying and balancing of the basic rights and liberties of the first principle of justice. The *Legislative Stage* is responsible for the specifying and balancing of the distributive aspects of the second principle of justice. Lastly the *Judicial Stage* would apply all of the above to actual specific situations. Once again, all of the steps are in hierarchical order and the veil of ignorance gets thinner as one goes from the constitutional stage to the legislative stage and finally to the judicial stage where there is no veil of ignorance. This "thinning" of the veil of ignorance is essential as the situations become more and more specific at each successive stage. This hierarchical ordering is a protective mechanism that makes sure that the basic rights and liberties, that are the necessary "goods" for the development of rational and reasonable citizens, are never infringed upon. Rawls does not believe that this is "The Theory of Justice" rather he held that this was only "A Theory of Justice" that would or could develop rational and reasonable citizens.

[5:9] In stage four, conventional morality is the result of the authority of the social contract that is actually in place, whereas in stage five, social contract theory is based purely on rational and reasonable arguments of an "ideal society". Critical reasoning that hypothetically promotes justice for all is the authority that outweighs any form of egoism and social conformity that is independent of such hypothetical processes.

[5:10] It is also the case that in stage three and four retributive and deterrence justice, i.e., social punishment, is considered necessary and is in fact demanded by society. Since stage 5 is ideally theoretical, punishment of any type becomes nonsense because the current social/political framework is flawed or may even be unjust. Promotion of the theoretical social contract, trumps the actual social contract that individuals find themselves in.

[5:11] Like the cynic in 4 1/2, in stage 5 the current imperfect social structures and authorities are also rejected, but unlike 4 1/2 in which they had no replacement for such rejections, stage 5 provides the rational and reasonable justifications of an ideal social framework that ought to replace the imperfect one. One criticism of this position is that that which is ideally perfect may not be practically expedient.

[5:12] Stage 5 is the "philosopher king" mentality in which social policy is directed and implemented by those who can grasp the ideal social contract and the ideal social ends.

Stage 6: Principlism: Autonomy, Beneficence, Nonmaleficence, and Justice (Practical)

[6:1] In stage six broad and general universal principles are practically recognized and applied to all sentient beings. Sentient beings are treated not solely as a means to personal and social ends, rather they are also considered to be ends in themselves. Lists of bureaucratic concrete rules are no longer appealed to, rather the process is that the broad and general principles are specified and balanced as the circumstances warrant.

[6:2] With regard to the IRB, 45CFR46 is no longer necessary for the protections of human subjects as decisions are now based on the abstract moral principles such as those found in The Belmont Report, not the codified bureaucratic rules and regulations found in 45CFR46. Abstract moral principles such as autonomy (informed consent), beneficence (do good), nonmaleficence (do no harm), and justice (be fair), are specified and balanced as the situation determines and may in fact outweigh the rules and regulations of the law as bureaucratic assessments can and often are quite different than moral assessments.

[6:3] Principlism, as a moral stage of development, arises through the synergistic reflective equilibrium process.

a. Intuitive Point of View

[6:4]

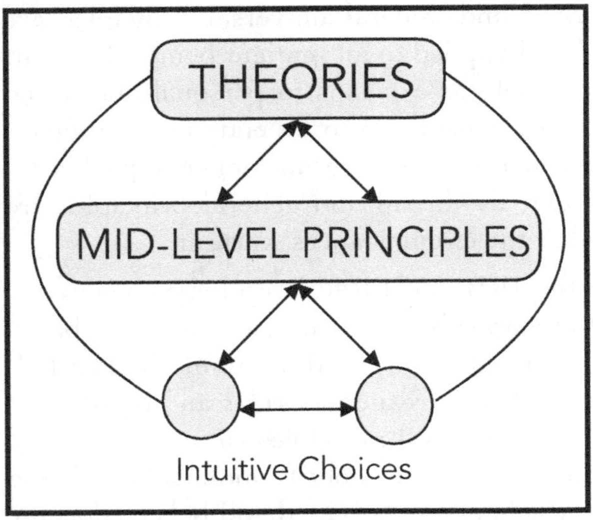

[6:5] Intuitive choices are decisions that are made without an appeal to principles, theory or any type of deductive processes of reasoning. For example, the intuitive determination that an action or inaction is "right" or "wrong" can be much like a clear and distinct idea is known to be true such as the law of identity A=A or other postulates and axioms of mathematics. Whether or not this intuition is based on patterned or imprinted punishment avoidance, self-interest, social conformity, social authority or even emotions and/or personal social relationships will not change the fact of the intuitive choice but may greatly influence the effects that will occur from the choice as they are indicative of an agent's moral stage of development. These intuitive determinations can effect other intuitive choices, mid-level principles, and moral theory.

[6:6] When an agent makes an intuitive choice, other future intuitive choices are also naturally effected both because of the environments and situations created by such choices, but also because of a matter of consistency. One of the major criticisms that can be made of intuitive choices is that they have a tendency to be much more variable and inconsistent than principles and theories. For example, it is not unusual to have a relational intuition of say love at one moment and experience quite a different relational intuition shortly thereafter.

[6:7] When an agent makes a series of intuitive choices, particular patterns start developing which creates the opportunity for the creation of mid-level principles and/or theories that will result in greater consistency and predictability. However, when a future intuitive choice is made that conflicts with a developed mid-level principle and/or theory then a resolution will have to occur. Either the principle and/or theory that has been developed by multiple previous intuitive choices will have to be modified or the current intuitive choice will have to be rejected in order to come into compliance with the more established principle and/or theory using the reflective equilibrium process. However, because the established principle and/or theory in question was created by evaluating many previous intuitive choices, to change the moral principle and/or theory would also mean that all the intuitive choices that were previously used to develop the principle and/or theory would also have to be reevaluated as to their consistency with the new modified principle and/or theory.

b. Theory Point of View

[6:9] Theories are cognitive constructs that attempt to explain mid-level principles and intuitive choices both descriptively and prescriptively. This of course is paradoxical. If theories are fundamentally based on intuitive choices and mid-level principles, then how can a theory claim explanation independently of such influences? Kohlberg's theory of moral stage development is a good example of this in that as a theory it is to be an explanation of moral development independent of moral decisions and yet at the same time his theory is totally based on actual moral decision-making practices. This criticism can also be made with regard to John Rawls' theory of justice, as presented in Stage 5, where it seems that his theoretical presuppositions of a free and equal pluralistic democratic constitutional society results in a theory that is the same as his presuppositions. This is true of mathematical theory as well in which the presupposed axioms and postulates result in a mathematical system that reflect those very axioms and postulates. If axioms and postulates are permissible in mathematics and other disciplines without weakening the resulting activity then it should also be acceptable with regard to the discipline of moral development as well.

[6:10] Once a theory or theories have been developed then the reflective equilibrium process will need to occur between multiple theories, intuitive choices and mid-level principles in an attempt to maximize each of the principles and to minimize existing inconsistencies. This reflective equilibrium activity is parallel to the activity of the Supreme Court whose responsibility includes the recognition of Constitutional rights and liberties and the elimination of laws that fail to recognize such rights and liberties.

[6:11] Lastly, just as moral agents appeal to various moral principles for moral decision-making so also a single moral agent may appeal to more than one theory for dealing with differing types of moral determinations, circumstances, and/or equilibrium harmonizing, such as Utilitarianism or Deontology.

c. Mid-Level Principles Point of View

[6:12] Mid-level principles from the theory point of view are heuristic shortcuts for moral decision-making. An example of a nonmoral heuristic principle might be "the clearer an object appears to be the closer it is." Although the heuristic principle works very well for most circumstances it can also result in heuristic errors when used under circumstances it was not meant to be used for, such as a hazy day, in which objects appear further away than they actually are because of lower visibility. Mid-level principles are similar heuristic devices that need to be specified and balanced. Specification is the taking of a broad and general principle and making it relevant to a specific event or situation. Balancing is the taking of two or more moral principles and harmonizing them as much as possible to a specific event or situation. Moral theory(s) only need to be addressed when there appears to be specification or balancing inconsistencies between two or more moral principles.

[6:13] Although there are no conflicting moral principles, moral dilemmas may occur in two forms: single principle and plural principles.

[6:14] The first form of a moral dilemma is when a single moral principle is specified for the making of a particular decision and it appears that the options available seem to both promote and not promote that single principle at the same time.

[6:15] The second form of a moral dilemma is when two or more moral principles are specified and balanced for the making of a particular decision and it appears that the options available seem to both promote and not promote two or more moral principles at the same time.

[6:16] However, having moral dilemmas does not mean that the principles conflict with each other, rather what it means is that the principles need to be specified and balanced with regard to each other. Principlism holds that a moral judgment can be made by the weighing and balancing of the principles as they relate to the particular circumstances. Unlike Rawls' political framework, moral principles are not in hierarchical order in that depending on the decision that is being made one or more principles may carry more weight than one or more other principles.

[6:17] Mid-level principles from the intuition point of view are also considered to be heuristic shortcuts in that they result in greater consistency and predictability than what intuitions alone are able to provide which is advantageous for social and political development in which the mid-level principles are often perceived as being "common ground" even within pluralistic societies.

[6:18] This descriptive moral model is synergistic because when all the parts are working together, the experience of the moral agent is that the whole is greater than the sum of the parts. Thus the name Synergistic Reflective Equilibrium Model.

[6:19] Although stage six individuals have few supporters with regard to their rejection of the moral reasoning of the earlier stages, independently of those stage rejections, the universal principles are derivable from, consistent with, or at least not in conflict with most theoretical and intuitional moral approaches. In other words, contrary to what Kohlberg argued, the principles found in Principlism, can be presented in such a way that others in the lower stages can accept them as being part of their own moral point of view.

[6:20] In this process of "inception" Principlism also recognizes that there can and will be incommensurable disagreements in beliefs and/or facts that will result in differing assessments as to the specification and balancing of these abstract moral principles, especially when agents from differing stages of moral development are making such assessments. However, such moral agreement on universal abstract principles, such as autonomy (informed consent), beneficence (do good), nonmaleficence (do no harm), and justice (be fair), is a great advancement for moral persuasion and compromise in practical reality.

Stage 6 is the "Moral considerability for all sentient beings" mentality.

Conclusion

[6:21] If Lawrence Kohlberg's stages of moral development are descriptively true, then it shouldn't be a surprise to find that most researchers and IRBs focus on codified bureaucratic rules and regulations and rarely address universal abstract moral principles that need to be specified and balanced in their evaluations of research proposals.

[6:22] 45CFR46 is often used at the exclusion of Principlism because 45CFR46 is based on the moral stages of 1 to 4, whereas The Belmont Report is based primarily on stage 6 reasoning called Principlism.

[6:23] Since researchers and IRB members are composed of individuals who vary with regard to moral stages, then it would seem that the lowest common denominator will prevail, i.e., the appeal to the codified bureaucratic rules and regulations of

45CFR46 at the expense of the specification and balancing judgments of moral Principlism as found in the Belmont Report.

[6:24] If stage six moral reasoning is the goal in the protection of research subjects, how is such a Principlistic method possible to implement with those who are functioning at a lower moral stage of development?

[6:25] According to Kohlberg such an implementation would be impossible because: 1. Moral stage development is invariant and sequential, and 2. It is impossible to comprehend moral reasoning more than one stage beyond where an individual currently is. Individuals in higher stages are able to comprehend the reasoning of lower stages but individuals in lower stages are never able to comprehend the reasoning of more than the next higher stage.

[6:26] However, as explained above, if Principlism is presented as derivable from, consistent with, or at least not in conflict with an agent or community's moral position, regardless of the moral stage, then it will be possible to present Principlism as being part of their own moral worldview in which there can arise personal and social ownership of the moral principles.

[6:27] Therefore, although it would be impossible for individuals to reject the moral stage they find themselves in, such as self, community, or hypothetical ideals, (stages 1-5), and although the higher stages transcend the comprehension of those in the lower stages, Principlism does offer the practical hope of being adopted by those in the lower stages as part of their own stage if properly presented.

[6:28] In the end, we will find ourselves at the beginning, for the very first time.

***

2. HONEYBEE DEMOCRACY

Abstract

[1]

Honeybee hives are composed of individual bees that through the mutual cooperation and division of labor function effectively as a superorganism. Beehive social organization has nothing related to human democratic decision-making, yet it has become popular to talk about "honeybee democracy." Democracy is usually associated with an authoritative centralized government in which an informed citizenry and/or representatives engage in adversarial debate. Beehives function without a centralized government, without an informed citizenry, and without adversarial debate and although there is nothing that honeybees can learn from us, there is plenty that we as social beings can learn from honeybees.

[2] *"In all these scenes of animal life which crossed before my eyes, I saw mutual aid and mutual support carried on to an extent which made me suspect in it a feature of the greatest importance for the maintenance of life, the preservation of each species and its further evolution."*

(Petr Kropotkin, *Mutual Aid: A Factor of Evolution*, 1902, p. xxxvii, ISBN: 0-87558-024-6.)

I. Evolutionary Misnomers

[3] Nature, through the process of natural selection, has been honing the stimulus response mechanisms of both the individual honeybee and the honeybee colony as a whole, to such a degree of accuracy that it now rivals some of the best rational approaches of contemporary decision-making, especially those decisions that are classified as democratic. However, it is becoming popular in some circles to refer to honeybee colony behavior as "honeybee democracy," and this label is an unfortunate anthropocentric misnomer. "Honeybee democracy" is a misnomer much like the "Big Bang" is a misnomer caused by a misunderstanding of the process of evolution. With regard to the "Big Bang," the beginning of the cosmos was neither "Big," as the universe arose from an infinitesimal point, nor was there a "Bang," as there existed no medium for "sound" nor was there any perceiving beings to experience a "Bang." "Honeybee democracy" is likewise a misnomer caused by both a misunderstanding of the process of natural selection as it relates to bees progeny of genetic traits, and also a misunderstanding as it relates to the progeny of cultural memes or more specifically the development of linguistic signals that promote effective bee cooperation. It is true that honeybee colonies do not have an informed central ruling administration, nor an informed monarchical figure such as a "queen" or "king." However, that fact in no way means that the honeybee colony must therefore be a democracy. The "queen bee" is another misnomer created from the anthropocentric concept of a type of centralized authority. Although it is true that the queen bee is the mother of all the brood in the nest, and although she uses her pheromones to keep the hive together and to signal the workers to not make any new "queen cells" she is not a central organizer, has no authority on the daily workings of the colony, and has no knowledge of the activities that are going on around her that are necessary for the hive to function as a superorganism.

[4] Usually when addressing the issue of democracy, and/or decision-making there is the assumption of information exchange, comparisons, and choice. For bees there is evidence that there is

some very rudimentary information exchange, but there is no evidence that bees are able to respond to stimuli in any other way than a cause effect deterministic manner. Therefore if democratic decision-making is based on nondeterministic information exchange, and if bee information exchange turns out to be mechanistically determined, then the criteria of democracy and decision-making would not be met and the term "honeybee democracy" or "honeybee decision-making" would be a misnomer at best and a fundamental misunderstanding at worst.

II. Passive Cues and Active Signals

[5] Since a necessary condition for democracy and decision-making is knowledge acquisition it is imperative to take a closer look at how honeybees acquire knowledge. Honeybees can be considered to have two types of information gathering means: passive cues and active signals.

[6] Passive cues are subtle environmental stimuli that result in adaptive responses by the perceiving bee. Environmental cues can provide either excitatory feedback, such as an excellent nectar source, or inhibitory feedback, such as too long a time to find a nectar receiver at the hive entrance. The pressures of natural selection cause the perceiving bee to adapt their responses to the passive environmental cues in such a way that the bee's responses are more advantageous than disadvantageous to the reproductive interests of the colony.

[7] Active signals are information bearing actions that involve the adaptive modification of both the stimulus (signal) and the response (receiver). Bees have limited communicative signals, three of them being: the waggle dance (informs location), the tremble dance (recruits nurse bees to become nectar storage bees,) and shaking (recruits nonforagers to become foraging bees). Natural selection of communicative signals generally occurs when environmental cues are not able to adequately or effectively convey necessary information creating natural selection pressure for the development of active communication signals. Active communicative signals are difficult to develop because they require the development of both the signal stimulus (cause) and the proper response (effect) of the perceiver. In contrast, passive cues cannot be defined as communicative language in that cues are passive and merely environmental states of affairs. Active signals clearly are a type of communicative language in that signals have both well developed causal stimuli and well developed subjective effects caused by the stimuli. Since democratic decision-making is a social affair that requires information exchange, it therefore appears that language is a necessary condition for democratic decision-making.

III. Different Language Perspectives

[8] There are several different language perspectives that can be adopted. Four of which are: 1. Language as sense data, 2. Language as thought, 3. Language as any subjective experience, and 4. Language as pluralistic frameworks.

A. Language as sense data

[9] If language signals are defined as being a type of sense data then they do not directly communicate the "idea" rather they represent the "idea" in a form that may have little if any resemblance at all to the idea. For example, in the waggle dance, the number of waggles represents the amount of energy output necessary for the bee to get to a particular location, i.e. distance. If so then the waggle signal itself (number of waggles) is only a representation that has little if any resemblance at all to the idea being communicated (distance based on energy output). Then the question arises as to whether or not the interpretation and/or response of the perceiver to the signal is determined. Mechanistic determinism of sense data is exemplified in the experience of say "green grass," in which the perceiver has no voluntary input as to the experience caused by wavelengths of light that stimulate the rods and cones in the eyes that create nerve impulses that stimulates the brain resulting in the subjective experience of "green" that only exists in the mind of the experiencer, i.e., "greenness" is an experience that is independent of the sense data causation. This experience is determined as made evidenced by the simple fact that perceivers of "green" grass cannot voluntarily choose to experience the grass as "red." Therefore it can be concluded that the experience of the quality of "green" is a determined experience for the perceiver that has little if any resemblance at all to the light wavelengths of 53,000 angstroms that is the causation of the subjective experience of "green." If the waggle signal is as such, then the waggles represents information which then stimulates the perceiving bee into having a particular experience resulting in a particular response. If this perspective of bee language is correct, then it would not support the notion of democ-

racy, or critical decision-making because all the responses are deterministically fixed and therefore no choices are being made.

B. Language as thought

[10] Another perspective on language would be to consider the language signals as being the very thought or idea itself. However the consequence of such a language perspective would be the conclusion that without language signals there would therefore be no thoughts or ideas and without thoughts or ideas there would be no language signals as they are one and the same. In other words, is the concept of democracy dependent on language symbols and concepts? Is it possible to have a thought of democracy without a language framework? The human perspective of democracy and decision-making seems to be very dependent on the language framework of a centralized constitutional government with individual rights and liberties defined. One benefit of such a viewpoint is that the transferring of the subjective thought would be direct for those who share the same verbal language framework as there would be no intermediary transformations such as for example sense data. It would also follow that the types of thoughts that are possible would be directly related to the complexity of the language framework used. Simple language frameworks would generally result in simpler thoughts and more complex language frameworks would have the potential of more complex thoughts. An example is the language of mathematics in which in proportion to the mastery of mathematical axioms, postulates, and proofs, there results the potential for a greater number of types and complexities of mathematical expressions. Bees in contrast have such a rudimentary or limited set of symbolic language, e.g., waggle, tremble and shake, that it is inconceivable to even think that those symbols would meet the necessary conditions for the development of the cognitive concepts necessary for democratic decision-making.

C. Language as any subjective experience

[11] If the notion of language were to be expanded to include all knowledge gained by the experiences of perceivable beings, e.g., symbols and cues, then language would be defined as any subjec-

tive experience. This definition of language would be either meaningless or at least tautological as all that can be known by definition is already a cognitive experience and language would therefore not provide any type of synthetic additive knowledge or communicative activity to the subjective experience. If language is a purely subjective cognitive experience, then language would no longer be the means of explaining how one subjective cognitive experiencer is able to communicate to another subjective cognitive experiencer which is a necessary condition for the concept of honeybee democracy and decision-making.

D. Language has pluralistic frameworks

[12] Clearly language is pluralistic in its form and function. For example, the waggle dance is useful in communicating distance and direction, the tremble dance is useful in recruiting storagers, and shaking helps recruit foragers. However, like the game of charades in which the body language framework attempts to communicate a verbal language framework, it is many times difficult, if not impossible, to use one language framework to communicate a thought or event that can only be communicated using a different language framework. For example, it would be impossible for a bee to use the tremble dance to communicate what the waggle dance communicates. The problem that arises is that if human democracy and decision-making depends on certain types of language frameworks and if bees do not have those language frameworks then it is unreasonable to conclude that bees are democratic decision-makers from a human linguistic point of view.

IV. Honeybees Are Cooperative Not Adversarial

[13] Democracies are generally understood to be adversarial and competitive, requiring an informed authoritative centralized government and a rational and informed citizenry. Honeybees in contrast are cooperative, not adversarial, and their social organization are based on a complex of individual responses, not based on any type of authority or centralized government. Honeybees appear to be neither rational nor informed in terms of having a plurality of options. Rather, their actions are determined by very sophisticated, and effective stimulus response mechanisms. Since democratic decision-making is founded on an adversarial centralized authoritative government with an informed and rational citizenry, and since beehives are cooperative in nature, not adversarial, and since beehives do not have a centralized authoritative government rather beehives are decentralized in structure, and since bees are not informed as to the states and conditions of the other individual bees or the beehive as a whole, it therefore follows that beehives do not operate anything like a human democracy.

V. Academic Limits

[14] Lastly, it is true that academics has significant epistemological limits as to what it can metaphysically establish. First of all, empirical evidence can only evaluate the evidence for that which does exists as the empirical evidence for that which does not exist would obviously not exist. In other words, just as it is impossible to empirically prove the nonexistence of something, such as Santa Claus the tooth fairy or God for that matter, it is likewise empirically impossible to prove that honeybees do not make democratic decisions. However, what can be empirically established is that the actions of honeybees can be best explained and understood as being determined by cooperative stimulus response mechanisms instead of being based on an adversarial democratic process. Currently, there is no empirical evidence that even remotely supports that bees experience democratic decision-making, let alone information acquisition that is a necessary condition for a centralized democratic adversarial debate. Secondly, statements of "facts" can never derive statements of "ought," as that would be to commit the "naturalistic fallacy." In other words, empirical facts can never establish purpose, ends, or any other type of moral claims. Such teleological and/or deontological claims are subjective determinations of experience, not empirical claims of facts. Lastly, it must also be recognized that all of reality has evolved into existence regardless of whether or not the subject is planetary systems, biological beings, or rational and moral principles. "Honeybee democracy" is clearly an anthropocentric misnomer, that must be eliminated if entomology is to continue to progress in its analysis and understanding of honeybee behavior.

VI. Lessons To Be Learned

[15] A beehive is a splendidly sophisticated superorganism with individual bees deterministically responding to various stimuli all the while behaving as a single cooperative organism. The lessons to be learned is not how honeybees function as democratic decision-makers, as they do not, rather the lessons to be learned is how human democratic decision-making can be improved by becoming less adversarial and authoritatively centralized and becoming more decentralized and cooperative, i.e., becoming more beelike—a superorganism that has evolved from individual solitary parts into a mutually cooperative organism resulting in the maximization of overall social and individual benefits and the minimization of burdens in a just and fair society—democracy and the honeybee.

[16] *In the practice of mutual aid, which we can retrace to the earliest beginnings of evolution, we thus find the positive and undoubted origin of our ethical conceptions; and we can affirm that in the ethical progress of man, mutual support—not mutual struggle—has had the leading part. In its wide extension, even at the present time, we also see the best guarantee of a still loftier evolution of our race.*

(Petr Kropotkin, *Mutual Aid: A Factor of Evolution*, 1902, p. 300 ISBN: 0-87558-024-6.)

***

3. FOOD PRODUCTION

An IRB Analysis

Abstract

[1:1]

Corn-fed beef will be used to illustrate how the Institutional Review Board—IRB criteria of Principlism can be practically applied as a regulatory model for food systems, just as Principlism is being practically applied as a regulatory model for research on human subjects. A partial solution to some of the most serious problems associated with the industrialization of food production will then be presented as a three-step process that argues that society ought to:

1. Implement stricter conflict of interest laws for government regulators,

2. Have Congress mandate that the Food and Drug Administration—FDA, the Environmental Protection Agency—EPA and the Food Safety and Inspection Service—FSIS adopt the Belmont Report principles that are currently used by the Department of Health and Human Services—HHS for regulating research on human subjects, and

3. Have HHS expand Title 45 Part 46 of the Code of Federal Regulations to include a Subpart F: Additional Considerations for Animal Husbandry and Agriculture.

Introduction

[1:2] Who are people more afraid of, a terrorist attack by some religious fanatic or Monsanto?

[1:3] Lacking statistical knowledge and lacking public examples of even who Monsanto is, and being able to identify and come up with multiple instances of dangerous terrorists, the availability heuristic model correctly concludes that most citizens have an excessive fear of a terrorist attack, and a lack of fear towards Monsanto, Cargill, and Archer's Daniels Midland—ADM.

[1:4] Heuristics are mental shortcuts that generally work well but they can also lead to systematic errors. The availability heuristic is the propensity to put higher probability of an event occurring on those events in which there is a higher availability of recollection, than those in which there are fewer recollections.

[1:5] Because most Americans have a higher recollection of terrorist activities than those of food producers they therefore have a disproportionate fear of terrorists. Outside of the food production industry, most people in society don't even know who Monsanto, Cargill or ADM are.

[1:6] Monsanto is the maker of DDT, PCBs, Aspartame, Agent Orange (also known as Round-Up), Bovine Growth Hormone (BGH), genetically engineered seeds, and Terminator Technology. Monsanto is well on its way to owning the majority of the world's seeds and they are affiliated with the world's largest seed developers and research companies. Together with Cargill—The largest privately held food conglomerate in the world, and ADM they own and/or control the majority of the western world's agriculture, animal husbandry, and food processing.

I. Principlism

A. Principlism's multiple criteria

[1:7] One approach that can be used to minimize such evaluative errors of threat is through the use of Principlism. Principlism is a practical approach for moral analysis and decision-making that is used by Institutional Review Boards—IRBs, for the protection of human research subjects. Principlism, as public policy, is meant to be compatible with, a variety of worldviews.

[1:8] Principlism has already proven its effectiveness in both the biomedical and the behavioral science fields in the protection of human research subjects. The origins of principlistic approach can be traced back to the Belmont Report, a Congressional mandate adopted by the Department of Health and Human Services—HHS.

[1:9] With Principlism there are the four principles of autonomy (informed consent), beneficence (do good), nonmaleficence (do no harm), and justice, be fair that are in nonhierarchical order, and each principle is to be specified and balanced with regard to each other in terms of applicability and importance as determined by the situation. This synergistic reflective equilibrium model provides the internal checks and balances that a single principle approach would not have.

[1:10] Principlism with its multiple principles, and its internal complexities, greatly expands its useful range of applicability.

B. Intersubjective Agreements

[1:11] Principlism provides a clear and distinct approach for the moral analysis of not only research on human subjects, but also for agricultural, animal husbandry and industrial food production in general.

[1:12] Historically philosophy has not been very effective in practically analyzing such topics because traditionally philosophy has been dependent on narrow incompatible worldviews. Practical solutions must recognize the benefits of diverse pluralistic societies and the need for diverse pluralistic public policy.

[1:13] Principlism is generally recognized as being derivable from, consistent with, or at least not in conflict with a multitude of worldviews as exemplified by theological and spiritual worldviews, scientific and naturalistic worldviews, and social and political worldviews.

[1:14] Principlism addresses the constructive dialogue between worldviews that have the intersubjective moral agreement of the broad and general principles of autonomy (informed consent), beneficence (do good), nonmaleficence (do no harm), and justice (be fair).

[1:15] However, the traditional moral justification and processes for making such political and corporate changes seem to be lacking or inadequate as they are dependent on agents who hold to differing worldviews agreeing on one particular worldview. When such mono-worldview approaches are used, "success" is usually defined by the dominant group "winning" through the progressive use of conflict, violence, and war.

[1:16] Principlism, provides the much-needed paradigm or framework for moral analysis and effective implementation of political and corporate changes in food systems within a pluralistic society that hold to many different types of worldviews.

C. Principlism Is Federal Law

[1:17] Principlism is federal law for all research on human subjects in which there is any type of direct or indirect federal funding.

[1:18] Every Institutional Review Board—IRB in the country must comply with the uniform criteria derived from the Belmont Report, here being referred to as Principlism.

[1:19] In response to the Belmont Report the Department of Health and Human Services—HHS revised and expanded its regulations for the protection of human research subjects.

D. Food Production Is Research

[1:20] The U.S. government defines Institutional research as follows:

INSTITUTIONAL RESEARCH
A systematic investigation, including research development, testing and evaluation, designed to develop or contribute to generalizable

[1:21] Although food systems and the human consumption of its products does not technically meet the above definition of "research" it is still not so far removed from being classified as a "type" of research on human subjects.

[1:22] When you consider the short term and long term consequences of genetically modified soybeans, corn, canola, and wheat cross pollinating with other traditional plants, or that of genetically modified Salmon that get loose and breed with the other wild Salmon, or the health consequences related to the consumption of corn-fed beef and highly processed and refined foods, then food science certainly can be classified as a "type" of research on human subjects. As research, the industrial food system violates all four principles of Principlism.

*** Principlism Evaluation: Research**

1. Autonomy:

[1:23] Consumers are not being informed as to the risks and harms of consuming the foods they purchase and therefore are not providing an informed consent which is a necessary condition for research—a violation of autonomy.

2. Beneficence:

[1:24] Consumers are not getting health benefits from much of the food that they consume which is a necessary condition for research—a violation of beneficence.

3. Nonmaleficence:

[1:25] Consumers are being exposed to significant risks and health burdens which is not allowed in research—a violation of nonmaleficence.

4. Justice:

[1:26] Many consumer groups have little economic choice but to consume the government subsidized cheap, empty calories that disproportionately affect the poor creating unequal distribution of subject burdens—a violation of justice.

[1:27] Food production is, under no uncertain terms, not only research on human subjects, but also research on the entire biota and environment. It is one thing for food production to negatively effect a current generation in which the harm was generated, but it is quite an entirely different matter when food systems negatively effect all future generations that had no part in the generation of the harm.

[1:28] Since food production has utterly failed in its ability to self-regulate, the government, whose prime directive is to protect individual rights and liberties in society, must compensate for that failure and regulate food production.

[1:29] However, the government has also failed to effectively regulate food production because corporate America, such as Monsanto, Cargill and ADM also have enormous economic interests and influence over government regulations. As a result the FDA, EPA and the Food Safety and Inspection Service—FSIS are being directed by individuals that have significant conflicts of interests in that they have either worked for, or are getting benefits from, Monsanto, Cargill and ADM, the very industrialized food producers that need to be regulated.

II. Feeding Corn To Cattle

A. Government Regulation

[2:1] The industrial food production giants, with their economic interests and lack of moral insight, and the DHH, FDA, EPA, and FSIS with there lack of being effective protective regulatory agencies, are unjustly exposing the public, biota and the environment to significant risks and harms without the public's consent.

[2:2] This is very similar to what happened with the for profit private pharmaceutical industry distribution of Thalidomide, "one of the biggest medical tragedies of modern times" which resulted in severe birth defects effecting up to 10,000 - 20,000 people, and the government human research Syphilis Study at Tuskegee, "arguably the most infamous biomedical research study in U.S. history" in which 399 impoverished black men were not informed that they had syphilis and were denied treatment when treatment was available.

[2:3] Those who were involved in the private distribution of drugs and those who were doing government research totally failed in the proper use of any reasonable moral reflectivity. Once exposed, the public outrage resulted in a congressional mandate that resulted in the Belmont Report—Principlism. HHS then adopted the moral principles of the Belmont Report, and mandated that every institution that received any direct or indirect federal funding, and performed any research on human subjects had to comply with the Belmont Report's principles. IRBs were then created in each institution in order to protect individuals who were research subjects. Government regulation, with the threat of loss of federal funding, became necessary in order to prevent the most outrageous forms of moral disregard.

[2:4] A credible threat of significant economic loss for noncompliance to reasonable moral reflectivity must also be made against food producers. An independent review board for moral analysis of food production activities using Principlism needs to be implemented, and enforced for the protection of food consumers, for those who are being consumed, and for the environment.

B. Anthropocentric Argument

[2:6] If the IRB criteria of Principlism were to be expanded to include agriculture and animal science, then not only would the treatment and welfare of human beings be improved, but the treatment and welfare of other species would also be indirectly improved.

[2:7] It can be argued that the indirect improvement of the treatment of other species is immoral as it is too anthropocentric—(human-centered) and that the improvement of the treatment of other species needs to be directly implemented by the recognition of their intrinsic worth from a biocentric or life-centered point of view.

[2:8] However, the reality of the matter is that our current society is not very receptive to biocentric—(life-centered), or naturalistic—(scientific-holism) standards. Most western people are anthropocentric, a point of view that has been perpetuated by theocentric—(God-centered) religious perspectives. Many people's theocentric worldviews are modified anthropocentric worldviews where God is anthropomorphized by attributing Him with both the image and attributes of man.

[2:9] In such a social context, the most effective arguments for the benefit of animals, are arguments that show that the conditions that make these animals suffer also results in unacceptable human harm and or human suffering.

[2:10] For example, feedlot cattle, in both the beef and dairy industries, results in cattle consuming very little grass, and a tremendous amount of corn, which their digestive rumen is not designed to digest.

[2:11] This corn diet results in the acidification of the rumen. The e-coli, which naturally exists in the colon of grass-fed cattle is usually destroyed by the acid in the human stomach making the e-coli harmless. However, corn in the cattle feed results in the acidification of the rumen, which normally has a pH between 6.0

- 6.2. This acidification of the rumen caused by the high starch corn diet resulted in the natural selection of the acid resistant strain Escherichia-coli O157:H7 that no one had seen before 1980. Now it is found in more than 40 percent of feedlot cattle and ingesting as few as ten of these microbes can cause a fatal infection to a human. E-coli 0157:H7 produces toxins that can destroy the human kidneys and no treatment is currently available for this type of food poisoning. If an infected person were to unfortunately be given antibiotics, then the antibiotics would kill the e-coli microbes but the resulting flood of toxins from the dead microbes could also destroy the kidneys and the patient as well.

[2:12] In addition, the rumen is also not designed for the acidic environment created by the eating of corn instead of grass and as a result the cattle develop painful ulcers and infections resulting in the need for the cattle to be treated with high doses of antibiotics or else they will slowly die, and in the case of dairy cattle, they would have an unacceptable amount of pus in the milk.

[2:13] This very high use of both preventative and therapeutic antibiotics for corn-fed beef is also the cause of the natural selection of strains of antibiotic resistant bacteria that also puts humans at significant health-risks when consumed.

[2:14] Therefore, the unnecessary and real risk of e-coli O157:H7, the pus filled antibiotic laden milk and cheese products, antibiotic resistant bacteria, the toxic runoff from the fertilizers used to grow the corn the cattle eat in which the nitrates convert to nitrites which binds to hemoglobin, compromising the blood's ability to carry oxygen to the brain, some of the ammonium nitrate evaporates and is transformed into nitrous oxide, an important greenhouse gas that contributes to global warming, and some of the fertilizers, herbicides and pesticides seep down contaminating the water table, the genetically modified corn and agricultural contamination that is spreading around the globe by pollination, and the contaminated animal sewage that is filled with heavy metals, chemicals, hormones, and other pharmaceuticals making the manure too toxic to be used even as fertilizers which inadvertently end up in waterways where downstream scientists have found fish and amphibians exhibiting abnormal sex characteristics, the nitrogen tides in the ocean that stimulates the excessive growth of algae creating a hypoxic dead zone, and the list of negative harmful effects to humans goes on and on, making it impossible to come to any other conclusion using the criteria of Principlism that such practices are anything but immoral, wrong and ought to be made illegal. The function of law is to prevent and protect citizens from such unnecessary human harms that affect not only the current generation but all future generations as well.

[2:15] Concentrated Animal Feeding Operations—CAFOs is one such unnecessary harmful activity that is usually done in order to maximize dairy production, or to quickly fatten up the cattle during the last six to eight months before slaughter. For beef cattle, because of the high proportion of corn that is being fed to them, 180 days is about the maximum amount of time that the toxic diet can be "tolerated" by the cattle before their abscessed livers are blown out.

[2:16] What makes this practice of grain-fed cattle even more outrageous is the fact that economically, the increased cost per cattle, if they were to be only grass-fed would only be around $25 per/head.

[2:17] Grass-fed beef is much more healthy in that it is leaner, has three times more omega-3 fatty acids, and for many people tastes better too. Scientific research now indicates that many of the health-related problems associated with the eating red meat is really a problem of eating corn-fed beef. Just as ruminants are ill adapted to eating corn so also humans are ill adapted to eating ruminants that eat corn.

[2:18] If the true cost of grain-fed beef were to include all the externalized costs to the consumers and environment, grain-fed beef would be prohibitively expensive.

*** Principlism Evaluation: Anthropocentric**

1. Autonomy:

[2:19] Since humans are being exposed to significant risks and burdensome consequences because of the consumption of corn-fed beef and dairy products, and because most human consumers are: a) being manipulated by culture and advertising, b) not being provided with full disclosure of what they are consuming, along with c) their inability to evaluate and act on scientific evidence of what good wholesome food choices are, it follows that most human consumers have not given an informed consent to the eating of corn-fed beef and dairy products. Therefore the feeding of corn to cattle is a violation of human autonomy.

2. Beneficence:

[2:20] Since it is more beneficial for humans to consume grass-fed beef and dairy products rather than corn-fed beef and dairy products it follows that the feeding of corn to cattle is a violation of beneficence.

3. Nonmaleficence:

[2:21] Since it is risky and harmful for humans to consume corn-fed beef and dairy products as compared to grass-fed beef and dairy products, the feeding of corn to cattle is a violation of nonmaleficence.

4. Justice:

[2:22] Since the human consumption of meat and dairy products from corn-fed cattle is currently cheaper than grass-fed cattle this has resulted in the unequal distribution of benefits and burdens across economic and educational classes. Corn-fed cattle products are more burdensome for the poor and uneducated than those who are more wealthy and educated because grass-fed cattle products are prohibitively expensive for the poor, and information as to the benefits and burdens of food choices are more difficult to acquire and understand for the uneducated than the educated. Therefore, the feeding of corn to cattle is a violation of justice.

[2:23] This anthropocentric argument that shows that it is a violation of autonomy (informed consent), beneficence (do good), nonmaleficence (do no harm), and justice (be fair), to feed cattle a high starch diet of corn is an effective argument for for the anthropocentric majority in which arguments for animal rights and animal welfare based on the pain and suffering of sentient beings has little to no effect on their food consumption.

C. Biocentric Argument

[2:25] Animal welfare and rights arguments, for the biocentric minority in society, would be that sentient beings avoid pain and suffering as much as possible and therefore it is not in their interest or preference to be subjected to pain and suffering. Therefore, it is morally wrong for human beings to unnecessarily inflict pain and suffering on any sentient being and to unnecessarily treat any subject-of-a-life solely as a means to an end, all of which is currently being done with regard to our meat and dairy production.

[2:26] From a biocentric point of view the feeding of corn to cattle results in the acidification of the rumen which results in painful ulcers, diarrhea, bloat, rumenitis, liver disease, and a general weakening of the immune system that leaves the animals vulnerable to feedlot diseases such as pneumonia, coccidiosis, enterotoxemia, feedlot polio, etc. The high starch corn diet would eventually kill the cattle because over time the acids eat away at the rumen wall, allowing bacteria to enter the animal's bloodstream. These microbes wind up in the liver, where they form abscesses and impair the liver's function. To keep the cattle alive long enough for slaughter at the CAFOs, which is about 180 days, the cattle are given prodigious amounts of antacids and antibiotics. In fact, most of the antibiotics sold in America today go into animal feed causing the natural selection of antibiotic resistant strains of bacteria. From this biocentric point of view, the feeding of corn to cattle is biologically unnatural and causes the sentient being to experience unacceptable amounts of pain and suffering.

*** Principlism Evaluation: Biocentric**

1. Autonomy:

[2:27] Cattle are herbivores that have one of the most evolved digestive systems of all living beings. However, their rumens are not adapted for high starch diets or animal flesh products. It follows that cattle have not and would not choose to eat high starch corn, meat, fat, blood, and the arsenal of pharmaceutical drugs that are necessary because of such a diet. It also follows that since cattle are sentient beings, they would never choose to be exposed to the pain and suffering that is associated with such diets and CAFO living arrangements. Therefore, the feeding of high starch diets such as corn to cattle is a violation of animal autonomy.

2. Beneficence:

[2:28] Since there is no personal benefit for cattle to be eating corn, meat, fat, blood, and the necessary arsenal of pharmaceutical drugs because of such a diet, and since being kept in a CAFO is also not in the cattle's best interests with regard to comfort, and communicable diseases, it follows that the feeding of high starch diets such as corn to cattle is a violation of beneficence.

3. Nonmaleficence:

[2:29] Since being kept in a CAFO and being fed a high starch diet of corn, meat, fat, blood, and the arsenal of pharmaceutical drugs that are necessary because of such a diet is harmful to the cattle and results in communicable diseases and unnecessary pain and suffering, it follows that the feeding of corn to cattle is a violation of nonmaleficence.

4. Justice:

[2:30] Since living in a CAFO and being fed the high starch diet of corn, meat, fat, blood, and the arsenal of pharmaceutical drugs that are necessary because of such a diet is unnatural and particularly burdensome for cattle, it follows that there is an unfair distribution of benefits and burdens. Therefore, the feeding of corn to cattle is a violation of justice.

[2:31] This biocentric argument that shows that it is a violation of autonomy, beneficence, nonmaleficence and justice to feed cattle a high starch diet of corn is an effective argument for those who have worldviews that are more biocentric and holistic.

D. Human Rights and Animal Rights

[2:32] If HHS, FDA, EPA, and FSIS were to subject agriculture and animal science to the criteria of Principlism then the feeding of corn to cattle would have to be both a human rights violation and an animal rights violation.

[2:33] Humans have a positive right to the accessibility of good wholesome food and a negative right of not being deceived into thinking that unwholesome foods are wholesome.

[2:34] Domesticated animals that are dependent on humans for sustenance have a positive right to be fed good wholesome food as determined by their biological species, and a negative right of not having their natural diets and habits unnecessarily interfered with when the burdens outweigh the benefits for the animal.

[2:35] The anthropocentric, biocentric, and holistic worldviews all conclude that the feeding of corn to cattle violates all four principles of autonomy, beneficence, nonmaleficence, and justice. It is also the case that human rights and animal rights, both positive and negative, are being violated by the feeding of corn to cattle. Therefore, the only logical conclusion for any rational human being, regardless of worldviews or perspectives, is that the feeding of high starch diets such as corn to cattle is immoral and wrong and ought to be prohibited.

III. Heuristic Biases

A. Availability Heuristic

[3:1] The availability heuristic is the propensity to put higher probability of an event occurring on those events in which there is a higher availability of recollection, than those in which there are fewer recollections. Often times this intuition works well, other times it doesn't work so well as exemplified by people being more afraid of a terrorist attack than Monsanto. Industrial food producers stay as invisible as possible as the less people know about them and what they do, the less they will object and the less they will be fearful. For example, with all the different name brand beef products at the supermarket, who would have thought that in this country Tyson subsidiary IBP, Cargill subsidiary Excel, Swift & Company, and National, slaughter and market four out of five beef. Most consumers haven't even heard of IBP, Excel, Swift & Company or National. This of course is intentional. If consumers don't know who produces the products they consume then there can be no distrust, fear, or blame attributed to them.

B. Adjustment Anchoring Heuristic

[3:2] Another heuristic bias is called adjustment anchoring where people are psychologically biased toward the probability of the initial starting point.

[3:3] For example, in complex systems where there are multiple components that all have a low probability of failure the complex system as a whole can in fact have a very high rate of failure. However, the intuitive heuristic error of adjustment anchoring is that people will have a tendency to underestimate the probabilities of failure in such complex systems. Food production and the human body are such complex systems, and when people ingest multiple "low risk" products, people intuitively conclude that the health risk is low, when in reality the health risk is very high. Consumption of such products can result in numerous kinds of system failures such as cancers, heart disease and Alzheimer's just to name a few. Unfortunately food producers and their regulators take economic advantage of this psychological propensity for consumers to use the heuristic bias of adjustment anchoring with the products they are consuming. It is not unusual for industrialized food products to have multiple "low risk" ingredients in a single product so that when an individual eats the product, or multiple products, the risks become compounded and the products can become dangerously unhealthy.

[3:4] Corporations in the food industry are capitalizing on these naturally occurring intuitive heuristic biases by becoming intimately involved in the creation and implementation of public policies. These public policies promote the interests of industrialized food production, at the expense of both the consumers and those who are being consumed.

*** Principlism Evaluation: Heuristic Errors**

1. Autonomy:

[3:5] Consumers are not being informed as to who is producing what, how they are being produced, and what the total risk is when consuming food products. Consumers because of the availability and adjustment anchoring heurists are therefore not providing an informed consent—a violation of autonomy.

2. Beneficence:

[3:6] Corporations are economically benefiting from consumers not being autonomous. Corporate food producers have very little regard towards providing good wholesome food to consumers. Therefore, corporations are not all that concerned for the best interests of the consumer and are capitalizing on the availability and adjustment anchoring heurists—a violation of beneficence.

3. Nonmaleficence:

[3:7] Consumers are being exposed to significant risks and health burdens by the foods they are consuming. Corporations are lacing food products with all types of toxic chemicals capitalizing on the availability and adjustment anchoring heurists—a violation of nonmaleficence.

4. Justice:

[3:8] Low economic consumers have very few options other than consuming that which the corporate giants provide them. This monopolistic imbalance of necessary basic needs is unacceptable in a democratic society and is accomplished by capitalizing on the availability and adjustment anchoring heurists—a violation of justice.

IV. Conflict of Interests

[4:1] One of the main responsibilities of the EPA, FDA, and Food Safety and Inspection Service is to effectively regulate harmful substances for human and animal consumption. In order for this to occur it is recognized that conflict of interests must be minimized as much as possible. However, it is often times the case that government policy, that is meant to regulate a particular corporation, is developed by that very corporation itself. This, of course, is a conflict of interests.

A. EPA

[4:2] The EPA is charged with the responsibility to protect human health and the environment, by writing and enforcing regulations based on laws passed by Congress.

[4:3] The EPA employs 17,000 people, has 10 regional offices and 27 laboratories. The main problem with the EPA is that the White House has direct control over the EPA and it enforcements are subject to whoever is in power. Republicans and Democrats differ in their approaches and concerns towards the environment.

[4:4] In April of 2008, the Union of Concerned Scientists said that more than half of the 1,600 EPA staff scientists reported that they had experienced political interference in their work. The highest number of complaints came from scientists who were involved in the determination of the risks of cancer by chemicals used in food and other aspects of everyday life.

[4:5] Part of the problem comes from the White House. Linda Fisher, for example, who was the appointed EPA Deputy Administrator from 2000–2003, was also Vice President of Government and Public Affairs for Monsanto from 1995–2000, one of the very companies the EPA needs to regulate, creating a serious conflict of interest.

B. FDA

[4:6] The FDA is no better. Margaret Miller was the Chemical Lab Supervisor for Monsanto from 1985–1989. She then became the FDA Branch Chief in 1989. When clinical trials showed that cows were getting mastitis—(pus in the milk), caused by dairy cattle consuming a high starch diet of corn and developing ulcers and infections, she changed the antibiotic protocol and increased the amounts of permissible antibiotic residues in milk by 100 times. As a result, when the Consumer's Union tested milk in the New York metropolitan area they found the presence of 52 different antibiotics in the milk samples. The Wall Street Journal did their own tests and confirmed those results.

[4:7] Monsanto executives are being appointed to leadership positions for the EPA and FDA without it being considered a conflict of interest. Michael Taylor was a King & Spaulding Lawyer from 1984–1991 and their primary client was Monsanto. He became the FDA Deputy Commissioner for Policy from 1991–1994 and oversaw the FDA's decision not to label genetically modified foods.

[4:8] After his FDA stint he then went back to Monsanto as Vice President for Public Policy from 1998–2000.

C. White House Council On Environmental Quality

[4:9] One last, of many possible examples of conflicts of interests, is Philip Cooney, former chief of staff for the Bush White House Council on Environmental Quality, and former lobbyist for the American Petroleum Institute.

[4:10] A June 2005 memo revealed that Cooney had personally edited documents, summarizing government research on climate change, before their release. Cooney resigned two days after the memo was published in *The New York Times* and then one week later he took a job at Exxon Mobil in their public affairs department.

* Principlism Evaluation: Conflict Of Interests

1. Autonomy:

[4:11] Democracies are based on the Jeffersonian principle of an informed electorate. Instead consumers are being kept uninformed for the economic gains of corporations. Corporations have successfully infiltrated government policy process in order to keep people as uninformed as possible—a violation of autonomy.

2. Beneficence:

[4:12] Government is to represent the best interests of its citizens. Instead the government is representing the best interest of corporations at the expense of consumers—a violation of beneficence.

3. Nonmaleficence:

[4:13] Government is meant to protect its citizens from unwanted risks and harms such as those presented by food producers. Corporations are lacing food products with all types of toxic chemicals just so that they can maximize profits—a violation of nonmaleficence.

4. Justice:

[4:14] Government has created a legislative environment in which corporations have a monopolistic influence on public policy. As a result consumers have very few options other than consuming that which the corporate giants provide them. This monopolistic imbalance of necessary basic needs is unacceptable in a democracy—a violation of justice.

V. Legislation

A. Conflict Of Interest Laws

[5:1] The DHH, EPA, FDA, FSIS has failed the American public by not paying close attention to conflicts of interests. Not only has the government increased profits for corporations at the expense of the consuming public, animals, agriculture, and ecosystem, but it has also failed to keep itself independent of legitimate conflicts of interests. As a result the government has failed to determine just what is "safe" both with regard to consumable products and with regard to agricultural, chemical, or environmental contaminants.

[5:2] What is necessary if government regulation is to work is the legislation of much stricter conflict of interest laws. Government protective agencies must not be unduly influenced by corporate and political influence and the government must promote the principles of autonomy, beneficence, nonmaleficence, and justice.

B. Subpart F: Animal Husbandry and Agriculture

[5:3] Society needs to expand the application of Principlism that is currently used by HHS to protect human research subjects to include more disciplines, other species, agriculture and the ecosystem as a whole. One logical way, that has historical precedence, would be for the Department of Health and Human Services—HHS to expand the legal scope of Title 45 Part 46: Protection of Human Subjects to include a Subpart F: Additional Considerations for Animal Husbandry and Agriculture.

[5:4]

[5:5] Subpart A is the basic HHS policy for the protection of human research subjects that establishes the IRB, and the Principlistic approach. The addition of Subpart F would significantly add to the protection of not only human subjects but it would also protect nonhuman sentient beings and indirectly plants and the environment as well. This added subpart would also be consistent with the other added Subparts as Subparts B, C, and D, already represent other vulnerable groups and those that are unable to represent themselves, i.e., pregnant women, fetuses, neonates, prisoners, and children. The added Subpart F proposed here would then add the vulnerable group of nonhuman sentient beings—NHSB who also cannot represent themselves as an entity per say. If Subpart F were to be adopted then Part 46 would probably also have to change its current title of Protection of Human Subjects to a more inclusive title such as Protection of Research Subjects.

Conclusion

[5:6] In conclusion, it has now become necessary to regulate and protect humans, animals, and agriculture from what is currently the most significant threat towards society, industrial food production. Although there isn't a single solution to the fact that the industrial food production industry has failed in its ability to self-regulate and to be regulated, the following would start the restorative process:

[5:7]

1. Implement stricter conflict of interest laws for government regulators,

2. Have Congress mandate that: the Food and Drug Administration—FDA, the Environmental Protection Agency—EPA and the Food Safety and Inspection Service—FSIS adopt the Belmont Report principles that are currently used by the Department of Health and Human Services—HHS for regulating research on human subjects, and

3. Have HHS expand Title 45 Part 46 of the Code of Federal Regulations to include a Subpart F: Additional Considerations for Animal Husbandry and Agriculture.

[5:8]

FOOD SYSTEM THREAT SOLUTION
I. Implement Stricter Conflict of Interest Laws II. Congress Must Mandate That The FDA, EPA, FSIS Adopt Principlism III. Expand 45CFR46 To Include Subpart F: Animal Husbandry and Agriculture

[5:9] It is well past the time for society to extend the implementation of Principlism to all areas of food production. Effective regulation, such as the prohibiting of the feeding of corn to cattle, will result in not only a more fair, equal and just society, but a safer society as well.

[5:11]

Proposal: Subpart F: Additional Considerations for Animal Husbandry and Agriculture.

CFR Title 45: Public Welfare, DHH, Part 46: Protection of Research Subjects

[5:12]

§46.601 To whom do these regulations apply?

(a) This subpart applies to all research involving nonhuman sentient beings. This includes all research conducted or supported by the Department of Health and Human Services.

(1) This includes research conducted by Department employees.

(2) It also includes research conducted or supported by the Department of Health and Human Services outside the United States.

(b) Nothing in this subpart shall be construed as indicating that compliance with the procedures set forth herein will authorize research involving nonhuman sentient beings as subjects, to the extent such research is limited or barred by applicable State or local law.

(c) Exemptions (Need to be written)

[5:13]

§46.602 Definition

The definition in §46.102 of subpart B shall be applicable to this subpart as well. In addition, as used in this subpart:

(a) *Sentient beings* are any living beings that can experience pain and or suffering either physically or mentally.

(b) *Nonhuman sentient being—NHSB* is any sentient being that is not a human being.

(c) *NHSB guardian* means an individual or group who is authorized under applicable State or local law to consent on behalf of the NHSB based on the promotion of the NHSB best interest.

[5:14]

§46.603 IRB duties

In addition to other responsibilities assigned to IRBs under this part, each IRB shall review research covered by this subpart and approve only research which satisfies the conditions of all applicable sections of this subpart.

[5:15]

§46.603 IRB duties

In addition to other responsibilities assigned to IRBs under this part, each IRB shall review research covered by this subpart and approve only research which satisfies the conditions of all applicable sections of this subpart.

[5:16]

§46.604 Research not involving greater than minimal risk.

HHS will conduct or fund research in which the IRB finds that no greater than minimal risk to nonhuman sentient beings is presented by an intervention or procedure that holds out the prospect of direct benefit for the being, or by a monitoring procedure that is likely to contribute to the subject's well-being, only if the IRB finds that:

(a) the risk is justified by the anticipated benefit to the subjects

(b) the relation of the anticipated benefit to the risk is at least as favorable to the subjects as that presented by available alternative approaches; and

(c) adequate provisions are made for soliciting permission of the NHSB guardians.

[5:17]

§46.406 Research involving greater than minimal risk and no prospect of direct benefit to individual subjects, but likely to yield generalizable knowledge about the subject's disorder or condition.

HHS will conduct or fund research in which the IRB finds that more than minimal risk to NHSB is presented by an intervention or procedure that does not hold out the prospect of direct benefit for the NHSB, or by a monitoring procedure which is not likely to contribute to the well-being of the subject, only if the IRB finds that:

(a) The risk represents a minor increase over minimal risk;

(b) The intervention or procedure presents experiences to subjects that are reasonably commensurate with those inherent in their actual or expected situations;

(c) The intervention or procedure is likely to yield generalizable knowledge about the subjects' disorder or condition which is of vital importance for the understanding or amelioration of the subjects' disorder or condition; and

(d) Adequate provisions are made for soliciting assent of the NHSB guardians.

[5:18]

§46.607 Research not otherwise approvable which presents an opportunity to understand, prevent, or alleviate a serious problem affecting the health or welfare of NHSB.

HHS will conduct or fund research that the IRB does not believe meets the requirements of §46.604, §46.605, §46.606 only if:

(a) The IRB finds that the research presents a reasonable opportunity to further the understanding, prevention, or alleviation of a serious problem affecting the health or welfare of the NHSB.

(b) The Secretary, after consultation with a panel of experts in pertinent disciplines (for example: science, medicine, ethics, law) and following opportunity for public review and comment, has determined either:

(1) That the research in fact satisfies the conditions of §46.604, §46.605, §46.606, as applicable, or (2) the following:

(i) the research presents a reasonable opportunity to further the understanding, prevention, or alleviation of a serious problem affecting the health or welfare of NHSB.

(ii) The research will be conducted in accordance with sound ethical principles; adequate provisions are made for soliciting the permission of the NHSB guardian.

[5:19]

§46.608 Requirements for permission by guardians.

Permissions by guardians shall be documented in accordance with and to the extent required by §46.117 of subpart A.

[5:20]

§46.609 Wards

(a) NHSB who are wards of the state or any other agency, institution, or entity can be included in research approved under §46.606, or §46.607 only if such research is related to their status as wards.

(b) If the research is approved under paragraph (a) of this section, the IRB shall require appointment of an advocate for each NHSB who is a ward, in addition to any other individual's action on behalf of the NHSB as guardian. One individual may serve as advocate for more than one NHSB. The advocate shall be an individual who has the background and experience to act in, and agrees to act in, the best interests of the NHSB for the duration of the NHSB participation in the research and who is not associated in any way (except in the role as advocate or member of the IRB) with the research, the investigator(s), or the guardian organization.

***

4. MEDICAL MARIJUANA

Case Study: Gonzalez v Raich

[1:1]

By a vote of 6-3 the U.S. Supreme Court ruled in June of 2005 that patients who use marijuana for medical purposes are not immune from federal prosecution. In Gonzalez v Raich the Court decreed that patients who possessed marijuana were liable to criminal prosecution by federal law enforcement personnel, even if the drug has been prescribed by a physician practicing in a state whose laws permit such prescriptions. Currently 36 states have laws that allow physicians to prescribe marijuana for seriously ill patients. The laws protect doctors and other care providers, as well as patients, from prosecution if the drug is prescribed/used to control pain and suffering. Most physicians who do prescribe marijuana report doing so after more traditional drugs have failed to provide relief. The medical use of marijuana has gained favor among patients with chronic nausea or anorexia (e.g., AIDS patients, patients undergoing cancer chemotherapy), chronic pain (e.g., glaucoma, migraine headaches), and muscle spasticity (e.g., multiple sclerosis and other neurological conditions). Patients who use marijuana to alleviate these symptoms typically report significant relief of pain and suffering, as well as an improved ability to live more normal lives. Such marked improvement, they argue, demonstrates that marijuana is a legitimate medical treatment that, like any other medical treatment, is the business of and only of patients and physicians. Gonzalez v Raich concerned two California women, Angel Raich and Diane Monson, who suffered from diverse serious medical problems, and had both used marijuana for several years, on their doctors' recommendations, to alleviate symptoms of their conditions. (Angel Raich's doctor expressed the opinion that without access to marijuana Ms Raich would experience excruciating pain that could prove fatal.) Ms Raich was provided marijuana at no charge by two of her caregivers, and Ms Monson cultivated her own marijuana plants. In 2002 agents from the federal Drug Enforcement Administration (DEA) enforced the 1970 federal Controlled Substances Act (CSA) against Ms Raich and Ms Monson, even though local (county) law enforcement officials had concluded that their use of marijuana was entirely legal under California law. In this regard, in 1976 California had enacted, by referendum, a law known as the Compassionate Use Act, designed to assure that severely ill patients have access to marijuana for medical purposes. There was one legal issue presented to the Supreme Court in Gonzalez v Raich—whether the enforcement of the CSA against Ms Raich and Ms Monson by DEA agents was constitutional under the commerce clause of the U.S. Constitution (Article 1, section 8), which confers upon Congress the power to regulate interstate commerce. Based upon a review of its prior cases interpreting the commerce clause, the Supreme Court concluded, by a 6-3 vote, that the DEA agents had acted within the scope of their legitimate legal authority. In announcing this conclusion, however, the Court also stated the following words, which describe the case as both difficult and troubling: [This] case is made difficult by [Ms Raich's and Ms Monson's] strong arguments that they will suffer irreparable harms [M]arijuana does have valid therapeutic purposes. The question before us, however, is not whether it is wise to enforce the [CSA] in these circumstances; rather, it is whether Congress' power to regulate interstate markets for medicinal substances encompasses the portions of those markets that are supplied with drugs produced and consumed locally. Well settled law controls our answer. The CSA is a valid exercise of federal power, even as applied to the troubling facts of this case.

Introduction

[1:2] Principlism is a practical approach for moral decision-making that focuses on four major principles: autonomy (informed consent), beneficence (do good), nonmaleficence (do no harm), and justice (be fair).

[1:3] The four principles that make up the principlistic approach are broad general concepts that most individuals and cultures share as important and vital for moral decision-making. These principles are derivable from, consistent with, or at least not in contradiction with most moral frameworks. This puts Principlism in a unique position in that its epistemic justification is not essential for the presentation of its moral evaluation. Principlism is also an excellent approach when dealing with pluralistic and diversified populations that are attempting to come to a shared moral consensus.

[1:4] Principlism is a nonhierarchical approach in that no one, or group of principles, is any more important than any other principle. It may be the case that one principle is more relevant for a particular case than the other principles, but that would have to be determined case by case.

[1:5] The Medical Marijuana case will be evaluated not by order of importance of the principles but rather by standard order of presentation of Autonomy, Beneficence, Nonmaleficence, and Justice.

I. Determine The Relevant Parties

[1:6] In this Medical Marijuana case we have at least three major competing parties that are each claiming sovereignty:

1. United States Federal Government

2. State Government

3. Individual Citizens

II. Autonomy

[2:1] Etymologically, autonomy comes from two Greek words of *autos*; meaning self, and *noumos*; meaning rule, i.e., self-rule. Historically, autonomy, or self-rule was used for the establishment of the sovereignty of countries. It was generally considered that a sovereign country was autonomous in that other countries were not to interfere with the self-rule of that country.

[2:2] In contemporary society, this autonomy of "states" or "countries" has been extended to individual "citizens," and "non-citizens" alike and due to international law autonomy is now considered a basic human right.

[2:3] What needs to be evaluated here is how to specify the principle of autonomy for each group and then how to balance the legitimate competing interests.

[2:4] To be autonomous it has generally been recognized that three necessary components must be met:

1. Intentionality

2. Knowledge

3. Freedom

[2:5] Intentionality is the actual activity of making a choice. It is not a matter of degree, rather the agent makes a choice of one type or the other.

[2:6] Knowledge and freedom, in contrast with intentionality, is a matter of degree as no agent can be totally informed and no action is in accord with total freedom. Therefore, the goal is to have substantial knowledge and substantial freedom.

Rights

[2:7] Autonomy, as a human right, results in certain social responsibilities with regard to the above three necessary conditions. When there is any kind of "right" it always means that others have some type of obligation that can be broken down under the following two categories:

1. Positive Rights:

When others have an obligation to provide something.

2. Negative Rights:

When others have an obligation to not interfere.

A. Intentionality Defined

[2:8] Intentionality is primarily a negative right, in that others have an obligation of not interfering with a person's choice. However, intentionality is also a positive right, especially with regard to healthcare, in that there are recognized responsibilities of others to provide services, medicine—i.e. medicinal marijuana, and other provisions that are necessary for the exercise of intention.

1) Federal Government

[2:9] With regard to intention in the Medical Marijuana case, the Federal Government has failed under both negative rights criteria and positive rights criteria as it interfered with the legitimate personal choices, and it did not provide for legitimate needs such as medical marijuana.

2) State Government

[2:10] It is inconclusive whether or not the State Government of California would have acted under justified intent as the law allowing the use of medical marijuana was passed by referendum in which the public forces a single issue vote by the public bypassing public politicians.

3) Individual Citizens

[2:11] Individual Citizens of the State of California, by virtue of their referendum forced the passing of legislation that respects both positive and negative rights by providing a means of dispensing medicinal marijuana without violating federal commerce laws and by not interfering with legitimate personal choices.

Conclusion on Intentionality

1) Federal Government

[2:12] Although the Federal Government, under the direction of Gonzalez and those political leaders who supported him, exercised intention, the intentional act will have to be considered as invalid and immoral as it is in direct contradiction to recognized basic human negative and positive rights and its resultant social responsibilities.

2) State Government

[2:13] Inconclusive

3) Individual Citizens

[2:14] Only the Individual Citizens in this case exercised a legitimate act of intention.

B. Knowledge

1) Federal Government

[2:15] "There was one legal issue presented to the Supreme Court in Gonzalez v Raich. Whether the enforcement of the federal Controlled Substances Act (CSA) against Ms Raich and Ms Monson by DEA agents was constitutional under the commerce clause of the U.S. Constitution (Article 1, section 8), which confers upon Congress the power to regulate interstate commerce. Based upon a review of its prior cases interpreting the commerce clause, the Supreme Court concluded, by a 6-3 vote, that the DEA agents had acted within the scope of their legitimate legal authority."

[2:16] Article I, Section 8, Clause 3 of the United States Constitution, known as the Commerce Clause, reads as follows: "The Congress shall have Power ...To regulate Commerce with foreign Nations, and among the several States, and with the Indian Tribes."

[2:17] However, "Ms Raich was provided marijuana at no charge by two of her caregivers, and Ms Monson cultivated her own marijuana plants. In 2002 agents from the federal Drug Enforcement Administration (DEA) enforced the 1970 federal Controlled Substances Act (CSA) against Ms Raich and Ms Monson, even though local (county) law enforcement officials had concluded that their use of marijuana was entirely legal under California law."

[2:18] Clearly, with the information that has been given by this case the foreign, state, and tribal commerce laws have little if any relation to this medical marijuana case. Therefore the Federal Government has failed the necessary condition of substantial knowledge for acting autonomously.

2) State Government

[2:19] Medicinal use of marijuana was legal in the state of residence of Ms. Raich. Since this law was implemented by a public referendum it is inconclusive whether or not the State Government would have met the necessary condition of substantial knowledge.

3) Individual Citizens

[2:20] "Angel Raich[1]s doctor expressed the opinion that without access to marijuana Ms Raich would experience excruciating pain that could prove fatal." Ms Raich was sufficiently informed about her condition by her doctor and therefore was acting with substantial understanding. Since no court, nor professional medical association ever questioned the competency of Ms Raich's doctor, we can only infer that his conclusions were reasonable with the information that he had.

Conclusion on Knowledge

1. Federal Government

[2:21] The Federal Government failed to make their case of a violation of interstate commerce and therefore failed in making a rational or "knowledgeable" case against Ms Raich and Ms Monson.

2. State Government

[2:22] Inconclusive

3. Individual Citizens

[2:23] Ms Raich and Ms Monson were acting with substantial understanding with regard to their condition and effects of medical marijuana.

C. Freedom

1) Federal Government

[2:24] Being that interstate commerce has little if anything to do with this case, and being that the best interests of Ms Raich was certainly not being considered, it is clear that the Federal Government, under the leadership of Mr. Gonzalez and his political supporters, were exercising powers with little or no concern for its citizens. This type of irrational behavior cannot be considered as substantial freedom for the purpose of autonomy especially considering the logical inconsistency with the spirit of freedom as outlined by the constitution and the violation of its citizen's positive and negative rights.

2) State Government

[2:25] Inconclusive

3) Individual Citizens

[2:26] Ms Raich and Ms Monson both were following prescribed medicinal use of marijuana in accord with their primary physician. Both patients did so making sure that they were not violating any state law or federal interstate commerce laws. The only effective treatment available—medicinal marijuana was maximizing both patient's medical best interests. All things considered it appears that Ms Raich and Ms Monson had made their decision based on substantial freedom as there appears to be no manipulation, coercion, or other illegitimate means of persuasion used on them.

Conclusion on Freedom

1) Federal Government

[2:27] Failed with regard to the legitimate exercise of freedom as it violated basic human rights of positive and negative rights.

2) State Government

[2:28] Inconclusive.

3) Individual Citizens

[2:29] Ms Raich and Ms Monson appear to have made an autonomous decision in full exercise of substantial freedom.

Conclusion on Autonomy

1) Federal Government

[2:30] The Federal Government has failed all three necessary conditions of legitimate intent, substantial knowledge and substantial freedom. As a result the Federal Government cannot be considered autonomous with regard to this case.

2) State Government

[2:31] Inconclusive

3) Individual Citizens

[2:32] Ms Raich and Ms Monson, and the Californian citizens met all three necessary conditions of autonomy with intent, substantial knowledge and substantial freedom. Therefore the Individual Citizens will have to be considered autonomous.

D. Informed Consent

[2:33] Autonomy as a practical application has been put forth both legally and as a basic human right in terms of Informed Consent. Informed Consent has two necessary conditions:

1. Autonomous Authorization

2. Institutional or Legal Authorization

[2:34] Failure to meet any one of the above necessary conditions will invalidate the "informed consent."

[2:35] The Autonomous Authorization condition is met when the agent has and understands the sufficient information necessary for making the decision, and has sufficient freedom to make the decision, and then through the exercise of intent, makes the decision.

[2:36] The Institutional or Legal Authorization, is the legal responsibility of an institution or agent as to what must be disclosed and or provisions provided to those who are in a position of making a decision. This is usually presented in the form of risks and burdens with a required signature indicating that the agent has read and understood the material presented. However, it is often times the case that the Institutional or legal authorization is completed without the autonomous authorization criteria being met as the agent has signed the legal authorization without substantial understanding or freedom.

[2:37] Informed consent is also based on the legal premise that the agent has decisional-capacity to make a decision. Competency is a term that means, "ability to perform a task." It is possible to have decisional-capacity in some areas of decision-making but lack decisional-capacity in other areas of decision-making. The necessary conditions for decisional-capacity are exactly the same as autonomy: intent, substantial knowledge, and substantial freedom. However, these necessary conditions are rarely verified for the purpose of legal consent. The interesting twist that results is that it is possible to be considered legally competent—e.g., based on being a citizen and of legal age, yet not be autonomous with regard to a particular decision. However, if a person or agent is autonomous, then that person or agent has decisional-capacity regardless of their legal standing.

Conclusion on Informed Consent

1. Federal Government

[2:38] The Federal Government would have to be considered both incompetent and in violation of informed consent with regard to medical marijuana. Incompetent as it failed on all three necessary conditions of decisional-capacity, and because of these failures it also failed to meet the autonomy conditions of all the Informed Consent conditions.

2. State of California

[2:39] The State of California moral position is inconclusive.

3. Individual Citizens

[2:40] The Individual Citizens—Ms Raich and Ms Monson would have to be considered Autonomous, Competent with decisional-capacity and meeting all the conditions of Informed Consent.

III. Nonmaleficence

[3:1] Nonmaleficence is the principle of minimizing burdens.

[3:2] Nonmaleficence is a:

1. Perfect obligation

a. specifies what the action or refrainment in question is, and

b. specifies to whom the action is or is not to be directed towards, (e.g., do not kill your brother)

2. Negative requirement of refrainment

3. Agent must be impartial

4. Failure to refrain often results in legal punishment

[3:3] It is possible to sufficiently live a life that fulfills the principle of nonmaleficence towards most people. Therefore failure to act nonmaleficently is considered immoral.

Conclusion on Nonmaleficence

1. Federal Government

[3:4] In the Medical Marijuana case the Federal Government under the direction of Gonzalez and the supporting political leaders failed with regard to the principle of nonmaleficence in that they had very little if any concern with regard to the minimization of burdens for Ms Raich or Ms Monson. The Federal Government negligently failed with regard to their perfect obligations. The Federal Government's attitude was that if Ms Raich and Ms Monson suffer more or if Ms Raich dies because of the Federal Government's interference in the medicinal use of marijuana then that would be just unfortunate.

[3:5] Since the failure to act nonmaleficently is considered as immoral the conclusion is that the Federal Government under the direction of Gonzalez and his supporters were acting immorally.

2. State Government

[3:6] Inconclusive

3. Individual Citizens

[3:7] Ms Raich and Ms Monson both were acting responsibly with regard to the principle of nonmaleficence. Medicinal use of marijuana was for the purpose of the minimization of medical burdens and since they were able to effectively fulfill their perfect obligations by minimizing their burdens they therefore acted morally.

IV. Beneficence

[4:1] Beneficence is the principle of maximizing benefits.

[4:2] Beneficence is a:

1. Imperfect obligation

a. does not specify what the action or refrainment in question is, and

b. does not specify to whom the action is or is not to be directed towards, (e.g., charity)

2. Positive requirement of action

3. Agent need not be impartial

4. Failure to act positively rarely results in legal punishment

[4:3] It is impossible to live a life that fulfills the principle of beneficence towards most people. Therefore failure to act beneficently is not necessarily considered immoral.

Conclusion on Beneficence

1. Federal Government

[4:4] In the Medical Marijuana case the Federal Government under the direction of Gonzalez and the supporting political leaders failed with regard to the principle of beneficence. The Federal Government negligently failed with regard to their imperfect obligations. There was little to no concern whatsoever with regard to the maximization of benefits for Ms Raich or Ms Monson.

[4:5] Under the principle of Beneficence the Federal Government negligently failed with regard to their imperfect obligations.

2. State Government

[4:6] Inconclusive

3. Individual Citizens

[4:7] Ms Raich and Ms Monson both were acting responsibly with regard to the principle of beneficence. Medicinal use of marijuana was for the purpose of maximizing benefits of health and since they were able to effectively fulfill their imperfect obligations by maximizing benefits they therefore acted morally.

V. Justice

[5:1] The formal definition of justice is harmony. Material definitions of justice attempt to specify what this harmony means and how to measure it. Historically this has been accomplished through the specification of :

a. distributions of benefits, and

b. acquisitions of burdens.

[5:2] Some historical examples of these are as follows:

Distributions of Benefits:

1. To each according to their need.

2. To each according to their merit.

3. To each according to their effort.

4. To each according to their contribution.

5. To each equally.

[5:3] **Acquisitions of Burdens:**

1. From each according to their ability.

2. From each according to their burden on society.

3. From those who are the least desirable.

4. From those who contribute the least.

5. From each equally.

[5:4] This list of distributions and acquisitions are not comprehensive and may be combined in a variety of combinations. Although these material principles are a specification of justice or harmony, they are still abstract enough that they will require further specification.

[5:5] One of most helpful descriptions of political positions is the political compass diagram based on the Cartesian Coordinate system.

[5:6] The top two quadrants are the authoritarian left and the authoritarian right and the bottom two quadrants are the libertarian left and the libertarian right. No one political position is necessarily right or wrong, rather where a person is on the "compass" is a matter of their political view of the role and function of government and their political view of the role and function of personal autonomy.

Justice Overview

1. Federal Government

[5:7] Gonzalez and his political supporters, i.e., President Bush, Vice President Cheney and the Republican Party are categorized as "Authoritarian Right." This position emphasizes both economic and moral governmental authority, usually in the form of trickle-down economics, and moral legislation. The focus, like the authoritarian left, is on the minimization of individual rights and liberties and the maximization of governmental authority. The authoritarian right is also usually manifested as totalitarian or fascist to the extent that there is a centralized government that controls both the economy and morality of a country while suppressing opposition. The Republican Party accomplishes this fascism, with its elimination of opposition, by its attempt to destroy any type of checks and balances as implemented by the competing branches of government. The goal of the Republican Party is to get a Republican President, and a republican majority in Congress, and in the House of Representative, and to appoint Supreme Court Judges that hold to the Republican ideology. With all three Branches of Government being held by a majority of Republicans along with Party Line Voting they will then be able to have total authority with no checks and balances, i.e., a fascist or totalitarian government. Under certain conditions this can in fact be the most practical political position when, for example,

a. citizens are not competent, and/or

b. not autonomous in their ability to maximize benefits and minimize burdens.

2. State Government

[5:8] The United States is at this point in time a two party government; Republican or Democrat. Both parties attempt to eliminate the branches of government both at the Federal Level and at the State level and therefore both Republicans and also the Democrats can be fairly categorized as fascists in intent. Likewise, under certain conditions this can in fact be the most practical political position when, for example,

a. citizens are not competent, and/or

b. not autonomous in their ability to maximize benefits and minimize burdens and/or

c. the government is in the best position to maximize benefits and minimize burdens for its citizens.

3. Individual Citizens

[5:9] Most citizens perceive themselves as competent and substantially autonomous in their ability to maximize benefits and minimize burdens and are in the best position for making that happen. As a result most citizens are primarily libertarian right (bottom right) or libertarian left, (bottom left).

[5:10] Libertarian right emphasizes both economic and moral autonomy through the implementation of fair procedures. The focus is on the minimization of governmental authority, and the maximization of personal autonomy. This personal autonomy is maximized by the establishment of individual rights and liberties and is implemented through the process of fair procedures.

[5:11] The libertarian left emphasizes both economic and moral autonomy through the implementation of fair procedures. The focus is on the minimization of governmental authority, and the maximization of personal autonomy. This personal autonomy is maximized by the establishment of individual rights and liberties and is implemented through the process of fair procedures. As the process of fair procedures determines economies they naturally tend towards a trickle-up egalitarian economy.

Conclusion on Justice

1. The Federal Government

[5:12] In this Medical Marijuana case the Federal Government is clearly acting from an authoritarian position. The problem is that the justification for authoritarianism is based on their ability to maximize benefits and minimize burdens. In this case, as seen in the evaluation of beneficence and nonmaleficence this is not the case. Therefore there is no justification for Government Authoritarianism as directed by Gonzalez or his republican cohorts with regard to Medical Marijuana.

2. State Government

[5:13] In this Medical Marijuana case the State Government is also more than likely acting from an authoritarian position, possibly in opposition with the public. The legalization process was in a sense high-jacked from the politicians through the referendum process where there is a forced vote by the public on a particular issue. Since the State Government did not bring up the referendum there is an indication that they were also holding a position of authority with no moral justification and therefore immoral. However, this is pure speculation with no empirical evidence given by the case study and therefore it is inconclusive whether the State's position is justified as there is not enough information.

3. Individual Citizens

[5:14] In this Medical Marijuana case it is clear that the general public is acting competently and autonomously with the referendum, with the practical result of maximizing overall individual and social benefits and minimizing overall individual and social burdens. Therefore, Ms. Raich and Ms Monson are morally justified.

VI. Balancing the Four Principles

1. Federal Government

[6:1] On many if not most moral decisions there will be a moral dilemma in that some principles will be justified by making one decision and other principles are justified by making an opposing decision. In those cases there will be a need for balancing the competing principles and coming to a compromise. What is interesting in this case, is that there is no such conflict of moral principles as the Federal Government failed on every moral principle and therefore requires no balancing.

2. State Government

[6:2] Inconclusive with the regard to the information as presented by the case study and therefore no balancing necessary.

3. Individual Citizens

[6:3] In this Medical Marijuana case Ms. Raich and Ms. Monson fulfilled every single moral principle and all the necessary conditions and the Federal Government failed every single moral principle, and the State of California is inconclusive. Therefore, there is no need to balance, rather the individual citizens, Ms. Raich and Ms. Monson are the only group that fulfilled any and all moral requirements and the Federal Government failed every single one of the moral requirements. As dominant as this position is, what is an even more interesting question is why there has been any controversy at all in regard to whose position had moral justification or weight.

Conclusion

1. Federal Government

[7:1] The Federal Government in regard to this Medical Marijuana case has failed every single moral principle and every single necessary condition, therefore the Federal Government was acting blatantly immoral. The Federal Government was clearly acting out of power with no regard towards morality. This should accentuate the positive need for independent branches of government controlled by an informed electorate.

2. State Government

[7:2] Inconclusive with the regard to the information as presented by the case study.

3. Individual Citizens

[7:3] In this Medical Marijuana case Ms. Raich and Ms. Monson fulfilled every single moral principle and all the necessary conditions and therefore there is no question or doubt that they were acting with clear moral justification.

***

5. APPLIED ETHICS

A Categorical Mistake

[1]

If applied ethics is being defined as practical ethics, and if practical ethics is being defined as suited for actual use then perhaps there is technically no problem with the term "applied ethics". However, if the term applied ethics is being used to describe an activity in which moral agents take specific ethical theories and "apply," like a band-aid, those theories to specific situations to see what the various results would be, then we are not describing how moral agents do in fact make moral decisions or even how they ought to make moral decisions. This "applied" approach seems to favor those approaches that are rights and/or duty based and tends to neglect casuistic, relational, and other types of decision-making. For example, the casuistic approach focuses on practical decision-making in particular cases and is skeptical of rules, rights, and theories divorced from history, precedent, and circumstances. Casuists maintain that some forms of moral reasoning and judgment make no appeal to principles, rules, rights, or virtues. Casuist's argue that just as case law develops incrementally from legal decisions in cases, so the moral law develops incrementally. The ethics of care approach is another perspective that cannot be "applied" to particular decision-making, as the emphasis is on the traits valued in intimate personal relationships. Like the casuistic approach the ethics of care does not necessarily focus on principles, rules, rights, or virtues that can be "applied" to a particular moral problem. Moral reasoning is instead a process that often blends appeals to principles, rules, rights, virtues, passions, analogies, paradigms, parables, narratives, and interpretations. Moral reasoning is not dependent on a single type of theory that is solely principle-based, virtue-based, rights-based, case-based, and so forth. Thus the idea of "applying" a theory or an approach to a moral problem seems to be too simplistic and a bit naive at best. There is no "applied ethics", rather what we have is "moral decision-making".

[2] Two of the most popular ethical theories that are typically thought of as being "applied" are those of Kant's *Metaphysics of Morals,* and Mill's *Utilitarianism*. However, most of the time this "application" is done so with mistaken notions. In this paper I will "show" how Kant defined "Ethics", express how he thought ethics could best be "taught", and pay attention to his emphasis on the casuistic approach.

[3] Kant in his introduction to the *Doctrine of Virtue* says the following:

> In ancient times "ethics" signified the doctrine of morals in general, which was also called the doctrine of duties. Later on it seemed better to reserve the name "ethics" for one part of moral philosophy, namely for the doctrine of those duties that do not come under external laws. Accordingly, the system of the doctrine of duties in general is now divided into the system of the doctrine of right which deals with duties that can be given by external laws, and the system of the doctrine of virtue, which treats of duties that cannot be so given. [6:379]

[4] The question that comes to my mind is that when addressing the philosophical issues of "Applied and Professional Ethics", to what extent are we actually addressing issues of "rights" and not issues of "ethics" as above described. For example, patient rights, or stockholder, manager, community, suppliers, employee and consumer rights.

[5] Kant, as a teleological ethicist, argues as follows:

> Now, I can indeed be constrained by others to perform actions that are directed as means to an end, but I can never be constrained by others to have an end: only I myself can make something my end. ... The doctrine of right dealt only with the formal condition of outer freedom, that is, with right". [6:380] "Any action, [or maxim], is right if it can coexist with everyone's freedom in accordance with universal law" [6:230] But ethics goes beyond this and provides a matter, an end of pure reason which it represents as an end that is also objectively necessary, that is, an

> end that, as far as human beings are concerned, it is a duty to have. [6:380-381] ... What are the ends that are also duties? They are one's own perfection and the happiness of others. [6:385]

[6] In the doctrine of right you adopt maxims on empirical grounds, in other words, you begin with whatever end you freely wish to choose and then you seek out the maxim of actions in conformity with duty, i.e., the maxim of action is still determined *a priori*, namely, that the freedom of the agent could coexist with the freedom of every other in accordance with a universal law, and thus enforceable by external laws of the land. [6:382] Kant says explicitly;

> In the doctrine of right an intentional untruth is called a lie only if it violates another's right. [6:429] "The only kind of untruth we want to call a lie, in the sense bearing upon rights, is one that directly infringes upon another's right, e.g., the false allegation that a contract has been concluded with someone, made in order to deprive him of what is his. [6:239] In the doctrine of right, freedom insofar as it can coexist with the freedom of every other in accordance with a universal law, is the only original right belonging to every man by virtue of his humanity. [6:237]
>
> [7] In the doctrine of virtue, or ethics, we establish maxims with respect to ends we ought to set for ourselves but which are not enforceable by external laws of the land. [6:382]

[8] Kant says that:

> Ethical duties are of Wide obligation, whereas duties of right are of narrow obligation ... The [subjective] law can prescribe only the maxim of actions, not actions themselves, this is a sign that it leaves a playroom for free choice in following or complying with the laws, that is, that the law cannot specify precisely in what way one is to act and how much one is to do by the action for an end that is also a duty. But a wide duty is not to be taken as permission to make exceptions to the maxim of actions but only as permission to limit one maxim of duty by another maxim of duty (e.g., love of one's neighbor in general by love of one's parent), by which in fact the field for the practice of virtue is widened. The wider the duty, therefore, the more imperfect is a man's obligation to action. ...

> Imperfect duties are, accordingly, only duties of virtue. [6:390]
>
> [9]… The doctrine of right has to do only with narrow duties whereas ethics has to do with wide duties. Hence the doctrine of right, which by its nature must determine duties strictly (precisely), has no more need of general direction (a method) as to how to proceed in judging than does pure mathematics; instead, it certifies its method by what it does. But ethics, because of the latitude it allows in its imperfect duties, unavoidably leads to questions that call upon judgment to decide how a maxim is to be applied in particular cases, and indeed in such a way that judgment provides another subordinate maxim. So ethics falls into a casuistry, which has no place in the doctrine of right. Casuistry is, accordingly, neither a science nor a part of a science; for in that case it would be dogmatics, and casuistry is not so much a doctrine about how to find something as rather a practice in how to seek truth. So it is woven into ethics in a fragmentary way, not systematically. [6:411]

[10] So as "teachers" of "Applied and Professional Ethics", how are we to go about doing our job? Kant's approach to "teaching" ethics is described in his last section of the *Doctrine of* Virtue, in his *Metaphysics of* Morals. He believes that in teaching ethics we should start out with the *Doctrine of Elements* and to proceed to *The Doctrine of Methods*. [6:413] In the *Doctrine of Elements* Kant first expounds on the *Duties of Virtue to Oneself* and then discusses our *Duties of Virtue to Others*. In the *Doctrine of Methods of Ethics* he first expounds on *Teaching Ethics* and then moves on to *Ethical Ascetics*.

[11] **THE DOCTRINE OF VIRTUE**

Doctrine of Elements of Ethics

A. On Ethical Duties to Oneself

1. Perfect Duties to Oneself as an Animal Being

- a. On Killing Oneself
  - Casuistical Questions
- b. On Defiling Oneself by Lust
  - Casuistical Questions
- c. On stupefying Oneself by the Excessive Use of Food or Drink
  - Casuistical Questions

2. Perfect Duties to Oneself as a Moral Being
a. On Lying
Casuistical Questions
b. On Avarice
Casuistical Questions
c. On Servility
Casuistical Questions
3. Duties to Oneself as your Own Innate Judge
4. Imperfect Duties to Oneself with Regard to His End
a. Natural Perfection
b. Moral Perfection
B. On Ethical Duties to Others
1. On the Duty of Love for Others
a. Benevolence
b. On the Duty of Beneficence
Casuistical Questions
c. On the Duty of Gratitude
d. Sympathetic Feeling Is Generally a Duty
Casuistical Questions
2. On the Duties of Respect for Others
On Vices that Violate the Duty of Respect
a. Arrogance
b. Defamation
Ridicule
c. Friendship
Doctrine of Methods of Ethics

A. Teaching Ethics

Ethical Ascetics

Conclusion of the Entire Ethics

[12] Focusing on Kant's *Teaching Ethics* he starts out by arguing that since virtue is acquired and not innate, virtues are therefore something that can be taught.

> As for the method of teaching … it can be set forth either by lectures, … or else by questions. … This erotetic method is, in turn, divided into the method of dialogue and that of catechism, depending on whether the teacher ad-

> dresses his questions to the pupil's reason or just to his memory. [6:478]

[13] Kant in addressing what the method of dialogue is for the teaching of virtue says the following:

> If the teacher wants to question his pupil's reason he must do this in a **dialogue** in which teacher and pupil question and answer each other in turn. The teacher, by his questions, guides his young pupil's course of thought merely by presenting him with cases in which his predisposition for certain concepts will develop (the teacher is the midwife of the pupil's thoughts). The pupil, who thus sees that he himself can think, responds with questions of his own about obscurities in the propositions admitted or about his doubts regarding them, and so provides occasions for the teacher himself to learn how to question skillfully, according to the saying 'by teaching we learn'. [6:478]

[14] Kant in addressing what the method of catechism is for the teaching of virtue says the following:

> For the beginning pupil the first and most essential instrument for teaching the doctrine of virtue is a moral catechism. This must precede a religious catechism … otherwise the professions of religions would be impure. … But pure moral catechism …developed from ordinary human reason, … needs only to be adapted to rules of teaching suited for the earliest instruction. The formal principle of such instruction does not, however, permit Socratic dialogue as the way of teaching for this purpose, since the pupil has no idea what questions to ask; and so the teacher alone does the questioning. … So the way of teaching by catechism differs from both the dogmatic way (in which only the teacher speaks) and the way of dialogue (in which both teacher and pupil question and answer each other). [6:479]

Fragment of a Moral Catechism

[15] The following is a teaching example given by Kant. [6:480-482]

> 1. Teacher: What is your greatest, in fact your whole, desire in life?
>
> Pupil: (is silent)

Teacher: That everything should always go the way you would like it to.

2. Teacher: What is such a condition called?

Pupil: (is silent)

Teacher: It is called happiness (continuous well-being, enjoyment of life, complete satisfaction with one's condition).

3. Teacher: Now, if it were up to you to dispose of all happiness (possible in the world), would you keep it all for yourself or would you share it with your fellow human beings?

Pupil: I would share it with others and make them happy and satisfied too.

4. Teacher: Now that proves that you have a good enough heart; but let us see whether you have a good head to go along with it.—Would you really give a lazy fellow soft cushions so that he could pass his life away in sweet idleness? Or would you see to it that a drunkard is never short of wine and whatever else he needs to get drunk? Would you give a swindler a charming air and manner to dupe other people? And would you give a violent man audacity and strong fists so that he could crush other people? Each of these things is a means that somebody wishes for in order to be happy in his own way.

Pupil: No, I would not.

5. Teacher: You see, then, that even if you had all happiness in your hands and, along with it, the best will, you would not give it without consideration to anyone who put out his hand for it; instead you would first try to find out to what extent each was worthy of happiness. But as for yourself, would you at least have no scruples about first providing yourself with everything that you count in your happiness?

Pupil: I would have none.

Teacher: But doesn't it occur to you to ask, again, whether you yourself are worthy of happiness?

...

[16] Kant concludes saying that:

> In this catechistic moral instruction it would be most helpful to the pupil's moral development to raise some casuistical questions in the analysis of every duty and to let the assembled children test their understanding by having each say how he would solve the tricky problem put to him. … Its advantage lies especially in the fact that it is natural for a human being to love a subject which he has, by his own handling, brought to a science (in which he is now proficient); and so, by this sort of practice, the pupil is drawn without noticing it to an interest in morality. But it is most important in this education not to present the moral catechism mixed with the religious (to combine them into one) or, what is worse yet, to have it follow upon the religious catechism. … For otherwise the religion that he afterwards professes will be nothing but hypocrisy; he will acknowledge duties out of fear and feign. [6:483-484]

[17] Kant's approach to teaching has the goal of helping the student develop their own moral reasoning skills. This can effectively be accomplished through the casuistic approach where one must personally weigh and balance various ethical duties. The ethical analysis of various wide duties in particular casuistic circumstances results in the mutual constrainment of various "competing" wide duties, e.g., the love of one's neighbor in general by the love of one's parents. As Kant said:

> A conflict of duties would be a relation between them in which one of them would cancel the other (wholly or in part). —But since duty and obligation are concepts that express the objective practical necessity of certain actions and two rules opposed to each other cannot be necessary at the same time, if it is a duty to act in accordance with one rule, to act in accordance with the opposite rule is not a duty but even contrary to duty; so a collision of duties and obligations is inconceivable. However, a subject may have, in a rule he prescribes to himself, two grounds of obligation one or the other of which is not sufficient to put him under obligation, so that one of them is not a duty. —When two such grounds conflict with each other, practical philosophy says, not that the stronger obligation takes precedence, but that the stronger ground of obligation prevails. [6:224]

[18] This is precisely where casuistry comes into play not only in the teaching of ethics but also in the making of life's decisions.

Casuistic decision-making is not the application of predetermined rules of action, rather, casuistic decision-making demands that moral reasoning and judgment be exercised in the fulfillment of one's wide obligations. Moral decision-making is not the application of ridged rules of conduct, like a Band-Aid, rather moral decision-making is a process of determining which stronger ground of obligation prevails in particular circumstances. As Kant says, over and over and over again:

> The law can prescribe only the maxim of actions, not actions themselves, this is a sign that it leaves a playroom for free choice in following the law, that is, that the law cannot specify precisely in what way one is to act and how much one is to do by the action for an end that is also a duty. [6:390] There is no law of reason for actions but only a law for maxims of action, which runs as follows: 'Cultivate your powers of mind and body so that they are fit to realize any ends you might encounter,' however uncertain you are which of them could sometime become yours. … The law, here again, prescribes only the maxim of the action … not the action itself. [6:392]

[19] The determination of how one is to act in a particular circumstance in compliance with one's self-legislative maxim often blends appeals to principles, rules, rights, virtues, passions, analogies, paradigms, parables, narratives, and interpretations. Even from a Kantian perspective we can now see that there is no "applied ethics", in the sense of prescribed actions, rather what we have is "moral decision-making" within the bounds of the maxims of wide obligations.

[20] However, it should be noted that if our "applied ethics" are really issues of rights, i.e. "applied rights", then we are talking about narrow duties in which the maxim of actions are adopted on empirical grounds in conformity with universal freedom. [6:385] The categorical mistake is the classification of the narrow duties of "rights" as wide duties of "ethics."

[21] When dealing with rights our duties are narrow and empirically precise. When dealing with ethics our duties are wide and casuistic.

6. THEORIES & CONCEPTS

I. Basic Epistemological Terms

Epistemology

[1] Theory of knowledge. The study of the origin, nature, and limits of knowledge, including especially the study of the nature of epistemic justification.

Empiricists

[2] All knowledge comes from experience—Locke, Berkeley and Hume.

Rationalists

[3] Some knowledge can be known to be true without empirical verification—Descartes, Spinoza, and Leibniz.

Primary Qualities

[4] Intrinsic characteristics of a physical object itself—solidity, extension, figure, motion/rest, and number. Primary qualities are ones that objects would continue to possess even if there were no perceiving beings in the world, for they are inseparable from the material object found in every part of it.

Secondary qualities

[5] Characteristics that exist only when sensed and then only "in the mind" of the one who senses them—color, taste, smell, sound, warmth, and cold, i.e., without minds, there would be no "secondary qualities".

Naïve Realism

[6] Position of "the ordinary man" who holds that both primary and secondary qualities have a real existence in material objects independently of perceiving minds.

Sophisticated Realism

[7] Sophisticated because it holds to the distinction of primary and secondary qualities; realism because it allows for the real existence of material objects independent of minds.

Representative Realism

[8] Ideas faithfully mirror or "represent" material objects to us in perception.

Realism

[9] The theory that the objects of our knowledge have an independent existence rather than being mind-dependent.

Causal Theory of Perception

[10] Material objects are the causes of ideas appearances, or sense data we have of them.

Substratum

[11] Is that which is distinct from its own secondary and primary qualities. It is simply posited as the unknowable.

Subjectivism

[12] The view that all knowledge is limited to the nature of objects as known through human experience, rather than objectively in themselves; it is impossible for us to transcend human subjectivity.

Subjective idealism (ideaism)

[13] World in which only perceiving minds (subjects) and their ideas (primary and secondary qualities) exist. The universe is purely mental.

II. Theories & Core Concepts

Universalizability, moral

[14] The principle of moral universalizabilty is derived from formal, rational, or *a priori* criteria.

The principle of universalizability is usually associated with the classic deontologist Immanuel Kant. Kant, in his Doctrine of Right, argues that:

> "Any action is right if it can coexist with everyone's freedom in accordance with a universal law, or if on its maxim the freedom of choice of each can coexist with everyone's freedom in accordance with a universal law." [6:230] Kant, in his Doctrine of Virtue, argues that: "The supreme principle of the doctrine of virtue is: act in accordance with a maxim of ends that it can be a universal law for everyone to have." [6:395]

The principle of universalizability is also evident with the classic utilitarian, John Stuart Mill. Mill, in his book Utilitarianism argues: "

> In the case of abstinences indeed—of things which people forbear to do from moral considerations, though the consequences in the particular case might be beneficial—it would be unworthy of an intelligent agent not to be consciously aware that the action is of a class which, if practiced generally, would be generally injurious, and that this is the ground of the obligation to abstain from it. ... [E]very systems of morals ... enjoin to abstain from whatever is manifestly pernicious to society." [Utilitarianism, John Stuart Mill, Chapter 2, Paragraph 18] Mill also argues: "In the golden rule of Jesus of Nazareth, we read the complete spirit of the ethics of utility. 'To do as you would be done by,' and 'to love your neighbor as yourself,' constitute the ideal perfection of utilitarian morality." [Utilitarianism, John Stuart Mill, Chapter 2, Paragraph 17]

Universality is represented by Kant as the principle of reciprocity and by Mill as equality.

Deontological Ethics

[15] Moral theories according to which certain acts must or must not be done, regardless, to some extent, of the consequences of

their performance or non-performance. (the Greek *dei* = one must, or duty). In contrast, teleology or consequentialism, as commonly understood, the rightness or wrongness of any act depends upon its consequences. Deontological theories either do not specify the good independently from the right or do not interpret the right as maximizing the good. (Note that deontology is not the same as absolutism, according to which certain acts are wrong whatever the consequences.) Two criticisms are, first, the difficulty of describing how we know which acts are wrong, and, second, the difficulty of drawing a sharp distinction between acts and omissions.

Systematic Exposition

[16] Presents the fundamental principles of right and wrong and shows how they yield all moral duties.

Intuitionism

[17] The standard model, **intuitionism**, is an axiomatic system of self-evident truths using not only first principles of a deductive system but also using principles whose truth can be seen immediately upon reflection.

Jural Justification

[18] Establishes the authority of the principles, legislative will, and so validates the moral code. Authority derives from the sovereignty of the person or collective whose will they are taken to express.

Divine Command Theory

[19] Moral principles are taken to be laws issued by God to humanity, and their authority thus derives from God's supremacy.

Formalism

[20] Moral principles are that which satisfy a formal criteria such as a "universal law". Authority is based on the formal criteria.

Contractarianism

[21] Moral principles represent the ideal terms of social cooperation for people who live together in fellowship, and regard each

other as "equals"—sociological fairness. Authority is based on group consensus.

Deontological Teleology

[22] Teleology is generally a category used in contrast with duty based systems. As a duty based system our fundamental teleological duty is to promote certain ends, and the principles of right and wrong organize and direct our efforts in this regard. Answers to questions about the ends we ought to pursue determine the principles of right and wrong. The general study of right action is therefore subordinate to the general study of "goodness", i.e., ends must be understood before we can act morally. The moral principles are authoritative in virtue of the wisdom of their prescriptions in attaining the ends or good.

Deontological Egoism

[23] Fundamental duty is to promote the good, i.e., one's own happiness—self-love.

Deontological Utilitarianism

[24] Utilitarianism, which is usually taken to be a paradigm consequentialist theory, can be expressed as deontological. The fundamental duty is to promote the good, e.g., happiness of sentient beings—benevolence. "Right" is that which promotes the good. Under this view, utilitarianism recognizes the "right" to be prior to the "good", in the sense that utilitarians can state that it is right to maximize the good, whatever the good turns out to be.

Kantian Morality

[25] Kant, 1724–1804, is the most famous of the deontological ethicists. Kant in his many writings wrote three treatises on ethics: *Groundwork of the Metaphysics of Morals*, 1785, *Critique of Practical Reason*, 1788, and *Metaphysics of Morals*, 1797. In the *Metaphysics of Morals*, Kant divides his text into two parts: Doctrine of Right, and the Doctrine of Virtue.

> [6:379] In ancient times "ethics" signified the doctrine of morality in general, which was also called the doctrine of duties. Later on it seemed better to reserve the name "ethics"[or virtue] for one part of moral philosophy, name-

ly for the doctrine of those duties that do not come under external laws. Accordingly, the system of the doctrine of duties in general is now divided into the system of the doctrine of right, which deals with duties that can be given by external laws, and the system of the doctrine of virtue/ethics, which treats of duties that cannot be so given.

Doctrine of Right

[26] The Doctrine of Right is Kant's social and political position on how the formal criteria of Universal Freedom ought to be used in the development of civil laws in order to attain the entire final end of social peace, as determined by reciprocity, and motivated by external coercion. That which is wrong is that which hinders the universal freedom of all, i.e., social rights, and that which is right is that which hinders the hindering of universal freedom, i.e., external coercion. The following are some excerpts from the Doctrine of Right.

> [6:312] It is not experience from which we learn of human beings' maxim of violence and of their malevolent tendency to attack one another before external legislation endowed with power appears. On the contrary, however well disposed and law abiding men might be, it still lies a priori in the rational idea of such a condition that before a public lawful condition is established individual human beings, peoples and states can never be secure against violence from one another, since each has its own right to do what seems right and good to it and not to be dependent upon another's opinion about this. ... [individual human beings] must leave the state of nature, in which each follows its own judgment, unite itself with all others, subject itself to a public lawful external coercion ... determined by law, ... i.e. ... a civil condition. ...
>
> It is true that the state of nature need not, just because it is natural, be a state of injustice, of dealing with one another only in terms of the degree of force each has. But it would still be a state devoid of justice, in which when rights are in dispute, there would be no judge competent to render a verdict having rightful force. Hence each may impel the other by force to leave this state and enter into a rightful condition. ...

Civil condition is thought of by pure rational concepts alone.

[6:354] Now morally practical reason pronounces in us its irresistible veto: there is to be no war. ...The question is no longer whether perpetual peace is something real or a fiction, ... Instead, we must act as if it is something real, though perhaps it is not; we must work toward establishing perpetual peace and the kind of constitution that seems to us most conducive to it in order bring about perpetual peace and put an end to the heinous waging of war...For this is our duty, ...

It can be said that establishing universal and lasting peace constitutes not merely a part of the doctrine of right but rather the entire final end of the doctrine of right within the limits of reason alone; for the condition of peace is the only condition in which what is mine and what is yours are secured under laws for a multitude of human beings living in proximity to one another and therefore under a constitution.

[6:230] Any action is right if it can coexist with everyone's freedom in accordance with a universal law, or if on its maxim the freedom of choice of each can coexist with everyone's freedom in accordance with a universal law.

[6:231] When one's aim is not to teach virtue but only to set forth what is right, one may not and should not represent that the law of right as itself the incentive to action. ... [coercion is].

[6:231] Resistance that counteract the hindering of an effect promotes this effect and is consistent with it. Now whatever is wrong is a hindrance to freedom in accordance with universal laws. Therefore, ... coercion that is opposed to this is consistent with freedom in accordance with universal law, that is, it is right. Hence there is connected with right by the principle of contradiction an authorization to coerce someone who infringes upon it.

[6:232] Strict right rests on the principle of its being possible to use external constraint that can coexist with the freedom of everyone in accordance with universal laws. ... Right and authorization to use coercion therefore mean one and the same thing.

The law of a reciprocal coercion necessarily in accord with the freedom of everyone under the principle of universal freedom is, as it were, the construction of that concept.

> [6:237] Freedom, insofar as it can coexist with the freedom of every other in accordance with a universal law, is the only original right belonging to every man by virtue of his humanity.
>
> [6:238] ...before [a human being] performs any act affecting rights he has done no wrong to anyone; being authorized to do to others anything that does not in itself diminish what is theirs.
>
> [6:256] I am therefore not under obligation to leave external objects belonging to others untouched unless everyone else provides me assurance that he will behave in accordance with the same principle with regard to what is mine. This assurance does not require a special act to establish a right, but is already contained in the concept of an obligation corresponding to an external right, since the universality, and with it the reciprocity, of obligation arises from a universal rule.

Doctrine of Virtue

[27] Kant in his Doctrine of Right argues for the necessity of a civil constitution, based on Universal Freedom and External Coercion, establishing the sole and final end of peace, as a principle of reciprocity.

Kant in his Doctrine of Virtue goes beyond the Doctrine of Right by arguing that *a priori* reasoning results in ends as duties that must be freely chosen, i.e., without any constraints. Those ends that are also duties are one's own perfection and the happiness of others.

> [6:380] The doctrine of right dealt only with the formal condition of outer freedom (the consistency of outer freedom with itself if its maxim were made universal law), that is, with right. But ethics goes beyond this and provides an object of free choice, an end of pure reason which it represents as an end that is also objectively necessary, that is, an end that, as far as human beings are concerned, it is a duty to have.
>
> [6:380] I can indeed be constrained by others to perform actions that are directed as means to an end, but I can never be constrained by others to have an end: only I myself can make something my end. ...That ethics contain duties that one cannot be constrained by other to fulfill

follows merely from its being a doctrine of ends, since coercion to ends is self-contradictory.

[6:382] One can think of the relation of end to duty in two ways: One can begin with the end [universal freedom, perpetual peace] and seek out the maxim of actions in conformity with duty [doctrine of right], or on the other hand, one can begin with the maxim of actions in conformity with duty and seek out the end that is also a duty [doctrine of virtue/ethics]. In the doctrine of right, what end anyone wants to set for his action is left to his free choice. The maxim of his action, however, is determined *a priori,* namely, that the freedom of the agent could coexist with the freedom of every other in accordance with a universal law.

But ethics takes the opposite way.

[6:383] what essentially distinguishes a duty of virtue from a duty of right is that external constraint to the latter kind of duty is morally possible, whereas the former is based only on free self-constraint.

[6:384] An end is an object of free choice. ... Every action, therefore, has its end; and since no one can have an end without himself making the object of his choice into an end, to have any end of action whatsoever is an act of freedom on the part of the acting subject, not an effect of nature. But because this act which determines an end is a practical principle that prescribes the end itself, not the means, it is a categorical imperative of pure practical reason. ... Since there are free actions there must also be ends to which, as their object these actions are directed. But among these ends there must be some that are also duties. —For were there no such ends, then all ends would hold for practical reason only as means to other ends; and since there can be no action without an end, a categorical imperative would be impossible. This would do away with any doctrine of morals.

What Are the Ends That Are Also Duties?

[6:385] They are one's own perfection and the happiness of others.

[6:387] One's own perfection...[qualitative (formal) perfection] as a concept belonging to teleology, it is taken to mean the harmony of a thing's properties with an end. ... cultivating one's faculties, the highest of which is understanding. At the same time this duty includes the cultivation of one's will. ... A human being (1) has a duty to diminish his ignorance, and (2) carry the cultivation of his will up to the purest virtuous disposition, in which the law becomes also the incentive to his actions that conform with duty and he obeys the law from duty. This disposition is inner morally practical perfection.

[6:389] Only the concept of an end that is also a duty, a concept that belongs exclusively to ethics, establishes a law for maxims of actions by subordinating the subjective end (that everyone has) to the objective end (that everyone ought to make his end). ... No free action is possible unless the agent also intend an end (which is the matter of choice.)

[6:390] ...[Ethical] laws can prescribe only the maxim of actions, not action themselves, this is a sign that it leaves a playroom for free choice in following (complying with) the [ethical] law, that is, that the law cannot specify precisely in what way one is to act and how much one is to do by the action for an end that is also a duty.—But a wide duty is not to be taken as permission to make exceptions to the maxim of actions but only as permission to limit one maxim of duty by another (e.g. , love of one's neighbor in general by love of one's parents)... The wider the duty, therefore, the more imperfect is man's obligation to action. ...

Imperfect duties are, accordingly, only duties of virtue.

[6:395] The supreme principle of the doctrine of virtue/ethics is: act in accordance with a maxim of ends that it can be a universal law for everyone to have.

[6:411] The doctrine of right has to do only with narrow duties, whereas ethics has to do with wide duties. Hence the doctrine of right, which by its nature must determine duties strictly (precisely), has no more need of general direction (a method) as to how to proceed in judging than does pure mathematics; instead, it certifies its method by what it does.—But ethics, because of the latitude it allows in its imperfect duties, unavoidably leads to questions that call upon judgment to decide how a maxim is to be applied in particular cases, and indeed in such a way that judgment provides another (subordinate) maxim. So ethics falls into a casuistry which has no place in the doctrine of right. ... Casuistry ... is not so much a doctrine about how to find something as rather a practice in how to seek truth.

In Conclusion, Kant's moral theory is divided into two parts; Doctrine of Rights, and Doctrine of Virtue. Doctrine of Rights is the construction of a Constitutional Government using the formal criteria of Universal Freedom of All for attaining the sole and final end of Social Peace mandated by legal coercion, i.e. narrow duties. Doctrine of Virtue are those ends that must be chosen freely and thus cannot be mandated by coercive law. Two wide duties that all have by virtue of *a priori* reasoning are one's own perfection and the happiness of others. We do not have a duty for our own happiness as everyone already pursues their own happiness by nature of their desires. We do not have a duty to perfect others as self-perfection is by definition a free choice of ends and thus a personal activity that cannot be coerced. However we can freely choose to perfect ourselves and we can freely choose to help others attain ends that they have determined will make them happy. This self-perfection and happiness of others is different for every person and every circumstance and thus ethics is a practice of casuistry, i.e., judgment.

Note: In both the doctrine of right and the doctrine of virtue, it is clear that Kant argues *a priori* for the defining of the "good/end", (i.e. universal freedom—peace, or self-perfection and happiness of others), as a necessary condition before a moral agent can define that which is "right", (i.e., justice, or virtue). Kant's Doctrine of Right is therefore teleological in that the "good/end" of "Peace" was determined through the *a priori* principle of Universal Freedom/Reciprocity. Kant's Doctrine of Virtue is also teleological, in that the "good/ends" of the duty of self-perfection and the happiness of others, is determined through the free choice, as choice of ends can only be done freely, of those ends that are duties.

Teleology, Consequentialism and Utilitarianism

[28] Teleology as a descriptive doctrine argues that all of nature, or at least intentional agents, are in fact goal directed or functionally organized. Teleology as a prescriptive doctrine argues that intentional agents ought to be goal directed.

The moral theory that falls under the category of teleology is consequentialism or Utilitarianism. Utilitarianism has two major divisions: 1) act utilitarianism, and 2) rule utilitarianism. Utilitarianism holds that the defining of "good" comes before the defining of "right". In other words, "good" is defined independently from the right, and the right is then defined as that which maximizes the good. If you wish to determine right actions you must first know the "good" or the "end" that you are trying to pursue, then you need to determine if the action that is being evaluated does in fact promote that end.

The "Good" or "End" is usually classified as either quantitative or qualitative. a) Quantitative goods or ends are those pleasures or satisfactions that maximize the number or units of ends. b) Qualitative goods or ends are those pleasures or satisfactions that you would not trade for any number of quantitative pleasures or satisfactions.

John Stuart Mill, 1806-1873

[29] John Stuart Mill is the classic utilitarian who's work, Utilitarianism, was published in three installments in Fraser's Magazine, 1861. Mill argued that quantitative goods or ends can become qualitative and that it is this psychological propensity that makes life interestingly diverse. Even power, money, and fame can become qualitative ends. However, virtue, Mill argues, is an unique end of which one cannot have too much of. All other quantitative ends, that become qualitative must be limited. Take for example money.

> Money's worth is solely that of the things to which it can buy ... but money is, in many cases, desired in and for itself; the desire to possess it is often stronger than the desire to use it. ... What was once desired as an instrument for the attainment of happiness has come to be desired for its own sake. In being desired for its own sake it is, however, desired as part of happiness. What was once desired as an instrument for the attainment of happiness has come to be desired for its own sake. ... Life would be a poor thing, very ill provided with sources of happiness, if there were not this provision of nature. ... Virtue is a good of this description. ... The difference between virtue and the

> love of money, power, or fame is that they may, and often do, render the individual noxious to the other members of society to which he belongs, whereas there is nothing which makes him so much a blessing to them as the cultivation of the disinterested love of virtue. (Utilitarianism, John Stuart Mill, Chapter 4, Paragraph 6)

Act Utilitarianism

[30] Act utilitarianism is the view that an act is morally obligatory if and only if it produces a greater balance of pleasure over pain, or of desired satisfaction, than any alternative action available to the agent. Acts are not right or obligatory because of their inherent character, their underlying motives, or their relation to divine or social dictates, but because of how much overall human or sentient well-being they produce.

Rule Utilitarianism

[31] Rule utilitarianism is the view that the rightness of an action depends on the consequences not of the action itself, but of various sets of rules.

Act & Rule Utilitarianism Combination

[32] Many Utilitarians use a combination of Act and Rule Utilitarianism. Mill's "rules" are manifested in his principles of justice such as personal liberty, property, desert, good faith, impartiality, and equality. Mill argues, like Hobbs, that personal security is the most vital of all social interests, one that no human being can do without.

> "The claim assumes that character of absoluteness, that apparent infinity and incommensurability with all other considerations which constitute the distinction between the feeling of right and wrong and that of ordinary expediency and inexpediency. The feelings concerned are so powerful, and we count so positively on finding a responsive feeling in others that ought and should grow into must, and recognized indispensability becomes a moral necessity, analogous to physical, and often not inferior to it in binding force." (Utilitarianism, John Stuart Mill, Chapter 5, Paragraph 23) "justice supposes two things—a rule of conduct and a sentiment which sanctions the rule." (Utilitarianism, John Stuart Mill, Chapter 5, Paragraph 21) "Justice is a name for certain moral requirements

> which, regarded collectively, stand higher in the scale of social utility, and are therefore of more paramount obligation, than any others, though particular cases may occur in which some other social duty is so important as to overrule any one of the general maxims of justice. Thus, to save a life, it may not only be allowable, but a duty, to steal or take by force the necessary food or medicine, or to kidnap and compel to officiate the only qualified medical practitioner. In such cases, as we do not call anything justice which is not a virtue, we usually say, not that justice must give way to some other moral principle, but that what is just in ordinary case is, by reason of that other principle, not just in the particular case." (Utilitarianism, John Stuart Mill, Chapter 5, Paragraph 37)

Some naïve criticisms of utilitarianism is that this moral theory could result in the justification of unjust actions such as enslaving 10% of the population for the greater benefit of 90% of the population, i.e., the "greatest good for the greatest amount of people". Mill would argue that personal liberty of everyone is an absolute rule and a necessary element for social structure, or social contract, and that the above argument is therefore a straw-man argument. Principles of justice, such as a constitution, are such absolute rules that are very rarely violated and if they are violated it is not on the basis of justification of unjust actions, rather what is just in one circumstance may be unjust in a different circumstance. Mill argues that these "absolute" rules of justice are in fact the necessary components for the "greatest good for the greatest amount of people".

III. Other Theories & Core Concepts

Free-will

[33] The deepest question that the student of moral agency must face is whether the capacity for free action is essential to moral agency, and whether free-will fits within a deterministic universe. Free-will position holds that certain decisions or choices can be made without a) any determination, or b) by a determination that can be considered to be "free". Problems with this view would be a) what would it mean to have an undetermined decision or choice?, i.e., would it random or chaos? b) what would it mean to have a determined free choice?

Determinism

[34] Determinism has three major divisions: 1) hard determinism, 2) soft determinism or compatibilism, and 3) indeterminism.

Hard Determinism

[35] Hard Determinism describes how all events, without exception, are effects following from previous causes, i.e., all events are necessitated by earlier events. In other words, it necessarily follows that all present and future events are as fixed and unalterable as the past is fixed and unalterable. If this position is in fact true, then many ethicists claim that then there can be no moral responsibility as moral responsibility is based on an agent's free will, and hard determinism is the claim that there is no free agency.

Soft Determinism

[36] Soft determinism is the view that determinism and free-will are compatible. Free agency, in this view, is a type of causation that does allow for moral responsibility.

Indeterminism

[37] Indeterminism is the view that some events are not caused. If determinism is false then its negation must be true, i.e., indeterminism must be true—successive events are not causally related. Indeterminism, like hard determinism, results in the conclu-

sion that if moral responsibility is based on an agent's free will, then there is no moral responsibility.

Intrinsic Worth

[38] Some philosophers believe that some "things" are "good" in themselves. Examples have included such "things" as life, happiness, pleasure, knowledge, virtue, friendship, beauty, and harmony. (This list can easily be extended.) One view would hold that there is intrinsic worth regardless of whether there are experiencers or not. This view would hold that intrinsic worth is a "primary quality" rather than a "secondary quality". Problem with this view is what would it mean to say that a value is a primary quality? How can a value be anything but a secondary quality? Another intrinsic worth viewpoint argues that intrinsic worth is in fact compatible with being agent relative, or a secondary quality. This view would hold that there can, and in fact are, different intrinsic values for different experiencers.

Extrinsic Worth

[39] This viewpoint argues that some or all values are instrumentally good. In other words, worth comes from its function or results and not by its nature of being. This view would hold that it makes no sense to think of a value that exists without a "valuer," or someone who values, i.e., value in this view is thought of as a secondary quality.

Altruism

[40] Altruism has two major divisions: 1) altruistic egoism, and 2) psychological altruism.

Altruistic Egoism

[41] Altruistic egoism prescribes how agents ought to act, i.e., agents ought to act without regard to their own self-interests. This position claims that if everyone were to act without regard to their own self-interests, life for the individual, and society at large, would in fact be a much more moral and better.

Psychological Altruism

[42] Psychological altruism describes how agents can in fact act, i.e., an agent can act without regard to their own self-interests. Psychological altruism and altruistic egoism are usually held concertedly.

Egoism

[43] Egoism has two major divisions: 1) ethical egoism, and 2) psychological egoism.

Ethical Egoism

[44] Ethical egoism prescribes how agents ought to act, i.e., agents ought to act according to their own self-interests. This position claims that if everyone were to act according to their own self-interests, life for the individual and society at large would in fact be a much more moral and better. Ethical egoism claims that not only is it immoral to act in ways that are incompatible with an agent's own self-interests, but acting outside of an agent's own self-interests, it is believed, would negatively effect both the agent and others in society.

Psychological Egoism

[45] Psychological egoism describes how agents do in fact act, i.e., agents will act according to their own self-interests. This position claims that regardless of a person's moral position, such as altruistic egoism, the person will always act according to their own self-interest. This position is unfalsifiable as even if the person thinks they are acting altruistically the psychological egoist will claim that the person actually has other, or even subconscious egoistic motivations. However, if psychological egoism claims to be an empirical scientific position, and if empirical scientific positions are by definition falsifiable, then it is questionable whether psychological egoism is a scientific fact.

Non-Teleological Morality

[46] The view that the study of right action is independent of the general study of ends or goodness as there are in fact no ends to be pursued. In this view, the principle of evolution perfectly illustrates this, i.e., nature is not evolving towards any particular end

or good, rather, change occurs simply as a process of natural selection.

Naturalism

[47] Ethical knowledge is empirical and accordingly it models morality on the paradigm of the natural sciences. Ethical concepts, on this view, concern natural phenomena.

Rationalism

[48] Ethical knowledge is *a priori* and accordingly it models morality on the paradigm of pure mathematics. Ethical concepts, on this view, concern morality understood as something completely distinct from, though applicable to, natural phenomena, something whose content and structure can be apprehended by reason independently of sensory inputs.

Noncognitivism

[49] Denies that ethics is a genuine branch of knowledge or takes it to be a branch of knowledge only in a qualified sense. Denies that ethics is properly modeled on science or mathematics. Some non-cognitivists argue that words like 'right', 'wrong', 'good', and 'evil' have no cognitive meaning but rather serve to vent feelings and emotions, to express decisions and commitments, or to influence attitudes and dispositions.

Moral Realism

[50] Affirms the real existence of ethical properties, independent of their being perceived. For moral realism, ethics is an objective discipline, a discipline that promises the discovery and confirmation of objective truths. At the same time, moral realists differ fundamentally on the question of the character of ethical properties. Plato, for example, regarded them as purely intellective and thus irreducibly distinct from empirical properties. Others, such as Aristotle, regarded them as empirical.

Moral Subjectivism

[51] Denies the real existence of ethical properties. Ethics is not a source of objective truth, rather, it is a projection of some feeling, impulse, or other state of mind onto the world, such as one

projects an emotion onto one's circumstances when one describes them as delightful or sad. In ancient philosophy this was advanced by the Sophists.

Naturalistic Fallacy

[52] Can there be a logically valid argument whose conclusion is a judgment of value and all of whose premises are statements of fact? In other words, can moral predicates represent properties that are explicable as complexes of empirical properties? A negative answer to these questions affirms the autonomy of ethics. A positive answer denies ethics' autonomy and implies that it is a branch of the natural sciences.

Moral Psychology

[53] It is generally recognized that an adequate understanding of desire, emotion, deliberation, choice, volition, character, and personality is indispensable to the theoretical treatment of human well-being, intrinsic value, and duty. On one view, moral agency consists in the power of reason to govern behavior, and being rational is thus sufficient for being responsible for one's actions. Another view is that moral agency consists of several things including reason, but also including a desire to act rightly and an aversion to acting wrongly that originate in natural desires and aversion. On this view, to be responsible for one's actions, one must not only be rational but also have certain desires and aversions whose acquisition is not guaranteed by the maturation of reason.

Ethical Relativism

[54] The view that there exists no point of view that is an "absolute" criteria of what is right or wrong. In support of their claims, the relativist usually appeals to cultural and historical diversity. Some practical problems are:

1. Moral Advancement

If ethical relativism is true then there could not be any moral advancement as that which is, is that which is moral.

2. Moral Revolutionaries

If ethical relativism is true then moral revolutionaries, e.g., Jesus, would have to be considered immoral as he promoted change.

3. Judging of Cultures

If ethical relativism is true then we could not judge other cultures as being moral or immoral, e.g. genocidal practices may have to be tolerated.

4. Tolerance of Intolerance

If ethical relativism is true then you may have to be tolerant towards an intolerant culture, which is not only logically inconsistent but also could be self-destructive. (Ethical relativism is frequently equated with toleration.)

***

7. HOMER TO KANT

A Short Moral History

Introduction

The history of philosophy has no beginning. Rather philosophy came about as a gradual change from an anthropomorphic and mythic point of view to a point of view that could be considered philosophical.

Homer

[2] One of the earliest extant writings of the western world is Homer, 8th century BCE. The Homeric heaven was an anthropomorphic reflection of the Greek City State. Homer's gods were the causal agents of all events and as long as events were attributed to the will of the gods, science, such as meteorology, was not possible.

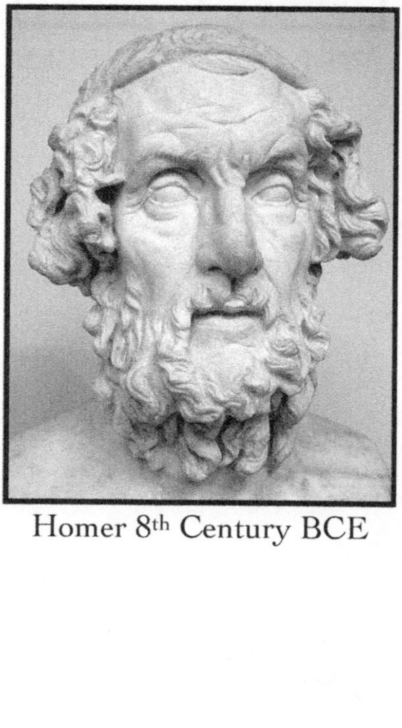

Homer 8th Century BCE

Thales

[3] Thales, lived sometime in the 620s - mid 540s BCE and is considered to be the first philosopher and the "father of science" as he attempted to explain the world independent of mythology. Thales is also considered to be the first mathematician and is reputed with also being the first person to scientifically predict a solar eclipse.

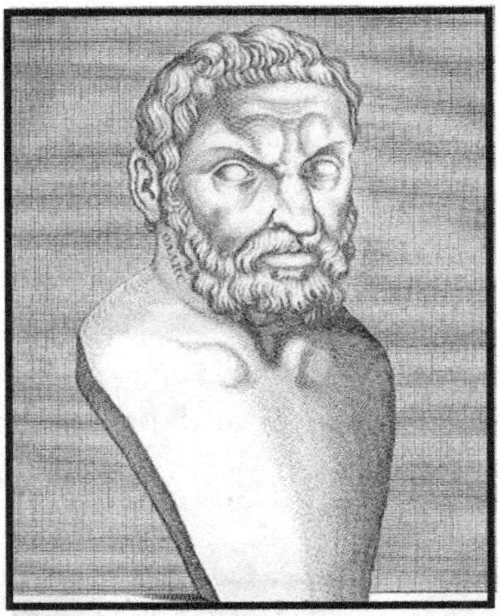

Thales 620s – 540s BCE

Anaximander

[4] Anaximander, lived sometime between 610 - 546 BCE he is considered to be the father of cosmology, and he presented the first rudimentary theory of evolutionary natural selection. Anaximander is also attributed to having recorded the first scientific experiment.

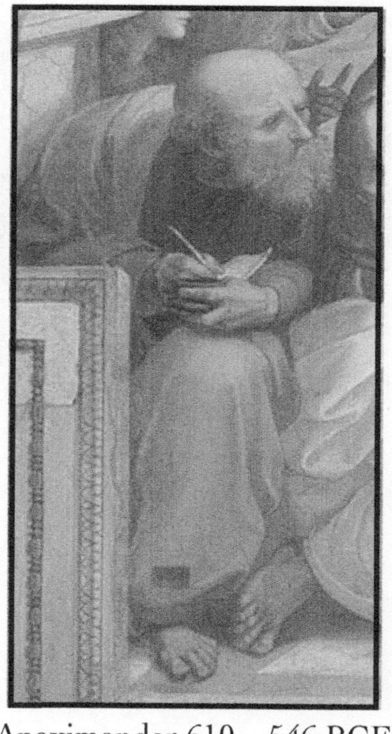

Anaximander 610 – 546 BCE

Heraclitus

[5] Heraclitus, 535 – 475 BCE, viewed the world as an ever changing process called logos. This change was also attributed to social arrangements in which tension and strife are necessary opposing forces for justice. Heraclitus had a significant influence on Plato with regard to his ever changing sense perceptions he called opinion.

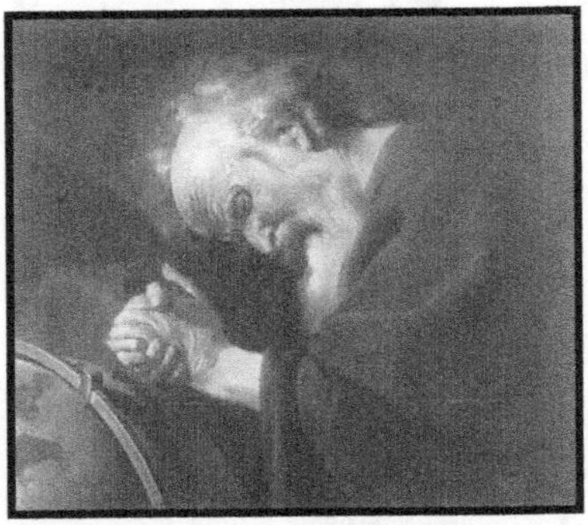

Heraclitus 535 – 475 BCE

Euclid

[6] Euclid, lived around 300 BCE and is known as the father of geometry. His axiomatic method uses logical reasoning from premises that are self-evidently true. Whereas the geometer reaches conclusions that agrees with sense experiences, physicists and cosmologists used the same geometric method to reach conclusion that were in contradiction with sense experience.

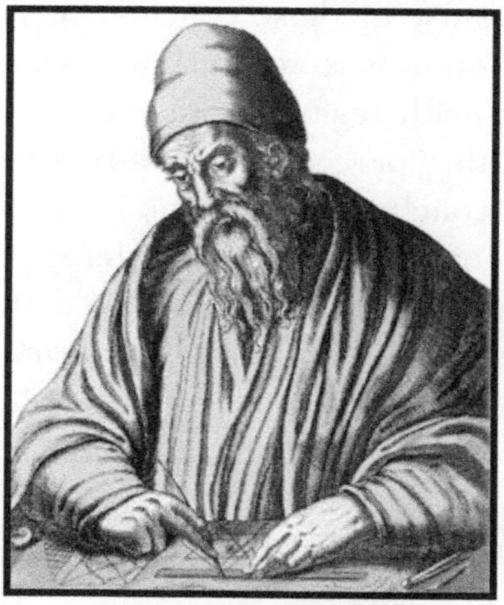

Euclid 300 BCE

Parmenides

[7] Parmenides, early 5th century BCE, argued that the perception of the world is false and deceptive. In addition to being a monist, which is the position that all of nature is of one substance, Parmenides held to two new premises: 1. "What is, is," and 2. "What is not, is not." From these he logically proved that whatever is, is 1. uncreated, 2., indestructible, 3. eternal, and 4. unchangeable. Because of these conclusions he believed that all was one and all motion was an illusion. Parmenides had a great influence on Plato with regard to his eternal unchanging forms, along with attributing perception as deceptive or mere opinion. Even though the conclusions they came up with seemed to go against common sense, Parmenides, Heraclitus, and Zeno did not become skeptics because that believed that rationality was universal, whereas perception, or empiricism, at best only gives information about particulars.

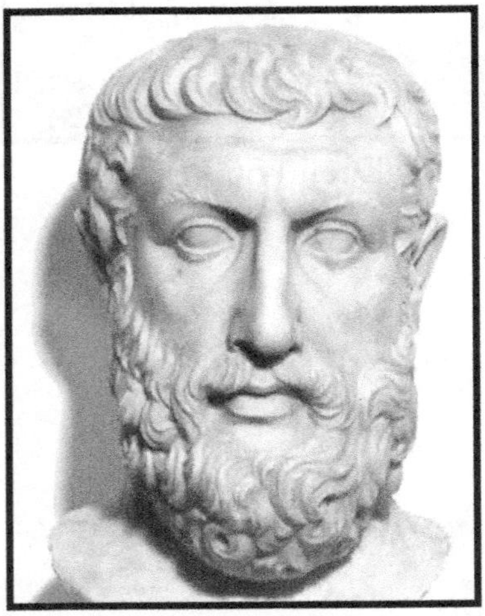

Parmenides Early 5th Century BCE

Zeno

[8] Zeno, 490 – 430 BCE, was Parmenides student and came up with paradoxes illustrating the problem of perceptual illusions. The most famous paradox is the story of the tortoise and the hare. Zeno with his paradoxes, was a start of the critique of the power of rationality.

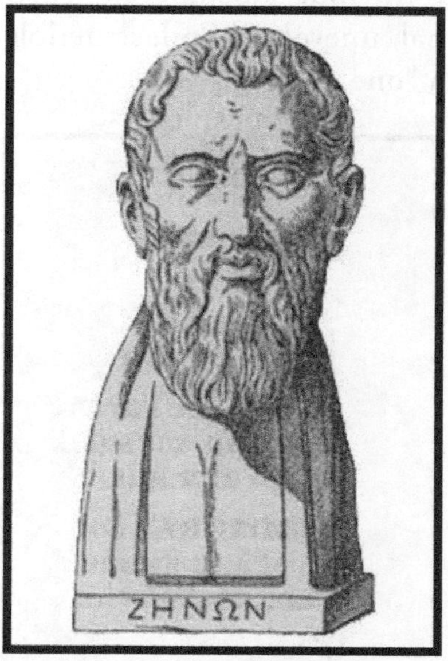

Zeno 490 – 430 BCE

Empedoles

[9] Empedocles, 490 - 430 BCE, like Anaximander, also anticipated modern evolutionary doctrines of random natural selection. Up to this time everyone was a monist, believing that all of reality was made of one substance. Empedocles was the first of the pluralists based on the notion that there was movement in the plenum. He held to the four substances of earth, air, fire, and water which are eternal, uncreated, indestructible, and unchanging, i.e., a Parmenidean "one."

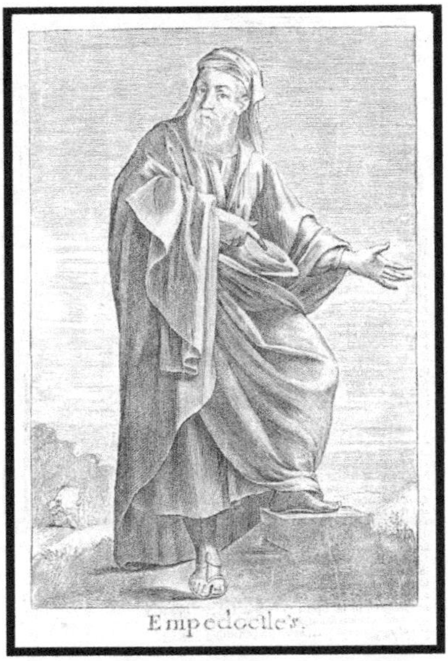

Empedocles 490 – 430 BCE

Pythagoras

[10] Pythagoras, 570 – 495 BCE, is of course most famous for the Pythagorean theorem which states that for any right triangle: $a^2 + b^2 = h^2$. Pythagoras was also known for continuing the cosmological notion of the circular motions of the cosmos, as well as the notion of sophrosyne or moderation between extremes for health. The Pythagoreans used music to purify their soul which they believe to be immortal and part of a cycle of reincarnation. Depending on how a person lived their life determined how they were to be reborn. For the Pythagoreans the moral goal was to be released from the cycle or wheel of birth and death and this could only be accomplished by attaining wisdom. Hence, the importance of "science." They cultivated science, as they cultivated music, as the means to spiritual redemption.

With the Pythagorean emphasis on mathematics, and the Atomists' view of nature, modern physics was in the making. The derailment of physics until the 17 century was partly because of Plato with his lack of interest in Atomism, and Christianity with its emphasis on otherworldliness.

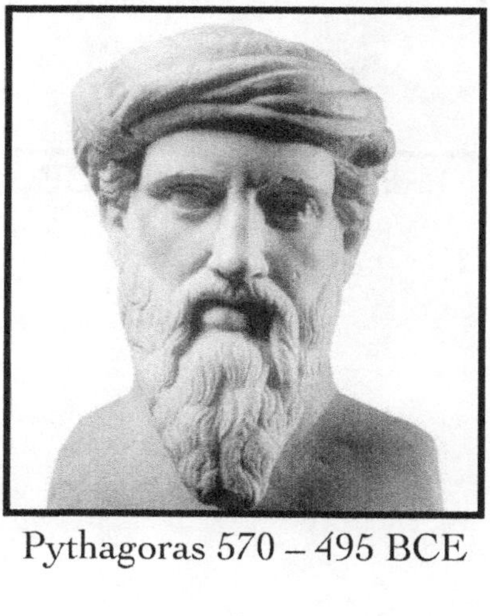

Pythagoras 570 – 495 BCE

Protagoras

[11] Sophists were neither scientists nor philosophers but were educators. As such, education shifted from the virtues of courage, loyalty, personal honor, and moderation to worldly talents of debate and oratorical skills. Protagoras one of the earliest Sophists argued that if the experience of color is a movement of sense organs and if we each have different sense organs then it follows that we each experience color differently from each other, i.e., color perception is relative. Radical skepticism became the norm because of the influence of these educators or so called sophists.

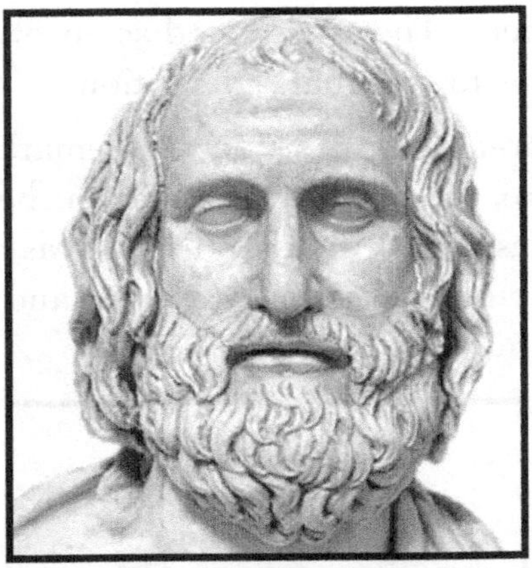

Protagoras 481-411 BCE

Democritus

Democritus, 460 – 370 BCE, believed that all of the world was made up of atoms and the void. Things differed only quantitatively, in shape and size, and things have no qualities. Democritus believed that what is perceived is totally different from the reality of the causation of the perception. Perception is never in a position to correct perception, rather only thought, by the means of the atomic theory, was able to correct the illusion of perception.

Epicurus thought that color was "out there" whereas Democritus thought that all that exists are atoms and the void and consequently was a hard determinist thinking that perception was totally illusory.

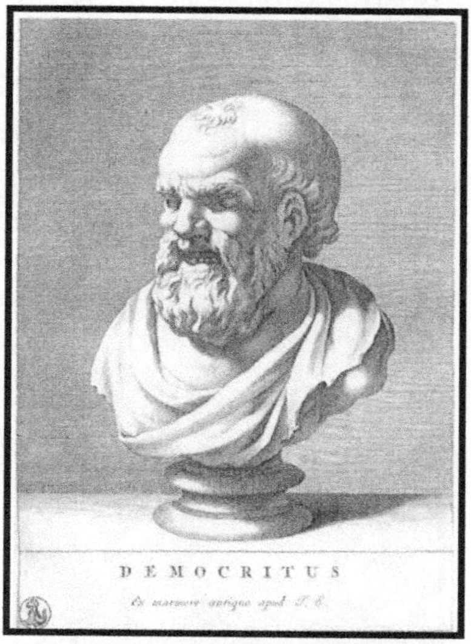

Democritus 460 – 370 BCE

Plato

[12] From Thales to Democritus the common assumption is that reality is material and that the material world is intelligible. However, the material world is intelligible only in terms of natural processes, not in teleological or supernatural terms.

Modern science has adopted this mechanistic nonteleological view of nature, which the Atomists were the first to formulate.

Plato, 428 – 347 BCE, synthesized Heraclitus' ever changing logos, and Parmenides' everything is one into a metaphysical dualism of the ever changing sense perceptions he called opinion and the immutable one of the world of the immaterial abstract Ideas or Forms.

Plato attempted to rid the subjective individual experience from relativism by arguing for a mystic preexistence of the eternal forms of which knowledge was simply a remembering of what the souls already new before the veil of ignorance covered the soul at incarnation. Unfortunately, Plato was the beginning of the regression of all the scientific progress of the presocratics.

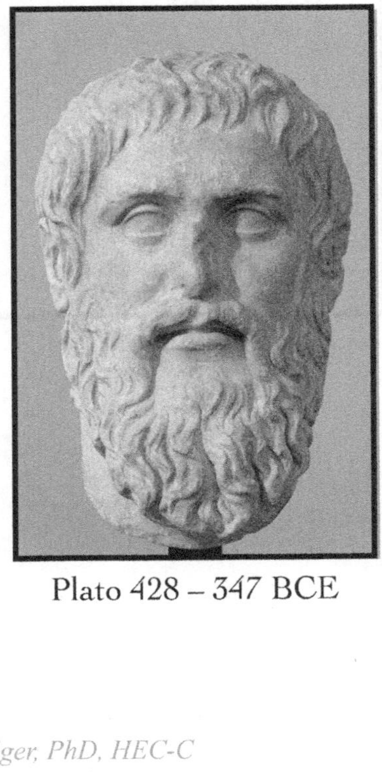

Plato 428 – 347 BCE

Aristotle

[13] Aristotle, 384 – 322 BCE, briefly stopped this backward Dark Age step by modifying Plato's mystic worldview by rejecting Plato's eternal immaterial ethereal forms and "grounding" the forms to potentiality and actuality. The acorn has the potential to be the oak tree and the oak tree is the actualization of the form of the acorn.

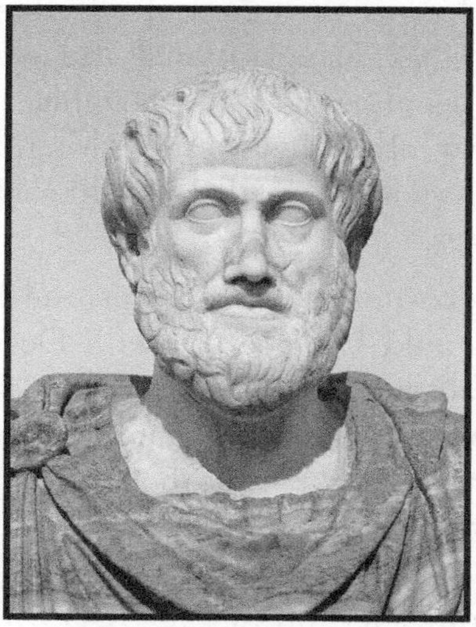

Aristotle 384 – 322 BCE

Descartes

[14] Then as a result of religious institutions, theocentrism became the thought of the day, throwing the western world back into the time of Homer, or what is now known as the Dark Ages.

Theology became the queen of the sciences. God as omniscient and omnipotent, controlled the universe. Science was considered to be unnecessary and unfaithful as the deity was in control of everything, and He was the cause of all effects. Instead of the science of meteorology using rational and empirical cause and effect prediction, people would, for example, pray to their deity to cause whatever weather they were desiring. Rational empirical science was dead, society was thinking like Homer, it was officially the Dark Ages.

After 1400 years or so of the Dark Ages, the Enlightenment began to arise in the mid 17th century with Descartes' "Discourse on Methods," published in 1637. Descartes is considered to be the father of modern philosophy and the creator of analytic geometry which was the key for the discovery of infinitesimal calculus which was part of Newton's "Principia Mathematica" published in 1687. In many respects science picked up from where the presocratics left off in 400 BCE with Democritus and his subjective rational-centric worldview. The enlightenment was a shift back to the importance of reason, and challenged the traditional values and social institutions that promoted values based on authority and faith. However, in this process Descartes started the anthropocentric movement in which only humans had experiences and therefore only humans had moral considerability. He devised what was to be called psychological dualism in which the physical world abides by the deterministic cause and effect relationships and the mental world of the soul was free and morally responsible. This was the first step in getting out of the Dark Ages as Descartes was able to argue that because of this psychological dualism, the mechanistic physical world could be given to the study of science, and the Church would still have full authority over the aspects of the immaterial human soul. However, since Descartes held that only humans had souls, it followed that animals were deterministic substances with no self-awareness.

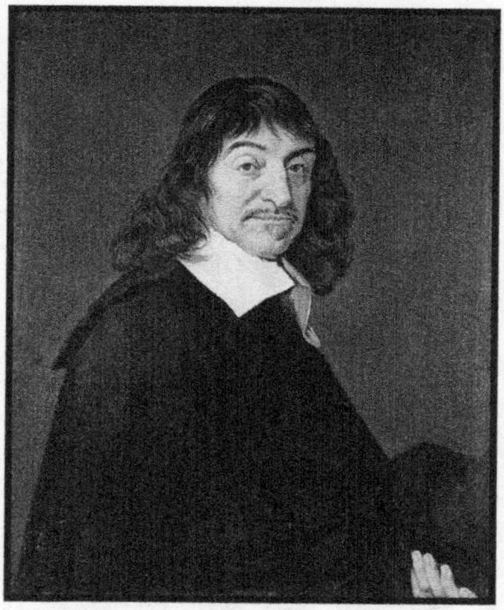

Descartes 1596 - 1650

Immanuel Kant

[15] Immanuel Kant, 1724 -1804 is considered to be the last influential thinker of the modern era culminating the study of epistemology of John Locke, George Berkeley, and David Hume. Kant in his book *Critique of Pure Reason* argues that the understanding of the world is based on *a priori* categories of the mind such as space and time. Experiences are subjective, yet humans share the same *a priori* categories of the mind.

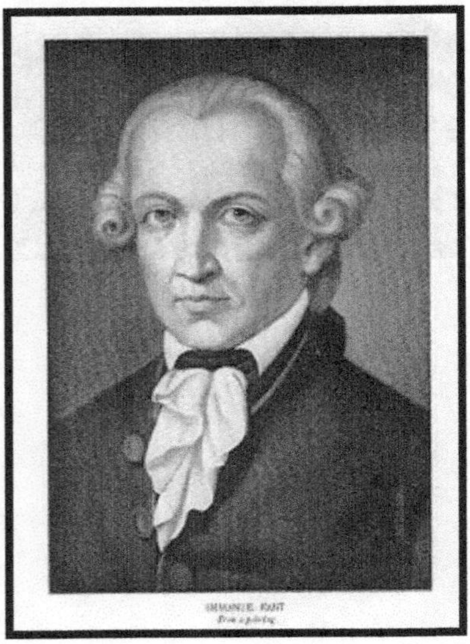

Immanuel Kant 1724 - 1804

***

VIII. UTILITARIANISM
John Stuart Mill

John Stuart Mill published Utilitarianism as a series of three articles in Fraser's Magazine in 1861, and they were compiled into a book in 1863.

Paragraphs have been numbered for easy referencing and for online orientation.

Chapter I: General Remarks

[1:1] There are few circumstances among those which make up the present condition of human knowledge more unlike what might have been expected, or more significant of the backward state in which speculation on the most important subjects still lingers, than the little progress which has been made in the decision of the controversy respecting the criterion of right and wrong.

[1:2] From the dawn of philosophy, the question concerning the *summum bonum*, or, what is the same thing, concerning the foundation of morality, has been accounted the main problem in speculative thought, has occupied the most gifted intellects and divided them into sects and schools carrying on a vigorous warfare against one another.

[1:3] And after more than two thousand years the same discussions continue, philosophers are still ranged under the same contending banners, and neither thinkers nor mankind at large seem nearer to being unanimous on the subject than when the youth Socrates listened to the old Protagoras and asserted (if Plato's dialogue be grounded on a real conversation) the theory of utilitarianism against the popular morality of the socalled sophist.

[1:4] It is true that similar confusion and uncertainty and, in some cases, similar discordance exist respecting the first principles of all the sciences, not excepting that which is deemed the most certain of them—mathematics, without much impairing, generally indeed without impairing at all, the trustworthiness of the conclusions of those sciences.

[1:5] An apparent anomaly, the explanation of which is that the detailed doctrines of a science are not usually deduced from, nor depend for their evidence upon, what are called its first principles.

[1:6] Were it not so, there would be no science more precarious, or whose conclusions were more insufficiently made out, than algebra, which derives none of its certainty from what are commonly taught to learners as its elements, since these, as laid down by some of its most eminent teachers, are as full of fictions as English law, and of mysteries as theology.

[1:7] The truths which are ultimately accepted as the first principles of a science are really the last results of metaphysical analysis practiced on the elementary notions with which the science is conversant; and their relation to the science is not that of foundations to an edifice, but of roots to a tree, which may perform their office equally well though they be never dug down to and exposed to light.

[1:8] But though in science the particular truths precede the general theory, the contrary might be expected to be the case with a practical art, such as morals or legislation.

[1:9] All action is for the sake of some end, and rules, of action, it seems natural to suppose, must take their whole character and color from the end to which they are subservient.

[1:10] When we engage in pursuit, a clear and precise conception of what we are pursuing would seem to be the first thing we need, instead of the last we are to look forward to.

[1:11] A test of right and wrong must be the means, one would think, of ascertaining what is right or wrong, and not a consequence of having already ascertained it.

[1:12] The difficulty is not avoided by having recourse to the popular theory of a natural faculty, a sense of instinct, informing us of right and wrong.

[1:13] For—besides that the existence of such a moral instinct is itself one of the matters in dispute—those believers in it who have any pretensions to philosophy have been obliged to abandon the idea that it discerns what is right or wrong in the particular case in hand, as our other senses discern the sight or sound actually present.

[1:14] Our moral faculty, according to all those of its interpreters who are entitled to the name of thinkers, supplies us only with the general principles of moral judgments; it is a branch of our reason, not of our sensitive faculty, and must be looked to for the abstract doctrines of morality, not for perception of it in the concrete.

[1:15] The intuitive, no less than what may be termed the inductive, school of ethics insists on the necessity of general laws.

[1:16] They both agree that the morality of an individual action is not a question of direct perception, but of the application of a law to an individual case.

[1:17] They recognize also, to a great extent, the same moral laws, but differ as to their evidence and the source from which they derive their authority.

[1:18] According to the one opinion, the principles of morals are evident *a priori*, requiring nothing to command assent except that the meaning of the terms be understood.

[1:19] According to the other doctrine, right and wrong, as well as truth and falsehood, are questions of observation and experience.

[1:20] But both hold equally that morality must be deduced from principles; and the intuitive school affirms as strongly as the inductive that there is a science of morals.

[1:21] Yet they seldom attempt to make out a list of the *a priori* principles which are to serve as the premises of the science; still more rarely do they make any effort to reduce those various principles to one first principle or common ground of obligation.

[1:22] They either assume the ordinary precepts of morals as of *a priori* authority, or they lay down as the common groundwork of those maxims some generality much less obviously authoritative than the maxims themselves, and which has never succeeded in gaining popular acceptance.

[1:23] Yet to support their pretensions there ought either to be some one fundamental principle or law at the root of all morality, or, if there be several, there should be a determinate order of precedence among them; and the one principle, or the rule for deciding between the various principles when they conflict, ought to be self evident.

[1:24] To inquire how far the bad effects of this deficiency have been mitigated in practice, or to what extent the moral beliefs of mankind have been vitiated or made uncertain by the absence of any distinct recognition of an ultimate standard, would imply a complete survey and criticism of past and present ethical doctrine.

[1:25] It would, however, be easy to show that whatever steadiness or consistency these moral beliefs have attained has been mainly due to the tacit influence of a standard not recognized.

[1:26] Although the nonexistence of an acknowledged first principle has made ethics not so much a guide as a consecration of men's actual sentiments, still, as men's sentiments, both of favor and of aversion, are greatly influenced by what they suppose to be the effects of things upon their happiness, the principle of utility, or, as Bentham latterly called it, the greatest happiness principle, has had a large share in forming the moral doctrines even of those who most scornfully reject its authority.

[1:27] Nor is there any school of thought which refuses to admit that the influence of actions on happiness is a most material and even predominant consideration in many of the details of morals, however unwilling to acknowledge it as the fundamental principle of morality and the source of moral obligation.

[1:28] I might go much further and say that to all those *a priori* moralists who deem it necessary to argue at all, utilitarian arguments are indispensable.

[1:29] It is not my present purpose to criticize these thinkers; but I cannot help referring, for illustration, to a systematic treatise by one of the most illustrious of them the *Metaphysics of Ethics* by Kant.

[1:30] This remarkable man, whose system of thought will long remain one of the landmarks in the history of philosophical speculation, does, in the treatise in question, lay down a universal first principle as the origin and ground of moral obligation; it is this: "So act that the rule on which thou actest would admit of being adopted as a law by all rational beings."

[1:31] But when he begins to deduce from this precept any of the actual duties of morality, he fails, almost grotesquely, to show that there would be any contradiction; any logical (not to say physical) impossibility, in the adoption by all rational beings of the most outrageously immoral rules of conduct.

[1:32] All he shows is that the consequences of their universal adoption would be such as no one would choose to incur.

[1:33] On the present occasion, I shall, without further discussion of the other theories, attempt to contribute something toward the understanding and appreciation of the "utilitarian" or "happiness" theory, and toward such proof as it is susceptible of.

[1:34] It is evident that this cannot be proof in the ordinary and popular meaning of the term.

[1:35] Questions of ultimate ends are not amenable to direct proof.

[1:36] Whatever can be proved to be good must be so by being shown to be a means to something admitted to be good without proof.

[1:37] The medical art is proved to be good by its conducing to health; but how is it possible to prove that health is good?

[1:38] The art of music is good, for the reason, among others, that it produces pleasure; but what proof is it possible to give that pleasure is good.

[1:39] If, then, it is asserted that there is a comprehensive formula, including all things which are in themselves good, and that whatever else is good is not so as an end but as a means, the formula may be accepted or rejected, but is not a subject of what is commonly understood by proof.

[1:40] We are not, however, to infer that its acceptance or rejection must depend on blind impulse or arbitrary choice.

[1:41] There is a larger meaning of the word "proof," in which this question is as amenable to it as any other of the disputed questions of philosophy.

[1:42] The subject is within the cognizance of the rational faculty; and neither does that faculty deal with it solely in the way of intuition.

[1:43] Considerations may be presented capable of determining the intellect either to give or withhold its assent to the doctrine; and this is equivalent to proof.

[1:44] We shall examine presently of what nature are these considerations; in what manner they apply to the case, and what rational grounds, therefore, can be given for accepting or rejecting the utilitarian formula.

[1:45] But it is a preliminary condition of rational acceptance or rejection that the formula should be correctly understood.

[1:46] I believe that the very imperfect notion ordinarily formed of its meaning is the chief obstacle which impedes its reception, and that, could it be cleared even from only the grosser misconceptions, the question would be greatly simplified and a large proportion of its difficulties removed.

[1:47] Before, therefore, I attempt to enter into the philosophical grounds which can be given for assenting to the utilitarian standard, I shall offer some illustrations of the doctrine itself, with the view of showing more clearly what it is, distinguishing it from what it is not, and disposing of such of the practical objections to it as either originate in, or are closely connected with, mistaken interpretations of its meaning.

[1:48] Having thus prepared the ground, I shall afterwards endeavor to throw such light as I can call upon the question considered as one of philosophical theory.

Chapter II: What Utilitarianism Is

[2:1] A passing remark is all that need be given to the ignorant blunder of supposing that those who stand up for utility as the test of right and wrong use the term in that restricted and merely colloquial sense in which utility is opposed to pleasure.

[2:2] An apology is due to the philosophical opponents of utilitarianism for even the momentary appearance of confounding them with anyone capable of so absurd a misconception; which is the more extraordinary, inasmuch as the contrary accusation, of referring everything to pleasure, and that too, in its grossest form, is another of the common charges against utilitarianism: and, as has been pointedly remarked by an able writer, the same sort of persons, and often the very same persons, denounce the theory "as impracticably dry when the word 'utility' precedes the word 'pleasure,' and as too practicably voluptuous when the word 'pleasure' precedes the word 'utility.' "

[2:3] Those who know anything about the matter are aware that every writer, from Epicurus to Bentham, who maintained the theory of utility meant by it, not something to be contradistinguished from pleasure, but pleasure itself, together with exemption from pain; and instead of opposing the useful to the agreeable or the ornamental, have always declared that the useful means these, among other things.

[2:4] Yet the common herd, including the herd of writers, not only in newspapers and periodicals, but in books of weight and pretension, are perpetually falling into this shallow mistake.

[2:5] Having caught up the word "utilitarian," while knowing nothing whatever about it but its sound, they habitually express by it the rejection or the neglect of pleasure in some of its forms: of beauty, of ornament, or of amusement.

[2:6] Nor is the term thus ignorantly misapplied solely in disparagement, but occasionally in complement, as though it implied superiority to frivolity and the mere pleasures of the moment.

[2:7] And this perverted use is the only one in which the word is popularly known, and the one from which the new generation are acquiring their sole notion of its meaning.

[2:8] Those who introduced the word, but who had for many years discontinued it as a distinctive appellation, may well feel themselves called upon to resume it if by doing so they can hope to contribute anything toward rescuing it from this utter degradation.

[2:9] The creed which accepts as the foundation of morals "utility" or the "greatest happiness principle," holds that actions are right in proportion as they tend to promote happiness; wrong as they tend to produce the reverse of happiness.

[2:10] By happiness is intended pleasure and the absence of pain; by unhappiness, pain and the privation of pleasure.

[2:11] To give a clear view of the moral standard set up by the theory, much more requires to be said; in particular, what things it includes in the ideas of pain and pleasure, and to what extent, is left an open question.

[2:12] But these supplementary explanations do not affect the theory of life on which this theory of morality is groundedname-ly, that pleasure and freedom from pain are the only things desirable as ends; and that all desirable things (which are as numerous in the utilitarian as in any other scheme) are desirable either for pleasure inherent in themselves or as means to the promotion of pleasure and the prevention of pain.

[2:13] Now such a theory of life excites in many minds, and among them in some of the most estimable in feeling and purpose, inveterate dislike.

[2:14] To suppose that life has (as they express it) no higher end than pleasure—no better and nobler object of desire and pursuit—they designate as utterly mean and groveling, as a doctrine worthy only of swine, to whom the followers of Epicurus were, at a very early period, contemptuously likened; and modern holders of the doctrine are occasionally made the subject of equally polite comparisons by its German, French, and English assailants.

[2:15] When thus attacked, the Epicureans have always answered that it is not they, but their accusers, who represent human nature in a degrading light, since the accusation supposes human beings to be capable of no pleasures except those of which swine are capable.

[2:16] If this supposition were true, the charge could not be gainsaid, but would then be no longer an imputation; for if the sources of pleasure were precisely the same to human beings and to swine, the rule of life which is good enough for the one would be good enough for the other.

[2:17] The comparison of the Epicurean life to that of beasts is felt as degrading, precisely because a beast's pleasures do not satisfy a human being's conceptions of happiness.

[2:18] Human beings have faculties more elevated than the animal appetites and, when once made conscious of them, do not regard anything as happiness which does not include their gratification.

[2:19] I do not indeed, consider the Epicureans to have been by any means faultless in drawing out their scheme of consequences from the utilitarian principle.

[2:20] To do this in any sufficient manner, many Stoic, as well as Christian, elements require to be included.

[2:21] But there is no known Epicurean theory of life which does not assign to the pleasures of the intellect, of the feelings and imagination, and of the moral sentiments a much higher value as pleasures than to those of mere sensation.

[2:22] It must be admitted, however, that utilitarian writers in general have placed the superiority of mental over bodily pleasures chiefly in the greater permanency, safety, uncostliness, etc., of the former—that is, in their circumstantial advantages rather than in their intrinsic nature.

[2:23] And on all these points utilitarians have fully proved their case; but they might have taken the other and, as it may be called, higher ground with entire consistency.

[2:24] It is quite compatible with the principle of utility to recognize the fact that some kinds of pleasure are more desirable and more valuable than others.

[2:25] It would be absurd that, while in estimating all other things quality is considered as well as quantity, the estimation of pleasure should be supposed to depend on quantity alone.

[2:26] If I am asked what I mean by difference of quality in pleasure, or what makes one pleasure more valuable than another, merely as a pleasure, except its being greater in amount, there is but one possible answer.

[2:27] Of two pleasures, if there be one to which all or almost all who have experience of both give a decided preference, irrespective of any feeling of moral obligation to prefer it, that is the more desirable pleasure.

[2:28] If one of the two is, by those who are competently acquainted with both, placed so far above the other that they prefer it, even though knowing it to be attended with a greater amount of discontent, and would not resign it for any quantity of the other pleasure which their nature is capable of, we are justified in ascribing to the preferred enjoyment a superiority in quality so far outweighing quantity as to render it, in comparison, of small account.

[2:29] Now it is an unquestionable fact that those who are equally acquainted with and equally capable of appreciating and enjoying both do give a most marked preference to the manner of existence which employs their higher faculties.

[2:30] Few human creatures would consent to be changed into any of the lower animals for a promise of the fullest allowance of a beast's pleasures; no intelligent human being would consent to be a fool, no instructed person would be an ignoramus, no person of feeling and conscience would be selfish and base, even though they should be persuaded that the fool, the dunce, or the rascal is better satisfied with his lot than they are with theirs.

[2:31] They would not resign what they possess more than he for the most complete satisfaction of all the desires which they have in common with him.

[2:32] If they ever fancy they would, it is only in cases of unhappiness so extreme that to escape from it they would exchange their lot for almost any other, however undesirable in their own eyes.

[2:33] A being of higher faculties requires more to make him happy, is capable probably of more acute suffering, and certainly accessible to it at more points, than one of an inferior type; but in spite of these liabilities, he can never really wish to sink into what he feels to be a lower grade of existence.

[2:34] We may give what explanation we please of this unwillingness; we may attribute it to pride, a name which is given indiscriminately to some of the most and to some of the least estimable feelings of which mankind are capable; we may refer it to the love of liberty and personal independence, an appeal to which was with the Stoics one of the most effective means for the inculcation of it; to the love of power or to the love of excitement, both of which do really enter into and contribute to it; but its most appropriate appellation is a sense of dignity, which all human beings possess in one form or other, and in some, though by no means in exact, proportion to their higher faculties, and which is so essential a part of the happiness of those in whom it is strong that nothing which conflicts with it could be otherwise than momentarily an object of desire to them.

[2:35] Whoever supposes that this preference takes place at a sacrifice of happiness—that the superior being, in anything like equal circumstances, is not happier than the inferior—confounds the two very different ideas of happiness and content.

[2:36] It is indisputable that the being whose capacities of enjoyment are low has the greatest chance of having them fully satisfied; and a highly endowed being will always feel that any happiness which he can look for, as the world is constituted, is imperfect.

[2:37] But he can learn to bear its imperfections, if they are at all bearable; and they will not make him envy the being who is indeed unconscious of the imperfections, but only because he feels not at all the good which those imperfections qualify.

[2:38] It is better to be a human being dissatisfied than a pig satisfied; better to be Socrates dissatisfied than a fool satisfied.

[2:39] And if the fool, or the pig, are of a different opinion, it is because they only know their own side of the question.

[2:40] The other party to the comparison knows both sides.

[2:41] It may be objected that many who are capable of the higher pleasures occasionally, under the influence of temptation, postpone them to the lower.

[2:42] But this is quite compatible with a full appreciation of the intrinsic superiority of the higher.

[2:43] Men often, from infirmity of character, make their election for the nearer good, though they know it to be the less valuable; and this no less when the choice is between two bodily pleasures than when it is between bodily and mental.

[2:44] They pursue sensual indulgences to the injury of health, though perfectly aware that health is the greater good.

[2:45] It may be further objected that many who begin with youthful enthusiasm for everything noble, as they advance in years, sink into indolence and selfishness.

[2:46] But I do not believe that those who undergo this very common change voluntarily choose the lower description of pleasures in preference to the higher.

[2:47] I believe that, before they devote themselves exclusively to the one, they have already become incapable of the other.

[2:48] Capacity for the nobler feelings is in most natures a very tender plant, easily killed, not only by hostile influences, but by mere want [lack] of sustenance; and in the majority of young persons it speedily dies away if the occupations to which their position in life has devoted them, and the society into which it has thrown them, are not favorable to keeping that higher capacity in exercise.

[2:49] Men lose their high aspirations as they lose their intellectual tastes, because they have not time or opportunity for indulging them; and they addict themselves to inferior pleasures, not because they deliberately prefer them, but because they are either the only ones to which they have access or the only ones which they are any longer capable of enjoying.

[2:50] It may be questioned whether anyone who has remained equally susceptible to both classes of pleasures ever knowingly and calmly preferred the lower, though many, in all ages, have broken down in an ineffectual attempt to combine both.

[2:51] From this verdict of the only competent judges, I apprehend there can be no appeal.

[2:52] On a question which is the best worth having of two pleasures, or which of two modes of existence is the most grateful to the feelings, apart from its moral attributes and from its consequences, the judgment of those who are qualified by knowledge of both, or, if they differ, that of the majority among them, must be admitted as final.

[2:53] And there needs be the less hesitation to accept this judgment respecting the quality of pleasures, since there is no other tribunal to be referred to even on the question of quantity.

[2:54] What means are there of determining which is the acutest of two pains, or the intensest of two pleasurable sensations, except the general suffrage of those who are familiar with both?

[2:55] Neither pains nor pleasures are homogeneous, and pain is always heterogeneous with pleasure.

[2:56] What is there to decide whether a particular pleasure is worth purchasing at the cost of a particular pain, except the feelings and judgment of the experienced?

[2:57] When, therefore, those feelings and judgment declare the pleasures derived from the higher faculties to be preferable *in kind*, apart from the question of intensity, to those of which the animal nature, disjoined from the higher faculties, is susceptible, they are entitled on this subject to the same regard.

[2:58] I have dwelt on this point as being part of a perfectly just conception of utility or happiness considered as the directive rule of human conduct.

[2:59] But it is by no means an indispensable condition to the acceptance of the utilitarian standard; for that standard is not the agent's own greatest happiness, but the greatest amount of happiness altogether; and if it may possibly be doubted whether a noble character is always the happier for its nobleness, there can be no doubt that it makes other people happier, and that the world in general is immensely a gainer by it.

[2:60] Utilitarianism, therefore, could only attain its end by the general cultivation of nobleness of character, even if each individual were only benefitted by the nobleness of others, and his own, so far as happiness is concerned, were a sheer deduction from the benefit.

[2:61] But the bare enunciation of such an absurdity as this last renders refutation superfluous.

[2:62] According to the greatest happiness principle, as above explained, the ultimate end, with reference to and for the sake of which all other things are desirable—whether we are considering our own good or that of other people—is an existence exempt as far as possible from pain, and as rich as possible in enjoyments, both in point of quantity and quality; the test of quality and the rule for measuring it against quantity being the preference felt by those who, in their opportunities of experience, to which must be added their habits of self-consciousness and self-observation, are best furnished with the means of comparison.

[2:63] This, being according to the utilitarian opinion the end of human action, is necessarily also the standard of morality, which may accordingly be defined "the rules and precepts for human conduct," by the observance of which an existence such as has been described might be, to the greatest extent possible, secured to all mankind; and not to them only, but, so far as the nature of things admits, to the whole sentient creation.

[2:64] Against this doctrine, however, arises another class of objectors who say that happiness, in any form, cannot be the rational purpose of human life and action; because, in the first place, it is unattainable; and they contemptuously ask, What right hast thou to be happy?—a question which Mr. Carlyle clinches by the addition, What right, a short time ago, hadst thou even *to be*?

[2:65] Next they say that men can do *without* happiness; that all noble human beings have felt this, and could not have become noble but by learning the lesson of *Entsagen*, or renunciation; which lesson, thoroughly learned and submitted to, they affirm to be the beginning and necessary condition of all virtue.

[2:66] The first of these objections would go to the root of the matter were it well founded; for if no happiness is to be had at all by human beings, the attainment of it cannot be the end of morality or of any rational conduct.

[2:67] Though, even in that case, something might still be said for the utilitarian theory, since utility includes not solely the pursuit of happiness, but the prevention or mitigation of unhappiness; and if the former aim be chimerical, there will be all the greater scope and more imperative need for the latter, so long at least as mankind think fit to live and do not take refuge in the simultaneous act of suicide recommended under certain conditions by Novalis.

[2:68] When, however, it is thus positively asserted to be impossible that human life should be happy, the assertion, if not something like a verbal quibble, is at least an exaggeration.

[2:69] If by happiness be meant a continuity of highly pleasurable excitement, it is evident enough that this is impossible.

[2:70] A state of exalted pleasure lasts only moments or in some cases, and with some intermissions, hours or days, and is the occasional brilliant flash of enjoyment, not its permanent and steady flame.

[2:71] Of this the philosophers who have taught that happiness is the end of life were as fully aware as those who taunt them.

[2:72] The happiness which they meant was not a life of rapture, but moments of such, in an existence made up of few and transitory pains, many and various pleasures, with a decided predominance of the active over the passive, and having as the foundation of the whole not to expect more from life than it is capable of bestowing.

[2:73] A life thus composed, to those who have been fortunate enough to obtain it, has always appeared worthy of the name of happiness.

[2:74] And such an existence is even now the lot of many during some considerable portion of their lives.

[2:75] The present wretched education and wretched social arrangements are the only real hindrance to its being attainable by almost all.

[2:76] The objectors perhaps may doubt whether human beings, if taught to consider happiness as the end of life, would be satisfied with such a moderate share of it.

[2:77] But great numbers of mankind have been satisfied with much less.

[2:78] The main constituents of a satisfied life appear to be two, either of which by itself is often found sufficient for the purpose: tranquillity and excitement.

[2:79] With much tranquillity, many find that they can be content with very little pleasure; with much excitement, many can reconcile themselves to a considerable quantity of pain.

[2:80] There is assuredly no inherent impossibility of enabling even the mass of mankind to unite both, since the two are so far from being incompatible that they are in natural alliance, the prolongation of either being a preparation for, and exciting a wish for, the other.

[2:81] It is only those in whom indolence amounts to a vice that do not desire excitement after an interval of response; it is only those in whom the need of excitement is a disease that feel the tranquillity which follows excitement dull and insipid, instead of pleasurable in direct proportion to the excitement which preceded it.

[2:82] When people who are tolerably fortunate in their outward lot do not find in life sufficient enjoyment to make it valuable to them, the cause generally is caring for nobody but themselves.

[2:83] To those who have neither public nor private affections, the excitements of life are much curtailed, and in any case dwindle in value as the time approaches when all selfish interests must be terminated by death; while those who leave after them objects of personal affection, and especially those who have also cultivated a fellow-feeling with the collective interests of mankind, retain as lively an interest in life on the eve of death as in the vigor of youth and health.

[2:84] Next to selfishness, the principal cause which makes life unsatisfactory is want [lack] of mental cultivation.

[2:85] A cultivated mind—I do not mean that of a philosopher, but any mind to which the fountains of knowledge have been opened, and which has been taught, in any tolerable degree, to exercise its faculties—finds sources of inexhaustible interest in all that surrounds it: in the objects of nature, the achievements of art, the imaginations of poetry, the incidents of history, the ways of mankind, past and present, and their prospects in the future.

[2:86] It is possible, indeed, to become indifferent to all this, and that too without having exhausted a thousandth part of it, but only when one has had from the beginning no moral or human interest in these things and has sought in them only the gratification of curiosity.

[2:87] Now there is absolutely no reason in the nature of things why an amount of mental culture sufficient to give an intelligent interest in these objects of contemplation should not be the inheritance of everyone born in a civilized country.

[2:88] As little is there an inherent necessity that any human being should be a selfish egotist, devoid of every feeling or care but those which center in his own miserable individuality.

[2:89] Something far superior to this is sufficiently common even now, to give ample earnest of what the human species may be made.

[2:90] Genuine private affections and a sincere interest in the public good are possible, though in unequal degrees, to every rightly brought up human being.

[2:91] In a world in which there is so much to interest, so much to enjoy, and so much also to correct and improve, everyone who has this moderate amount of moral and intellectual requisites is capable of an existence which may be called enviable; and unless such a person, through bad laws or subjection to the will of others, is denied the liberty to use the sources of happiness within his reach, he will not fail to find this enviable existence, if he escapes the positive evils of life, the great sources of physical and mental suffering—such as indigence, disease, and the unkindness, worthlessness, or premature loss of objects of affection.

[2:92] The main stress of the problem lies, therefore, in the contest with these calamities from which it is a rare good fortune entirely to escape; which, as things now are, cannot be obviated, and often cannot be in any material degree mitigated.

[2:93] Yet no one whose opinion deserves a moment's consideration can doubt that most of the great positive evils of the world are in themselves removable, and will, if human affairs continue to improve, be in the end reduced within narrow limits.

[2:94] Poverty, in any sense implying suffering, may be completely extinguished by the wisdom of society combined with the good sense and providence of individuals.

[2:95] Even that most intractable of enemies, disease, may be indefinitely reduced in dimensions by good physical and moral education and proper control of noxious influences, while the progress of science holds out a promise for the future of still more direct conquests over this detestable foe.

[2:96] And every advance in that direction relieves us from some, not only of the chances which cut short our own lives, but, what concerns us still more, which deprive us of those in whom our happiness is wrapped up.

[2:97] As for vicissitudes of fortune and other disappointments connected with worldly circumstances, these are principally the effect either of gross imprudence, of ill-regulated desires, or of bad or imperfect social institutions.

[2:98] All the grand sources, in short, of human suffering are in a great degree, many of them almost entirely, conquerable by human care and effort; and though their removal is grievously slow —though a long succession of generations will perish in the breach before the conquest is completed, and this world becomes all that, if will and knowledge were not wanting, it might easily be made—yet every mind sufficiently intelligent and generous to bear a part, however small and inconspicuous, in the endeavor will draw a noble enjoyment from the contest itself, which he would not for any bribe in the form of selfish indulgence consent to be without.

[2:99] And this leads to the true estimation of what is said by the objectors concerning the possibility; and the obligation of learning to do without happiness.

[2:100] Unquestionably it is possible to do without happiness; it is done involuntarily by nineteen-twentieths of mankind, even in those parts of our present world which are least deep in barbarism; and it often has to be done voluntarily by the hero or the martyr, for the sake of something which he prizes more than his individual happiness.

[2:101] But this something, what is it, unless the happiness of others or some of the requisites of happiness?

[2:102] It is noble to be capable of resigning entirely one's own portion of happiness, or chances of it; but, after all, this self-sacrifice must be for some end; it is not its own end; and if we are told that its end is not happiness but virtue, which is better than happiness, I ask, would the sacrifice be made if the hero or martyr did not believe that it would earn for others immunity from similar sacrifices?

[2:103] Would it be made if he thought that his renunciation of happiness for himself would produce no fruit for any of his fellow creatures, but to make their lot like his and place them also in the condition of persons who have renounced happiness?

[2:104] All honor to those who can abnegate for themselves the personal enjoyment of life when by such renunciation they contribute worthily to increase the amount of happiness in the world; but he who does it or professes to do it for any other purpose is no more deserving of admiration than the ascetic mounted on his pillar.

[2:105] He may be an inspiriting proof of what men *can* do, but assuredly not an example of what they *should.*

[2:106] Though it is only in a very imperfect state of the world's arrangements that anyone can best serve the happiness of others by the absolute sacrifice of his own, yet, so long as the world is in that imperfect state, I fully acknowledge that the readiness to make such a sacrifice is the highest virtue which can be found in man.

[2:107] I will add that in this condition of the world, paradoxical as the assertion may be, the conscious ability to do without happiness gives the best prospect of realizing such happiness as is attainable.

[2:108] For nothing except that consciousness can raise a person above the chances of life by making him feel that, let fate and fortune do their worst, they have not power to subdue him; which, once felt, frees him from excess of anxiety concerning the evils of life and enables him, like many a Stoic in the worst times of the Roman Empire, to cultivate in tranquillity the sources of satisfaction accessible to him, without concerning himself about the uncertainty of their duration any more than about their inevitable end.

[2:109] Meanwhile, let utilitarians never cease to claim the morality of self-devotion as a possession which belongs by as good a right to them as either to the Stoic or to the Transcendentalist.

[2:110] The utilitarian morality does recognize in human beings the power of sacrificing their own greatest good for the good of others.

[2:111] It only refuses to admit that the sacrifice is itself a good.

[2:112] A sacrifice which does not increase or tend to increase the sum total of happiness, it considers as wasted.

[2:113] The only self-renunciation which it applauds is devotion to the happiness, or to some of the means of happiness, of others, either of mankind collectively or of individuals within the limits imposed by the collective interests of mankind.

[2:114] I must again repeat what the assailants of utilitarianism seldom have the justice to acknowledge, that the happiness which forms the utilitarian standard of what is right in conduct is not the agent's own happiness but that of all concerned.

[2:115] As between his own happiness and that of others, utilitarianism requires him to be as strictly impartial as a disinterested and benevolent spectator.

[2:116] In the golden rule of Jesus of Nazareth, we read the complete spirit of the ethics of utility.

[2:117] "To do as you would be done by," and "to love your neighbor as yourself," constitute the ideal perfection of utilitarian morality.

[2:118] As the means of making the nearest approach to this ideal, utility would enjoin, first, that laws and social arrangements should place the happiness or (as, speaking practically, it may be called) the interest of every individual as nearly as possible in harmony with the interest of the whole; and, secondly, that education and opinion, which have so vast a power over human character, should so use that power as to establish in the mind of every individual an indissoluble association between his own happiness and the good of the whole, especially between his own happiness and the good of the whole, especially between his own happiness and the practice of such modes of conduct, negative and positive, as regard for the universal happiness prescribes; so that not only he may be unable to conceive the possibility of happiness to himself, consistently with conduct opposed to the general good, but also that a direct impulse to promote the general good may be in every individual one of the habitual motives of action, and the sentiments connected therewith may fill a large and prominent place in every human being's sentient existence.

[2:119] If the impugners of the utilitarian morality represented it to their own minds in this its true character, I know not what recommendation possessed by any other morality they could possibly affirm to be wanting to it; what more beautiful or more exalted developments of human nature any other ethical system can be supposed to foster, or what springs of action, not accessible to the utilitarian, such systems rely on for giving effect to their mandates.

[2:120] The objectors to utilitarianism cannot always be charged with representing it in a discreditable light.

[2:121] On the contrary, those among them who entertain anything like a just idea of its disinterested character sometimes find fault with its standard as being too high for humanity.

[2:122] They say it is exacting too much to require that people shall always act from the inducement of promoting the general interest of society.

[2:123] But this is to mistake the very meaning of a standard of morals and confound the rule of action with the motive of it.

[2:124] It is the business of ethics to tell us what are our duties, or by what test we may know them; but no system of ethics requires that the sole motive of all we do shall be a feeling of duty; on the contrary, ninety-nine hundredths of all our actions are done from other motives, and rightly so done if the rule of duty does not condemn them.

[2:125] It is the more unjust to utilitarianism that this particular misapprehension should be made a ground of objection to it, inasmuch as utilitarian moralists have gone beyond almost all others in affirming that the motive has nothing to do with the morality of the action, though much with the worth of the agent.

[2:126] He who saves a fellow creature from drowning does what is morally right, whether his motive be duty or the hope of being paid for his trouble; he who betrays the friend that trusts him is guilty of a crime, even if his object be to serve another friend to whom he is under greater obligations.

[2:127] But to speak only of actions done from the motive of duty, and in direct obedience to principle: it is a misapprehension of the utilitarian mode of thought to conceive it as implying that people should fix their minds upon so wide a generality as the world, or society at large.

[2:128] The great majority of good actions are intended not for the benefit of the world, but for that of individuals, of which the good of the world is made up; and the thoughts of the most virtuous man need not on these occasions travel beyond the particular persons concerned, except so far as is necessary to assure himself that in benefiting them he is not violating the rights, that is, the legitimate and authorized expectations, of anyone else.

[2:129] The multiplication of happiness is, according to the utilitarian ethics, the object of virtue: the occasions on which any person (except one in a thousand) has it in his power to do this on an extended scale—in other words, to be a public benefactor—are but exceptional and on these occasions alone is he called on to consider public utility; in every other case, private utility, the interest or happiness of some few persons, is all he has to attend to.

[2:130] Those alone the influence of whose actions extends to society in general need concern themselves habitually about so large an object.

[2:131] In the case of abstinences indeed—of things which people forbear to do from moral considerations, though the consequences in the particular case might be beneficial—it would be unworthy of an intelligent agent not to be consciously aware that the action is of a class which, if practiced generally, would be generally injurious, and that this is the ground of the obligation to abstain from it.

[2:132] The amount of regard for the public interest implied in this recognition is no greater than is demanded by every system of morals, for they all enjoin to abstain from whatever is manifestly pernicious to society.

[2:133] The same considerations dispose of another reproach against the doctrine of utility, founded on a still grosser misconception of the purpose of a standard of morality and of the very meaning of the words "right" and "wrong."

[2:134] It is often affirmed that utilitarianism renders men cold and unsympathizing; that it chills their moral feelings toward individuals; that it makes them regard only the dry and hard consideration of the consequences of actions, not taking into their moral estimate the qualities from which those actions emanate.

[2:135] If the assertion means that they do not allow their judgment respecting the rightness or wrongness of an action to be influenced by their opinion of the qualities of the person who does it, this is a complaint not against utilitarianism, but against any standard or morality at all; for certainly no known ethical standard decided an action to be good or bad because it is done by a good or bad man, still less because done by an amiable, a brave, or a benevolent man, or the contrary.

[2:136] These considerations are relevant, not to the estimation of actions, but of persons; and there is nothing in the utilitarian theory inconsistent with the fact that there are other things which interest us in persons besides the rightness and wrongness of their actions.

[2:137] The Stoics, indeed, with the paradoxical misuse of language which was part of their system, and by which they strove to raise themselves above all concern about anything but virtue, were fond of saying that he who has that has everything; that he, and only he, is rich, is beautiful, is a king.

[2:138] But no claim of this description is made for the virtuous man by the utilitarian doctrine.

[2:139] Utilitarians are quite aware that there are other desirable possessions and qualities besides virtue, and are perfectly willing to allow to all of them their full worth.

[2:140] They are also aware that a right action does not necessarily indicate a virtuous character, and that actions which are blamable often proceed from qualities entitled to praise.

[2:141] When this is apparent in any particular case, it modifies their estimation, not certainly of the act, but of the agent.

[2:142] I grant that they are, notwithstanding, of opinion that in the long run the best proof of a good character is good actions; and resolutely refuse to consider any mental disposition as good of which the predominant tendency is to produce bad conduct.

[2:143] This makes them unpopular with many people, but it is an unpopularity which they must share with everyone who regards the distinction between right and wrong in a serious light; and the reproach is not one which a conscientious utilitarian need be anxious to repel.

[2:144] If no more be meant by the objection than that many utilitarians look on the morality of actions, as measured by the utilitarian standards, with too exclusive a regard, and do not lay sufficient stress upon the other beauties of character which go toward making a human being lovable or admirable, this may be admitted.

[2:145] Utilitarians who have cultivated their moral feelings, but not their sympathies, nor their artistic perceptions, do fall into this mistake; and so do all other moralists under the same conditions.

[2:146] What can be said in excuse for other moralists is equally available for them, namely, that, if there is to be any error, it is better that it should be on that side.

[2:147] As a matter of fact, we may affirm that among utilitarians, as among adherents of other systems, there is every imaginable degree of rigidity and of laxity in the application of their standard; some are even puritanically rigorous, while others are as indulgent as can possibly be desired by sinner or by sentimentalist.

[2:148] But on the whole, a doctrine which brings prominently forward the interest that mankind have in the repression and prevention of conduct which violates the moral law is likely to be inferior to no other in turning the sanctions of opinion against such violations.

[2:149] It is true, the question "What does violate the moral law?" is one on which those who recognize different standards of morality are likely now and then to differ.

[2:150] But difference of opinion on moral questions was not first introduced into the world by utilitarianism, while that doctrine does supply, if not always an easy, at all events a tangible and intelligible, mode of deciding such difference.

[2:151] It may not be superfluous to notice a few more of the common misapprehensions of utilitarian ethics, even those which are so obvious and gross that it might appear impossible for any person of candor and intelligence to fall into them; since persons, even of considerable mental endowment, often give themselves so little trouble to understand the bearings of any opinion against which they entertain a prejudice, and men are in general so little conscious of this voluntary ignorance as a defect that the vulgarest misunderstandings of ethical doctrines are continually met with in the deliberate writings of persons of the greatest pretensions both to high principle and to philosophy.

[2:152] We not uncommonly hear the doctrine of utility inveighed against as a *godless* doctrine.

[2:153] If it be necessary to say anything at all against so mere an assumption, we may say that the question depends upon what idea we have formed of the moral character of the Deity.

[2:154] If it be a true belief that God desires, above all things, the happiness of his creatures, and that this was his purpose in their creation, utility is not only not a godless doctrine, but more profoundly religious than any other.

[2:155] If it be meant that utilitarianism does not recognize the revealed will of God as the supreme law of morals, I answer that a utilitarian who believes in the perfect goodness and wisdom of *God* necessarily believes that whatever God has thought fit to reveal on the subject of morals must fulfill the requirements of utility in a supreme degree.

[2:156] But others besides utilitarians have been of opinion that the Christian revelation was intended, and is fitted, to inform the hearts and minds of mankind with a spirit which should enable them to find for themselves what is right, and incline them to do it when found, rather than to tell them, except in a very general way, what it is; and that we need a doctrine of ethics, carefully followed out, to *interpret* to us the will of God.

[2:157] Whether this opinion is correct or not, it is superfluous here to discuss; since whatever aid religion, either natural or revealed, can afford to ethical investigation is as open to the utilitarian moralist as to any other.

[2:158] He can use it as the testimony of God to the usefulness or hurtfulness of any given course of action by as good a right as others can use it for the indication of a transcendental law having no connection with usefulness or with happiness.

[2:159] Again, utility is often summarily stigmatized as an immoral doctrine by giving it the name of "expediency;" and taking advantage of the popular use of that term to contrast it with principle.

[2:160] But the expedient, in the sense in which it is opposed to the right, generally means that which is expedient for the particular interest of the agent himself; as when a minister sacrifices the interests of his country to keep himself in place.

[2:161] When it means anything better than this, it means that which is expedient for some immediate object, some temporary purpose, but which violates a rule whose observance is expedient in a much higher degree.

[2:162] The expedient, in this sense, instead of being the same thing with the useful, is a branch of the hurtful.

[2:163] Thus it would often be expedient, for the purpose of getting over some momentary embarrassment, or attaining some object immediately useful to ourselves or others, to tell a lie.

[2:164] But inasmuch as the cultivation in ourselves of a sensitive feeling on the subject of veracity is one of the most useful, and the enfeeblement of that feeling one of the most hurtful, things to which our conduct can be instrumental; and inasmuch as any, even unintentional, deviation from truth does that much toward weakening the trustworthiness of human assertion, which is not only the principal support of all present social well-being, but the insufficiency of which does more than any one thing that can be named to keep back civilization, virtue, everything on which human happiness on the largest scale depends—we feel that the violation, for a present advantage, of a rule of such transcendent expediency is not expedient, and that he who, for the sake of convenience to himself or to some other individual, does what depends on him to deprive mankind of the good, and inflict upon them the evil, involved in the greater or less reliance which they can place in each other's words, acts the part of one of their worst enemies.

[2:165] Yet that even this rule, sacred as it is, admits of possible exceptions is acknowledged by all moralists; the chief of which is when the withholding of some fact (as of information from a malefactor, or of bad news from a person dangerously ill) would save an individual (especially an individual other than oneself) from great and unmerited evil, and when the withholding can only be effected by denial.

[2:166] But in order that the exception may not extend itself beyond the need, and may have the least possible effect in weakening reliance on veracity, it ought to be recognized and, if possible, its limits defined; and, if the principle of utility is good for anything, it must be good for weighing these conflicting utilities against one another and marking out the region within which one or the other preponderates.

[2:167] Again, defenders of utility often find themselves called upon to reply to such objections as this—that there is not time, previous to action, for calculating and weighing the effects of any line of conduct on the general happiness.

[2:168] This is exactly as if anyone were to say that it is impossible to guide our conduct by Christianity because there is not time, on every occasion on which anything has to be done, to read through the Old and New Testaments.

[2:169] The answer to the objection is that there has been ample time, namely, the whole past duration of the human species.

[2:170] During all that time mankind have been learning by experience the tendencies of actions; on which experience all the prudence as well as all the morality of life are dependent.

[2:171] People talk as if the commencement of this course of experience had hitherto been put off, and as if, at the moment when some man feels tempted to meddle with the property or life of another, he had to begin considering for the first time whether murder and theft are injurious to human happiness.

[2:172] Even then I do not think that he would find the question very puzzling; but, at all events, the matter is now done to his hand.

[2:173] It is truly a whimsical supposition that, if mankind were agreed in considering utility to be the test of morality, they would remain without any agreement as to what *is* useful, and would take no measures for having their notions on the subject taught to the young and enforced by law and opinion.

[2:174] There is no difficulty in proving any ethical standard whatever to work ill if we suppose universal idiocy to be conjoined with it; but on any hypothesis short of that, mankind must by this time have acquired positive beliefs as to the effects of some actions on their happiness; and the beliefs which have thus come down are the rules of morality for the multitude, and for the philosopher until he has succeeded in finding better.

[2:175] That philosophers might easily do this, even now, on many subjects; that the received code of ethics is by no means of divine right; and that mankind have still much to learn as to the effects of actions on the general happiness, I admit or rather earnestly maintain.

[2:176] The corollaries from the principles of utility, like the precepts of every practical art, admit of indefinite improvement, and, in a progressive state of the human mind, their improvement is perpetually going on.

[2:177] But to consider the rules of morality as improvable is one thing; to pass over the intermediate generalization entirely and endeavor to test each individual action directly by the first principle is another.

[2:178] Men really ought to leave off talking a kind of nonsense on this subject, which they would neither talk nor listen to on other matters of practical concernment.

[2:179] Nobody argues that the art of navigation is not founded on astronomy because sailors cannot wait to calculate the Nautical Almanac.

[2:180] Being rational creatures, they go to sea with it ready calculated; and all rational creatures go out upon the sea of life with their minds made up on the common questions of right and wrong, as well as on many of the far more difficult questions of wise and foolish.

[2:181] And this, as long as foresight is a human quality, it is to be presumed they will continue to do.

[2:182] Whatever we adopt as the fundamental principle of morality, we require subordinate principles to apply it by; the impossibility of doing without them, being common to all systems, can afford no argument against any one in particular; but gravely to argue as if no such secondary principles could be had, and as if mankind had remained till now, and always must remain, without drawing any general conclusions from the experience of human life is as high a pitch, I think, as absurdity has ever reached in philosophical controversy.

[2:183] The remainder of the stock arguments against utilitarianism mostly consist in laying to its charge the common infirmities of human nature, and the general difficulties which embarrass conscientious persons in shaping their course through life.

[2:184] We are told that a utilitarian will be apt to make his own particular case an exception to moral rules, and, when under temptation, will see a utility in the breach of a rule, greater than he will see in its observance.

[2:185] But is utility the only creed which is able to furnish us with excuses for evil-doing and means of cheating our own conscience?

[2:186] They are afforded in abundance by all doctrines which recognize as a fact in morals the existence of conflicting considerations, which all doctrines do that have been believed by sane persons.

[2:187] It is not the fault of any creed, but of the complicated nature of human affairs, that rules of conduct cannot be so framed as to require no exceptions, and that hardly any kind of action can safely be laid down as either always obligatory or always condemnable.

[2:188] There is no ethical creed which does not temper the rigidity of its laws by giving a certain latitude, under the moral responsibility of the agent, for accommodation to peculiarities of circumstances; and under every creed, at the opening thus made, self-deception and dishonest casuistry get in.

[2:189] There exists no moral system under which there do not arise unequivocal cases of conflicting obligation.

[2:190] These are the real difficulties, the knotty points both in the theory of ethics and in the conscientious guidance of personal conduct.

[2:191] They are overcome practically, with greater or with less success, according to the intellect and virtue of the individual; but it can hardly be pretended that anyone will be the less qualified for dealing with them, from possessing an ultimate standard to which conflicting rights and duties can be referred.

[2:192] If utility is the ultimate source of moral obligations, utility may be invoked to decide between them when their demands are incompatible.

[2:193] Though the application of the standard may be difficult, it is better than none at all; while in other systems, the moral laws all claiming independent authority, there is no common umpire entitled to interfere between them; their claims to precedence one over another rest on little better than sophistry, and, unless determined, as they generally are, by the unacknowledged influence of consideration of utility, afford a free scope for the action of personal desires and partialities.

[2:194] We must remember that only in these cases of conflict between secondary principles is it requisite that first principles should be appealed to.

[2:195] There is no case of moral obligation in which some secondary principle is not involved; and if only one, there can seldom be any real doubt which one it is, in the mind of any person by whom the principle itself is recognized.

Chapter III: Of The Ultimate Sanction Of The Principle Of Utility

[3:1] The question is often asked, and properly so, in regard to any supposed moral standard—What is its sanction? what are the motives to obey? or, more specifically, what is the source of its obligation? whence does it derive its binding force?

[3:2] It is a necessary part of moral philosophy to provide the answer to this question, which, though frequently assuming the shape of an objection to the utilitarian morality, as if it had some special applicability to that above others, really arises in regard to all standards.

[3:3] It arises, in fact, whenever a person is called on to *adopt* a standard, or refer morality to any basis on which he has not been accustomed to rest it.

[3:4] For the customary morality, that which education and opinion have consecrated, is the only one which presents itself to the mind with the feeling of being *in itself* obligatory; and when a person is asked to believe that this morality *derives* its obligation from some general principle round which custom has not thrown the same halo, the assertion is to him a paradox; the supposed corollaries seem to have a more binding force than the original theorem; the superstructure seems to stand better without than with what is represented as its foundation.

[3:5] He says to himself, I feel that I am bound not to rob or murder, betray or deceive; but why am I bound to promote the general happiness?

[3:6] If my own happiness lies in something else, why may I not give that the preference?

[3:7] If the view adopted by the utilitarian philosophy of the nature of the moral sense be correct, this difficulty will always present itself until the influences which form moral character have taken the same hold of the principle which they have taken of some of the consequences—until, by the improvement of education, the feeling of unity with our fellow creatures shall be (what it cannot be denied that Christ intended it to be) as deeply rooted in our character, and to our own consciousness as completely a part of our nature, as the horror of crime is in an ordinarily well brought up young person.

[3:8] In the meantime, however, the difficulty has no peculiar application to the doctrine of utility, but is inherent in every attempt to analyze morality and reduce it to principles; which, unless the principle is already in men's minds invested with as much sacredness as any of its applications, always seems to divest them of a part of their sanctity.

[3:9] The principle of utility either has, or there is no reason why it might not have, all the sanctions which belong to any other system of morals.

[3:10] Those sanctions are either external or internal.

[3:11] Of the external sanctions it is not necessary to speak at any length.

[3:12] They are the hope of favor and the fear of displeasure from our fellow creatures or from the Ruler of the universe, along with whatever we may have of sympathy or affection for them, or of love and awe of Him, inclining us to do His will independently of selfish consequences.

[3:13] There is evidently no reason why all these motives for observance should not attach themselves to the utilitarian morality as completely and as powerfully as to any other.

[3:14] Indeed, those of them which refer to our fellow creatures are sure to do so, in proportion to the amount of general intelligence; for whether there be any other ground of moral obligation than the general happiness or not, men do desire happiness; and however imperfect may be their own practice, they desire and commend all conduct in others toward themselves by which they think their happiness is promoted.

[3:15] With regard to the religious motive, if men believe, as most profess to do, in the goodness of God, those who think that conduciveness to the general happiness is the essence or even only the criterion of good must necessarily believe that it is also that which God approves.

[3:16] The whole force therefore of external reward and punishment, whether physical or moral, whether proceeding from God or from our fellow men, together with all that the capacities of human nature admit of disinterested devotion to either, become available to enforce the utilitarian morality, in proportion as that morality is recognized; and the more powerfully, the more the appliances of education and general cultivation are bent to the purpose.

[3:17] So far as to external sanctions.

[3:18] The internal sanction of duty, whatever our standard of duty may be, is one and the same—a feeling in our own mind; a pain, more or less intense, attendant on violation of duty, which in properly cultivated moral natures rises, in the more serious cases, into shrinking from it as an impossibility.

[3:19] This feeling, when disinterested and connecting itself with the pure idea of duty, and not with some particular form of it, or with any of the merely accessory circumstances, is the essence of conscience; though in that complex phenomenon as it actually exists, the simple fact is in general all encrusted over with collateral associations derived from sympathy, from love, and still more from fear; from all the forms of religious feeling; from the recollections of childhood and of all our past life; from self-esteem, desire of the esteem of others, and occasionally even self-abasement.

[3:20] This extreme complication is, I apprehend, the origin of the sort of mystical character which, by a tendency of the human mind of which there are many other examples, is apt to be attributed to the idea of moral obligation, and which leads people to believe that the idea cannot possibly attach itself to any other objects than those which, by a supposed mysterious law, are found in our present experience to excite it.

[3:21] Its binding force, however, consists in the existence of a mass of feeling which must be broken through in order to do what violates our standard of right, and which, if we do nevertheless violate that standard, will probably have to be encountered afterwards in the form of remorse.

[3:22] Whatever theory we have of the nature or origin of conscience, this is what essentially constitutes it.

[3:23] The ultimate sanction, therefore, of all morality (external motives apart) being a subjective feeling in our own minds, I see nothing embarrassing to those whose standard is utility in the question, What is the sanction of that particular standard?

[3:24] We may answer, the same as of all other moral standards—the conscientious feelings of mankind.

[3:25] Undoubtedly this sanction has no binding efficacy on those who do not possess the feelings it appeals to; but neither will these persons be more obedient to any other moral principle than to the utilitarian one.

[3:26] On them morality of any kind has no hold but through the external sanctions.

[3:27] Meanwhile the feelings exist, a fact in human nature, the reality of which, and the great power with which they are capable of acting on those in whom they have been duly cultivated, are proved by experience.

[3:28] No reason has ever been shown why they may not be cultivated to as great intensity in connection with the utilitarian as with any other rule of morals.

[3:29] There is, I am aware, a disposition to believe that a person who sees in moral obligation a transcendental fact, an objective reality belonging to the province of "things in themselves," is likely to be more obedient to it than one who believes it to be entirely subjective, having its seat in human consciousness only.

[3:30] But whatever a person's opinion may be on this point of ontology, the force he is really urged by is his own subjective feeling, and is exactly measured by its strength.

[3:31] No one's belief that duty is an objective reality is stronger than the belief that God is so; yet the belief in God, apart from the expectation of actual reward and punishment, only operates on conduct through, and in proportion to, the subjective religious feeling.

[3:32] The sanction, so far as it is disinterested, is always in the mind itself; and the notion, therefore, of the transcendental moralists must be that this sanction will not exist *in* the mind unless it is believed to have its root out of the mind; and that if a person is able to say to himself, "That which is restraining me and which is called my conscience is only a feeling in my own mind," he may possibly draw the conclusion that when the feeling ceases the obligation ceases, and that if he finds the feeling inconvenient, he may disregard it and endeavor to get rid of it.

[3:33] But is this danger confined to the utilitarian morality?

[3:34] Does the belief that moral obligation has its seat outside the mind make the feeling of it too strong to get rid of?

[3:35] The fact is so far otherwise that all moralists admit and lament the ease with which, in the generality of minds, conscience can be silenced or stifled.

[3:36] The question, "Need I obey my conscience?" is quite as often put to themselves by persons who never heard of the principle of utility as by its adherents.

[3:37] Those whose conscientious feelings are so weak as to allow of their asking this question, if they answer it affirmatively, will not do so because they believe in the transcendental theory, but because of the external sanctions.

[3:38] It is not necessary, for the present purpose, to decide whether the feeling of duty is innate or implanted.

[3:39] Assuming it to be innate, it is an open question to what objects it naturally attaches itself for the philosophic supporters of that theory are now agreed that the intuitive perception is of principles of morality and not of the details.

[3:40] If there be anything innate in the matter, I see no reason why the feeling which is innate should not be that of regard to the pleasures and pains of others.

[3:41] If there is any principle of morals which is intuitively obligatory, I should say it must be that.

[3:42] If so, the intuitive ethics would coincide with the utilitarian, and there would be no further quarrel between them.

[3:43] Even as it is, the intuitive moralists, though they believe that there are other intuitive moral obligations, do already believe this to be one; for they unanimously hold that a large *portion* of morality turns upon the consideration due to the interests of our fellow creatures.

[3:44] Therefore, if the belief in the transcendental origin of moral obligation gives any additional efficacy to the internal sanction, it appears to me that the utilitarian principle has already the benefit of it.

[3:45] On the other hand, if, as is my own belief, the moral feelings are not innate but acquired, they are not for that reason the less natural.

[3:46] It is natural to man to speak, to reason, to build cities, to cultivate the ground, though these are acquired faculties.

[3:47] The moral feelings are not indeed a part of our nature in the sense of being in any perceptible degree present in all of us; but this, unhappily, is a fact admitted by those who believe the most strenuously in their transcendental origin.

[3:48] Like the other acquired capacities above referred to, the moral faculty, if not a part of our nature, is a natural outgrowth from it; capable, like them, in a certain small degree, of springing up spontaneously; and susceptible of being brought by cultivation to a high degree of development.

[3:49] Unhappily it is also susceptible, by a sufficient use of the external sanctions and of the force of early impressions, of being cultivated in almost any direction, so that there is hardly anything so absurd or so mischievous that it may not, by means of these influences, be made to act on the human mind with all the authority of conscience.

[3:50] To doubt that the same potency might be given by the same means to the principle of utility, even if it had no foundation in human nature, would be flying in the face of all experience.

[3:51] But moral associations which are wholly of artificial creation, when the intellectual culture goes on, yield by degrees to the dissolving force of analysis; and if the feeling of duty, when associated with utility; would appear equally arbitrary; if there were no leading department of our nature, no powerful class of sentiments, with which that association would harmonize, which would make us feel congenial and incline us not only to foster it in others (for which we have abundant interested motives), but also to cherish it in ourselves—if there were not, in short, a natural basis of sentiment for utilitarian morality, it might well happen that this association also, even after it had been implanted by education, might be analyzed away.

[3:52] But there *is* this basis of powerful natural sentiment; and that it is which, when once the general happiness is recognized as the ethical standard, will constitute the strength of the utilitarian morality.

[3:53] This firm foundation is that of the social feelings of mankind—the desire to be in unity with our fellow creatures, which is already a powerful principle in human nature and happily one of those which tend to become stronger, even without express inculcation, from the influences of advancing civilization.

[3:54] The social state is at once so natural, so necessary, and so habitual to man, that, except in some unusual circumstances or by an effort of voluntary abstraction, he never conceives himself otherwise than as a member of a body; and this association is riveted more and more, as mankind are further removed from the state of savage independence.

[3:55] Any condition, therefore, which is essential to a state of society becomes more and more an inseparable part of every person's conception of the state of things which he is born into, and which is the destiny of a human being.

[3:56] Now society between human beings, except in the relation of master and slave, is manifestly impossible on any other footing than that the interests of all are to be consulted.

[3:57] Society between equals can only exist on the understanding that the interests of all are to be regarded equally.

[3:58] And since in all states of civilization, every person, except an absolute monarch, has equals, everyone is obliged to live on these terms with somebody; and in every age some advance is made toward a state in which it will be impossible to live permanently on other terms with anybody.

[3:59] In this way people grow up unable to conceive as possible to them a state of total disregard of other people's interests.

[3:60] They are under a necessity of conceiving themselves as at least abstaining from all the grosser injuries, and (if only for their own protection) living in a state of constant protest against them.

[3:61] They are also familiar with the fact of cooperating with others and proposing to themselves a collective, not an individual, interest as the aim (at least for the time being) of their actions.

[3:62] So long as they are cooperating, their ends are identified with those of others; there is at least a temporary feeling that the interest of others are their own interests.

[3:63] Not only does all strengthening of social ties, and all healthy growth of society, give to each individual a stronger personal interest in practically consulting the welfare of others, it also leads him to identify his *feelings* more and more with their good, or at least with an even greater degree of practical consideration for it.

[3:64] He comes, as though instinctively, to be conscious of himself as a being who *of course* pays regard to others.

[3:65] The good of others becomes to him a thing naturally and necessarily to be attended to, like any of the physical conditions of our existence.

[3:66] Now, whatever amount of this feeling a person has, he is urged by the strongest motives both of interest and of sympathy to demonstrate it, and to the utmost of his power encourage it in others; and even if he has none of it himself, he is as greatly interested as anyone else that others should have it.

[3:67] Consequently the smallest germs of the feeling are laid hold of and nourished by the contagion of sympathy and the influences of education; and a complete web of corroborative association is woven round it by the powerful agency of the external sanctions.

[3:68] This mode of conceiving ourselves and human life, as civilization goes on, is felt to be more and more natural.

[3:69] Every step in political improvement renders it more so, by removing the sources of opposition of interest and leveling those inequalities of legal privilege between individuals or classes, owing to which there are large portions of mankind whose happiness it is still practicable to disregard.

[3:70] In an improving state of the human mind, the influences are constantly on the increase which tend to generate in each individual a feeling of unity with all the rest; which, if perfect, would make him never think of, or desire, any beneficial condition for himself in the benefits of which they are not included.

[3:71] If we now suppose this feeling of unity to be taught as a religion, and the whole force of education, of institutions, and of opinion directed, as it once was in the case of religion, to make every person grow up from infancy surrounded on all sides both by the profession and the practice of it, I think that no one who can realize this conception will feel any misgiving about the sufficiency of the ultimate sanction for the happiness morality.

[3:72] To any ethical student who finds the realization difficult, I recommend, as a means of facilitating it, the second of M. Comte's two principal works, the *Traite' de politique positive.*

[3:73] I entertain the strongest objections to the system of politics and morals set forth in that treatise, but I think it has superabundantly shown the possibility of giving to the service of humanity, even without the aid of belief in a Providence, both the psychological power and the social efficacy of a religion, making it take hold of human life, and color all thought, feeling, and action in a manner of which the greatest ascendancy ever exercised by any religion may be but a type and foretaste; and of which the danger is, not that it should be insufficient, but that it should be so excessive as to interfere unduly with human freedom and individuality.

[3:74] Neither is it necessary to the feeling which constitutes the binding force of the utilitarian morality on those who recognize it to wait for those social influences which would make its obligation felt by mankind at large.

[3:75] In the comparatively early state of human advancement in which we now live, a person cannot, indeed, feel that entireness of sympathy with all others which would make any real discordance in the general direction of their conduct in life impossible, but already a person in whom the social feeling is at all developed cannot bring himself to think of the rest of his fellow creatures as struggling rivals with him for the means of happiness, whom he must desire to see defeated in their object in order that he may succeeded in his.

[3:76] The deeply rooted conception which every individual even now has of himself as a social being tends to make him feel it one of his natural wants that there should be harmony between his feelings and aims and those of his fellow creatures.

[3:77] If differences of opinion and of mental culture make it impossible for him to share many of their actual feelings—perhaps make him denounce and defy those feelings—he still needs to be conscious that his real aim and theirs do not conflict; that he is not opposing himself to what they really wish for, namely their own good, but is, on the contrary, promoting it.

[3:78] This feeling in most individuals is much inferior in strength to their selfish feelings, and is often wanting altogether.

[3:79] But to those who have it, it possesses all the characters of a natural feeling.

[3:80] It does not present itself to their minds as a superstition of education or a law despotically imposed by the power of society, but as an attribute which it would not be well for them to be without.

[3:81] This conviction is the ultimate sanction of the greatest happiness morality.

[3:82] This it is which makes any mind of well-developed feelings work with, and not against, the outward motives to care for others, afforded by what I have called the external sanctions; and, when those sanctions are wanting or act in an opposite direction, constitutes in itself a powerful internal binding force, in proportion to the sensitiveness and thoughtfulness of the character, since few but those whose mind is a moral blank could bear to lay out their course of life on the plan of paying no regard to others except so far as their own private interest compels.

Chapter IV: Of What Sort Of Proof The Principle Of Utility Is Susceptible

[4:1] It has already been remarked that questions of ultimate ends do not admit of proof, in the ordinary acceptation of the term.

[4:2] To be incapable of proof by reasoning is common to all first principles, to the first premises of our knowledge, as well as to those of our conduct.

[4:3] But the former, being matters of fact, may be the subject of a direct appeal to the faculties which judge of fact—namely, our senses and our internal consciousness.

[4:4] Can an appeal be made to the same faculties on questions of practical ends?

[4:5] Or by what other faculty is cognizance taken of them?

[4:6] Questions about ends are, in other words, questions what things are desirable.

[4:7] The utilitarian doctrine is that happiness is desirable, and the only thing desirable, as an end; all other things being only desirable as means to that end.

[4:8] What ought to be required of this doctrine, what conditions is it requisite that the doctrine should fulfill—to make good its claim to be believed?

[4:9] The only proof capable of being given that an object is visible is that people actually see it.

[4:10] The only proof that a sound is audible is that people hear it; and so of the other sources of our experience.

[4:11] In like manner, I apprehend, the sole evidence it is possible to produce that anything is desirable is that people do actually desire it.

[4:12] If the end which the utilitarian doctrine proposes to itself were not, in theory and in practice, acknowledged to be an end, nothing could ever convince any person that it was so.

[4:13] No reason can be given why the general happiness is desirable, except that each person, so far as he believes it to be attainable, desires his own happiness.

[4:14] This, however, being a fact, we have not only all the proof which the case admits of, but all which it is possible to require, that happiness is a good, that each person's happiness is a good to that person, and the general happiness, therefore, a good to the aggregate of all persons.

[4:15] Happiness has made out its title as *one* of the ends of conduct and, consequently, one of the criteria of morality.

[4:16] But it has not, by this alone, proved itself to be the sole criterion.

[4:17] To do that, it would seem, by the same rule, necessary to show, not only that people desire happiness, but that they never desire anything else.

[4:18] Now it is palpable that they do desire things which, in common language, are decidedly distinguished from happiness.

[4:19] They desire, for example, virtue and the absence of vice no less really than pleasure and the absence of pain.

[4:20] The desire of virtue is not as universal, but it is an authentic a fact as the desire of happiness.

[4:21] And hence the opponents of the utilitarian standard deem that they have a right to infer that there are other ends of human action besides happiness, and that happiness is not the standard of approbation and disapprobation.

[4:22] But does the utilitarian doctrine deny that people desire virtue, or maintain that virtue is not a thing to be desired?

[4:23] The very reverse.

[4:24] It maintains not only that virtue is to be desired, but that it is to be desired disinterestedly, for itself.

[4:25] Whatever may be the opinion of utilitarian moralists as to the original conditions by which virtue is made virtue, however they may believe (as they do) that actions and dispositions are only virtuous because they promote another end than virtue, yet this being granted, and it having been decided, from considerations of this description, what *is* virtuous, they not only place virtue at the very head of the things which are good as means to the ultimate end, but they also recognize as a psychological fact the possibility of its being, to the individual, a good in itself, without looking to any end beyond it; and hold that the mind is not in a right state, not in a state conformable to utility, not in the state most conducive to the general happiness, useless it does love virtue in this manner—as a thing desirable in itself, even although, in the individual instance, it should not produce those other desirable consequences which it tends to produce, and on account of which it is held to be virtue.

[4:26] This opinion is not, in the smallest degree, a departure from the happiness principle.

[4:27] The ingredients of happiness are very various, and each of them is desirable in itself, and not merely when considered as swelling an aggregate.

[4:28] The principle of utility does not mean that any given pleasure, as music, for instance, or any given exemption from pain, as for example health, is to be looked upon as means to a collective something termed happiness, and to be desired on that account.

[4:29] They are desired and desirable in and for themselves; besides being means, they are a part of the end.

[4:30] Virtue, according to the utilitarian doctrine, is not naturally and originally part of the end, but it is capable of becoming so; and in those who live it disinterestedly it has become so, and is desired and cherished, not as a means to happiness, but as a part of their happiness.

[4:31] To illustrate this further, we may remember that virtue is not the only thing originally a means, and which if it were not a means to anything else would be and remain indifferent, but which by association with what it is a means to comes to be desired for itself, and that too with the utmost intensity.

[4:32] What, for example, shall we say of the love of money?

[4:33] There is nothing originally more desirable about money than about any heap of glittering pebbles.

[4:34] Its worth is solely that of the things which it will buy; the desires for other things than itself, which it is a means of gratifying.

[4:35] Yet the love of money is not only one of the strongest moving forces of human life, but money is, in many cases, desired in and for itself; the desire to possess it is often stronger than the desire to use it, and goes on increasing when all the desires which point to ends beyond it, to be compassed by it, are falling off.

[4:36] It may, then, be said truly that money is desired not for the sake of an end, but as part of the end.

[4:37] From being a means to happiness, it has come to be itself a principal ingredient of the individual's conception of happiness.

[4:38] The same may be said of the majority of the great objects of human life; power, for example, or fame, except that to each of these there is a certain amount of immediate pleasure annexed, which has at least the semblance of being naturally inherent in them—a thing which cannot be said of money.

[4:39] Still, however, the strongest natural attraction, both of power and of fame, is the immense aid they give to the attainment of our other wishes; and it is the strong association thus generated between them and all our objects of desire which gives to the direct desire of them the intensity it often assumes, so as in some characters to surpass in strength all other desires.

[4:40] In these cases the means have become a part of the end, and a more important part of it than any of the things which they are means to.

[4:41] What was once desired as an instrument for the attainment of happiness has come to be desired for its own sake.

[4:42] In being desired for its own sake it is, however, desired as *part* of happiness.

[4:43] The person is made, or thinks he would be made, happy by its mere possession; and is made unhappy by failure to obtain it.

[4:44] The desire of it is not a different thing from the desire of happiness any more than the love of music or the desire of health.

[4:45] They are included in happiness.

[4:46] They are some of the elements of which the desire of happiness is made up.

[4:47] Happiness is not an abstract idea but a concrete whole; and these are some of its parts.

[4:48] And the utilitarian standard sanctions and approves their being so.

[4:49] Life would be a poor thing, very ill provided with sources of happiness, if there were not this provision of nature by which things originally indifferent, but conducive to, or otherwise associated with, the satisfaction of our primitive desires, become in themselves sources of pleasure more valuable than the primitive pleasures, both in permanency, in the space of human existence that they are capable of covering, and even in intensity.

[4:50] Virtue, according to the utilitarian conception, is a good of this description.

[4:51] There was no original desire of it, or motive to it, save its conduciveness to pleasure, and especially to protection from pain.

[4:52] But through the association thus formed it may be felt a good in itself, and desired as such with as great intensity as any other good; and with this difference between it and the love of money, of power, or of fame—that all of these may, and often do, render the individual noxious to the other members of the society to which he belongs, whereas there is nothing which makes him so much a blessing to them as the cultivation of the disinterested love of virtue.

[4:53] And consequently, the utilitarian standard, while it tolerates and approves those other acquired desires, up to the point beyond which they would be more injurious to the general happiness than promotive of it, enjoins and requires the cultivation of the love of virtue up to the greatest strength possible, as being above all things important to the general happiness.

[4:54 It results from the preceding considerations that there is in reality nothing desired except happiness.

[4:55] Whatever is desired otherwise than as a means to some end beyond itself, and ultimately to happiness, is desired as itself a part of happiness, and is not desired for itself until it has become so.

[4:56] Those who desire virtue for its own sake desire it either because the consciousness of it is a pleasure, or because the consciousness of being without it is a pain, or for both reason united; as in truth the pleasure and pain seldom exist separately, but almost always together—the same person feeling pleasure in the degree of virtue attained, and pain in not having attained more.

[4:57] If one of these gave him no pleasure, and the other no pain, he would not love or desire virtue, or would desire it only for the other benefits which it might produce to himself or to persons whom he cared for.

[4:58] We have now, then, an answer to the question, of what sort of proof the principle of utility is susceptible.

[4:59] If the opinion which I have now stated is psychologically true—if human nature is so constituted as to desire nothing which is not either a part of happiness or a means of happiness—we can have no other proof, and we require no other, that these are the only things desirable.

[4:60] If so, happiness is the sole end of human action, and the promotion of it the test by which to judge of all human conduct; from whence it necessarily follows that it must be the criterion of morality, since a part is included in the whole.

[4:61] And now to decide whether this is really so, whether mankind do desire nothing for itself but that which is a pleasure to them, or of which the absence is a pain, we have evidently arrived at a question of fact and experience, dependent, like all similar questions, upon evidence.

[4:62] It can only be determined by practiced self-consciousness and self-observation, assisted by observation of others.

[4:63] I believe that these sources of evidence, impartially consulted, will declare that desiring a thing and finding it pleasant, aversion to it and thinking of it as painful, are phenomena entirely inseparable or, rather, two parts of the same phenomenon—in strictness of language, two different modes of naming the same psychological fact; that to think of an object as desirable (unless for the sake of its consequences) and to think of it as pleasant are one and the same thing; and that to desire anything except in proportion as the idea of it is pleasant is a physical and metaphysical impossibility.

[4:64] So obvious does this appear to me that I expect it will hardly be disputed; and the objection made will be, not that desire can possibly be directed to anything ultimately except pleasure and exemption from pain, but that the will is a different thing from desire; that a persons of confirmed virtue or any other person whose purposes are fixed carries out his purposes without any thought of the pleasure he has in contemplating them or expects to derive from their fulfillment, and persists in acting on them, even though these pleasures are much diminished by changes in his character or decay of his passive sensibilities, or are outweighed by the pains which the pursuit of the purposes may bring upon him.

[4:65] All this I fully admit and have stated it elsewhere as positively and emphatically as anyone.

[4:66] Will, the active phenomenon, is a different thing from desire, the state of passive sensibility, and, though originally an offshoot from it, may in time take root and detach itself from the parent stock, so much so that in the case of a habitual purpose, instead of willing the thing because we desire it, we often desire it only because we will it.

[4:67] This, however, is but an instance of that familiar fact, the power of habit, and is nowise confined to the case of virtuous actions.

[4:68] Many indifferent things which men originally did from a motive of some sort they continue to do from habit.

[4:69] Sometimes this is done unconsciously, the consciousness coming only after the action; at other times with conscious volition, but volition which has become habitual and is put in operation by the force of habit, in opposition perhaps to the deliberate preference, as often happens with those who have contracted habits of vicious or hurtful indulgence.

[4:70] Third and last comes the case in which the habitual act of will in the individual instance is not in contradiction to the general intention prevailing at other times, but in fulfillment of it, as in the case of the person of confirmed virtue and of all who pursue deliberately and consistently any determinate end.

[4:71] The distinction between will and desire thus understood is an authentic and highly important psychological fact; but the fact consists solely in this—that will, like all other parts of our constitution, is amenable to habit, and that we may will from habit what we no longer desire for itself, or desire only because we will it.

[4:72] It is not the less true that will, in the beginning, is entirely produced by desire, including in that term the repelling influence of pain as well as the attractive one of pleasure.

[4:73] Let us take into consideration no longer the person who has a confirmed will to do right, but him in whom that virtuous will is still feeble, conquerable by temptation, and not to be fully relied on; by what means can it be strengthened?

[4:74] How can the will to be virtuous, where it does not exist in sufficient force, be implanted or awakened?

[4:75] Only by making the person *desire* virtue—by making him think of it in a pleasurable light, or of its absence in a painful one.

[4:76] It is by associating the doing right with pleasure, or the wrong with pain, or by eliciting and impressing and bringing home to the person's experience the pleasure naturally involved in the one or the pain in the other, that it is possible to call forth that will to be virtuous which, when confirmed, acts without any thought of either pleasure or pain.

[4:77] Will is the child of desire, and passes out of the dominion of its parent only to come under that of habit.

[4:78] That which is the result of habit affords no presumption of being intrinsically good; and there would be no reason for wishing that the purpose of virtue should become independent of pleasure and pain were it not that the influence of the pleasurable and painful associations which prompt to virtue is not sufficiently to be depended on for unerring constancy of action until it has acquired the support of habit.

[4:79] Both in feeling and in conduct, habit is the only thing which imparts certainty; and it is because of the importance to others of being able to rely absolutely on one's feelings and conduct, and to oneself of being able to rely on one's own, that the will to do right ought to be cultivated into this habitual independence.

[4:80] In other words, this state of the will is a means to good, not intrinsically a good; and does not contradict the doctrine that nothing is a good to human beings but in so far as it is either itself pleasurable or a means of attaining pleasure or averting pain.

[4:81] But if this doctrine be true, the principle of utility is proved.

[4:82] Whether it is so or not must now be left to the consideration of the thoughtful reader.

{**Bulger's Note:** In the *Metaphysics of Morals* [6:409] Kant argues that maxims ... cannot be based on habit ... as the subject would suffer loss to that freedom ... necessary for duty.}

{**Bulger's Note:** In the *Metaphysics of Morals* [6:225] Kant argues that nothing is good in and of itself except a good will. Good will is not free, rather it is the self-legislative consciousness, i.e., laws for maxims of actions. Choice is that which is free to obey maxims of actions, i.e., negative property, of not being necessitated to act by sensible determining grounds. What Mill is calling will Kant calls choice.}

Chapter V: On The Connection Between Justice And Utility

[5:1] In all ages of speculation one of the strongest obstacles to the reception of the doctrine that utility or happiness is the criterion of right and wrong has been drawn from the idea of justice.

[5:2] The powerful sentiment and apparently clear perception which that word recalls with a rapidity and certainty resembling an instinct have seemed to the majority of thinkers to point to an inherent quality in things; to show that the just must have an existence in nature as something absolute, generically distinct from every variety of the expedient and, in idea, opposed to it, though (as is commonly acknowledged) never, in the long run, disjoined from it in fact.

[5:3] In the case of this, as of our other moral sentiments, there is no necessary connection between the question of its origin and that of its binding force.

[5:4] That a feeling is bestowed on us by nature does not necessarily legitimate all its promptings.

[5:5] The feeling of justice might be a peculiar instinct, and might yet require, like our other instincts, to be controlled and enlightened by a higher reason.

[5:6] If we have intellectual instincts leading us to judge in a particular way, as well as animal instincts that prompt us to act in a particular way, there is no necessity that the former should be more infallible in their sphere than the latter in theirs; it may as well happen that wrong judgments are occasionally suggested by those, as wrong actions by these.

[5:7] But though it is one thing to believe that we have natural feelings of justice, and another to acknowledge them as an ultimate criterion of conduct, these two opinions are very closely connected in point of fact.

[5:8] Mankind are always predisposed to believe that any subjective feeling, not otherwise accounted for, is a revelation of some objective reality.

[5:9] Our present object is to determine whether the reality to which the feeling of justice corresponds is one which needs any such special revelation, whether the justice or injustice of an action is a thing intrinsically peculiar and distinct from all its other qualities or only a combination of certain of those qualities presented under a peculiar aspect.

[5:10] For the purpose of this inquiry it is practically important to consider whether the feeling itself, of justice and injustice, is *sui generis* like our sensations of color and taste or a derivative feeling formed by a combination of others.

[5:11] And this it is the more essential to examine, as people are in general willing enough to allow that objectively the dictates of justice coincide with a part of the field of general expediency; but inasmuch as the subjective mental feeling of justice is different from that which commonly attaches to simple expediency, and, except in the extreme cases of the latter, is far more imperative in its demands, people find it difficult to see in justice only a particular kind or branch of general utility, and think that its superior binding force requires a totally different origin.

[5:12] To throw light upon this question, it is necessary to attempt to ascertain what is the distinguishing character of justice, or of injustice; what is the quality, or whether there is any quality, attributed in common to all modes of conduct designated as unjust (for justice, like many other moral attributes, is best defined by its opposite), and distinguishing them from such modes of conduct as are disapproved, but without having that particular epithet of disapprobation applied to them.

[5:13] If in everything which men are accustomed to characterize as just or unjust some one common attribute or collection of attributes is always present, we may judge whether this particular attribute or combination of attributes would be capable of gathering round it a sentiment of that peculiar character and intensity by virtue of the general laws of our emotional constitution, or whether the sentiment is inexplicable and requires to be regarded as a special provision of nature.

[5:14] If we find the former to be the case, we shall, in resolving this question, have resolved also the main problem; if the latter, we shall have to seek for some other mode of investigating it.

[5:15] To find the common attributes of a variety of objects, it is necessary to begin by surveying the objects themselves in the concrete.

[5:16] Let us therefore advert successively to the various modes of action and arrangements of human affairs which are classed, by universal or widely spread opinion, as just or as unjust.

[5:17] The things well known to excite the sentiments associated with those names are of a very multifarious character.

[5:18] I shall pass them rapidly in review, without studying any particular arrangement.

[5:19] In the first place, it is mostly considered unjust to deprive anyone of his personal liberty, his property, or any other thing which belongs to him by law.

[5:20] Here, therefore, is one instance of the application of the terms "just" and "unjust" in a perfectly definite sense, namely, that it is just to respect, unjust to violate, the *legal rights* of anyone.

[5:21] But this judgment admits of several exceptions, arising from the other forms in which the notions of justice and injustice present themselves.

[5:22] For example, the person who suffers the deprivation may (as they phrase is) have *forfeited* the rights which he is so deprived of—a case to which we shall return presently.

[5:23] But also—

[5:24] Secondly, the legal rights of which he is deprived may be rights which *ought* not to have belonged to him; in other words, the law which confers on him these rights may be a bad law.

[5:25] When it is so or when (which is the same thing for our purpose) it is supposed to be so, opinions will differ as to the justice or injustice of infringing it.

[5:26] Some maintain that no law, however bad, ought to be disobeyed by an individual citizen; that his opposition to it, if shown at all, should only be shown in endeavoring to get it altered by competent authority.

[5:27] This opinion (which condemns many of the most illustrious benefactors of mankind, and would often protect pernicious institutions against the only weapons which, in the state of things existing at the time, have any chance of succeeding against them) is defended by those who hold it on grounds of expediency, principally on that of the importance to the common interest of mankind, of maintaining inviolate the sentiment of submission to law.

[5:28] Other persons, again, hold the directly contrary opinion that any law, judged to be bad, may blamelessly be disobeyed, even though it be not judged to be unjust but only inexpedient, while others would confine the license of disobedience to the case of unjust laws; but, again, some say that all laws which are inexpedient are unjust, since every law imposes some restriction on the natural liberty of mankind, which restriction is an injustice unless legitimated by tending to their good.

[5:29] Among these diversities of opinion it seems to be universally admitted that there may be unjust laws, and that law, consequently, is not the ultimate criterion of justice, but may give to one person a benefit, or impose on another an evil, which justice condemns.

[5:30] When, however, a law is thought to be unjust, it seems always to be regarded as being so in the same way in which a breach of law is unjust, namely, by infringing somebody's right, which, as it cannot in this case be a legal right, receives a different appellation and is called a moral right.

[5:31] We may say, therefore, that a second case of injustice consists in taking or withholding from any person that to which he has a *moral right*.

[5:32] Thirdly, it is universally considered just that each person should obtain that (whether good or evil) which he *deserves*, and unjust that he should obtain a good or be made to undergo an evil which he does not deserve.

[5:33] This is, perhaps, the clearest and most emphatic form in which the idea of justice is conceived by the general mind.

[5:34] As it involves the notion of desert, the question arises what constitutes desert?

[5:35] Speaking in a general way, a person is understood to deserve good if he does right, evil if he does wrong; and in a more particular sense, to deserve good from those to whom he does or has done good, and evil from those to whom he does or has done evil.

[5:36] The precept of returning good for evil has never been regarded as a case of the fulfillment of justice, but as one in which the claims of justice are waived, in obedience to other considerations.

[5:37] Fourthly, it is confessedly unjust to *break faith* with anyone: to violate an engagement, either express or implied, or disappoint expectations raised by our own conduct, at least if we have raised those expectations knowingly and voluntarily.

[5:38] Like the other obligations of justice already spoken of, this one is not regarded as absolute, but as capable of being overruled by a stronger obligation of justice on the other side, or by such conduct on the part of the person concerned as is deemed to absolve us from our obligation to him and to constitute a *forfeiture* of the benefit which he has been led to expect.

[5:39] Fifthly, it is, by universal admission, inconsistent with justice to be *partial*—to show favor or preference to one person over another in matters to which favor and preference do not properly apply.

[5:40] Impartiality, however, does not seem to be regarded as a duty in itself, but rather as instrumental to some other duty; for it is admitted that favor and preference are not always censurable, and, indeed, the cases in which they are condemned are rather the exception than the rule.

[5:41] A person would be more likely to be blamed than applauded for giving his family or friends no superiority in good offices over strangers when he could do so without violating any other duty; and no one thinks it unjust to seek one person in preference to another as a friend, connection, or companion.

[5:42] Impartiality where rights are concerned is of course obligatory, but this is involved in the more general obligation of giving to everyone his right.

[5:43] A tribunal, for example, must be impartial because it is bound to award, without regard to any other consideration, a disputed object to the one of two parties who has the right to it.

[5:44] There are other cases in which impartiality means being solely influenced by desert, as with those who, in the capacity of judges, preceptors, or parents, administer reward and punishment as such.

[5:45] There are cases, again, in which it means being solely influenced by consideration for the public interest, as in making a selection among candidates for a government employment.

[5:46] Impartiality, in short, as an obligation of justice, may be said to mean being exclusively influenced by the considerations which it is supposed ought to influence the particular case in hand, and resisting solicitation of any motives which prompt to conduct different from what those considerations would dictate.

[5:47] Nearly allied to the idea of impartiality is that of *equality*, which often enters as a component part both into the conception of justice and into the practice of it, and, in the eyes of many persons, constitutes its essence.

[5:48] But in this, still more than in any other case, the notion of justice varies in different persons, and always conforms in its variations to their notion of utility.

[5:49] Each person maintains that equality is the dictate of justice, except where he thinks that expediency requires inequality.

[5:50] The justice of giving equal protection to the rights of all is maintained by those who support the most outrageous inequality in the rights themselves.

[5:51] Even in slave countries it is theoretically admitted that the rights of the slave, such as they are, ought to be as sacred as those of the master, and that a tribunal which fails to enforce them with equal strictness is wanting in justice; while, at the same time, institutions which leave to the slave scarcely any rights to enforce are not deemed unjust because they are not deemed inexpedient.

[5:52] Those who think that utility requires distinctions of rank do not consider it unjust that riches and social privileges should be unequally dispensed; but those who think his inequality inexpedient think it unjust also.

[5:53] Whoever thinks that government is necessary sees no injustice in as much inequality as is constituted by giving to the magistrate powers not granted to other people.

[5:54] Even among those who hold leveling doctrines, there are differences of opinion about expediency.

[5:55] Some communists consider it unjust that the produce of the labor of the community should be shared on any other principle than that of exact equality; others think it just that those should receive most whose wants are greatest; while others hold that those who work harder, or who produce more, or whose services are more valuable to the community, may justly claim a larger quota in the division of the produce.

[5:56] And the sense of natural justice may be plausibly appealed to in behalf of every one of these opinions.

[5:57] Among so many diverse applications of the term "justice," which yet is not regarded as ambiguous, it is a matter of some difficulty to seize the mental link which holds them together, and on which the moral sentiment adhering to the term essentially depends.

[5:58] Perhaps, in this embarrassment, some help may be derived from the history of the word, as indicated by its etymology.

[5:59] In most if not in all languages, the etymology of the word which corresponds to "just" points distinctly to an origin connected with the ordinances of law.

[5:60] *Justum* is a form of *jussum,* that which has been ordered.

[5:61] *Dikaion* comes directly from *dike,* a suit at law.

[5:62] *Recht,* from which came *right* and *righteous,* is synonymous with law.

[5:63] The courts of justice, the administration of justice, are the courts and the administration of law.

[5:64] *La justice,* in French, is the established term for judicature.

[5:65] I am not committing the fallacy, imputed with some show of truth to Horne Tooke, of assuming that a word must still continue to mean what it originally meant.

[5:66] Etymology is slight evidence of what the idea now signified is, but the very best evidence of how it sprang up.

[5:67] There can, I think, be no doubt that the *idée mère,* the primitive element, in the formation of the notion of justice was conformity to law.

[5:68] It constituted the entire idea among the Hebrews, up to the birth of Christianity; as might be expected in the case of a people whose laws attempted to embrace all subjects on which precepts were required, and who believed those laws to be a direct emanation from the Supreme Being.

[5:69] But other nations, and in particular the Greeks and Romans, who knew that their laws had been made originally, and still continued to be made, by men, were not afraid to admit that those men might make bad laws; might do, by law, the same things, and from the same motives, which if done by individuals without the sanction of law would be called unjust.

[5:70] And hence the sentiment of injustice came to be attached, not to all violations of law, but only to violations of such laws as *ought* to exist, including such as ought to exist but do not, and to laws themselves if supposed to be contrary to what ought to be law.

[5:71] In this manner the idea of law and of its injunctions was still predominant in the notion of justice, even when the laws actually in force ceased to be accepted as the standard of it.

[5:72] It is true that mankind consider the idea of justice and its obligations as applicable to many things which neither are, nor is it desired that they should be, regulated by law.

[5:73] Nobody desires that laws should interfere with the whole detail of private life; yet everyone allows that in all daily conduct a person may and does show himself to be either just or unjust.

[5:74] But even here, the idea of the breach of what ought to be law still lingers in a modified shape.

[5:75] It would always give us pleasure, and chime in with our feelings of fitness, that acts which we deem unjust should be punished, though we do not always think it expedient that this should be done by the tribunals.

[5:76] We forego that gratification on account of incidental inconveniences.

[5:77] We should be glad to see just conduct enforced and injustice repressed, even in the minutest details, if we were not, with reason, afraid of trusting the magistrate with so unlimited an amount of power over individuals.

[5:78] When we think that a person is bound in justice to do a thing, it is an ordinary form of language to say that he ought to be compelled to do it.

[5:79] We should be gratified to see the obligation enforced by anybody who had the power.

[5:80] If we see that its enforcement by law would be inexpedient, we lament the impossibility, we consider the impunity given to injustice as a evil, and strive to make amends for it by bringing a strong expression of our own and the public disapprobation to bear upon the offender.

[5:81] Thus the idea of legal constraint is still the generating idea of the notion of justice, though undergoing several transformations before that notion as it exists in an advanced state of society becomes complete.

[5:82] The above is, I think, a true account, as far as it goes, of the origin and progressive growth of the idea of justice.

[5:83] But we must observe that it contains as yet nothing to distinguish that obligation from moral obligation in general.

[5:84] For the truth is that the idea of penal sanction, which is the essence of law, enters not only into the conception of injustice, but into that of any kind of wrong.

[5:85] We do not call anything wrong unless we mean to imply that a person ought to be punished in some way or other for doing it—if not by law, by the opinion of his fellow creatures; if not by opinion, by the reproaches of his own conscience.

[5:86] This seems the real turning point of the distinction between morality and simple expediency.

[5:87] It is a part of the notion of duty in every one of its forms that a person may rightfully be compelled to fulfill it.

[5:88] Duty is a thing which may be *exacted* from a person, as one exacts a debt.

[5:89] Unless we think that it may be exacted from him, we do not call it his duty.

[5:90] Reasons of prudence, or the interest of other people, may militate against actually exacting it, but the person himself, it is clearly understood, would not be entitled to complain.

[5:91] There are other things, on the contrary, which we wish that people should do, which we like or admire them for doing, perhaps dislike or despise them for not doing, but yet admit that they are not bound to do; it is not a case of moral obligation; we do not blame them, that is, we do not think that they are proper objects of punishment.

[5:92] How we come by these ideas of deserving and not deserving punishment will appear, perhaps, in the sequel; but I think there is no doubt that this distinction lies at the bottom of the notions of right and wrong; that we call any conduct wrong, or employ, instead, some other term of dislike or disparagement, according as we think that the person ought, or ought not, to be punished for it; and we say it would be right to do so and so, or merely that it would be desirable or laudable, according as we would wish to see the person whom it concerns compelled, or only persuaded and exhorted, to act in that manner.

[5:93] This, therefore, being the characteristic difference which marks off, not justice, but morality in general from the remaining provinces of expediency and worthiness, the character is still to be sought which distinguishes justice from other branches of morality.

[5:94] Now it is known that ethical writers divide moral duties into two classes, denoted by the ill-chosen expressions, duties of perfect and of imperfect obligation; the latter being those in which, though the act is obligatory, the particular occasions of performing it are left to our choice, as in the case of charity or beneficence, which we are indeed bound to practice but not toward any definite person, nor at any prescribed time.

[5:95] In the more precise language of philosophic jurists, duties of perfect obligation are those duties in virtue of which a correlative *right* resides in some person or persons; duties of imperfect obligation are those moral obligations which do not give birth to any right.

[5:96] I think it will be found that this distinction exactly coincides with that which exists between justice and the other obligations of morality.

[5:97] In our survey of the various popular acceptations of justice, the term appeared generally to involve the idea of a personal right—a claim on the part of one or more individuals, like that which the law gives when it confers a proprietary or other legal right.

[5:98] Whether the injustice consists in depriving a person of a possession, or in breaking faith with him, or in treating him worse than he deserves, or worse than other people who have no greater claims—in each case the supposition implies two things: a wrong done, and some assignable person who is wronged.

[5:99] Injustice may also be done by treating a person better than others; but the wrong in this case is to his competitors, who are also assignable persons.

[5:100] It seems to me that this feature in the case—a right in some person, correlative to the moral obligation—constitutes the specific difference between justice and generosity or beneficence.

[5:101] Justice implies something which it is not only right to do, and wrong not to do, but which some individual person can claim from us as his moral right.

[5:102] No one has a moral right to our generosity or beneficence because we are not morally bound to practice those virtues toward any given individual.

[5:103] And it will be found with respect to this as to every correct definition that the instances which seem to conflict with it are those which most confirm it.

[5:104] For if a moralist attempts, as some have done, to make out that mankind generally, though not any given individual, have a right to all the good we can do them, he at once, by that thesis, includes generosity and beneficence within the category of justice.

[5:105] He is obliged to say that our utmost exertions are *due* to our fellow creatures, thus assimilating them to a debt; or that nothing less can be a sufficient *return* for what society does for us, thus classing the case as one of gratitude; both of which are acknowledged cases of justice, and not of the virtue of beneficence; and whoever does not place the distinction between justice and morality in general, where we have now placed it, will be found to make no distinction between them at all, but to merge all morality in justice.

[5:106] Having thus endeavored to determine the distinctive elements which enter into the composition of the idea of justice, we are ready to enter on the inquiry whether the feeling which accompanies the idea is attached to it by a special dispensation of nature, or whether it could have grown up, by any known laws, out of the idea itself; and, in particular, whether it can have originated in considerations of general expediency.

[5:107] I conceive that the sentiment itself does not arise from anything which would commonly or correctly be termed an idea of expediency, but that, though the sentiment does not, whatever is moral in it does.

[5:108] We have seen that the two essential ingredients in the sentiment of justice are the desire to punish a person who has done harm and the knowledge or belief that there is some definite individual or individuals to whom harm has been done.

[5:109] Now it appears to me that the desire to punish a person who has done harm to some individual is a spontaneous outgrowth from two sentiments, both in the highest degree natural and which either are or resemble instincts: the impulse of self-defense and the feeling of sympathy.

[5:110] It is natural to resent and repel or retaliate any harm done or attempted against ourselves or against those with whom we sympathize.

[5:111] The origin of this sentiment it is not necessary here to discuss.

[5:112] Whether it be an instinct or a result of intelligence, it is, we know, common to all animal nature; for every animal tries to hurt those who have hurt, or who it thinks are about to hurt, itself or its young.

[5:113] Human beings, on this point, only differ from other animals in two particulars.

[5:114] First, in being capable of sympathizing, not solely with their offspring, or, like some of the more noble animals, with some superior animal who is kind to them, but with all human, and even with all sentient, beings; secondly, in having a more developed intelligence, which gives a wider range to the whole of their sentiments, whether self-regarding or sympathetic.

[5:115] By virtue of his superior intelligence, even apart from his superior range of sympathy, a human being is capable of apprehending a community of interest between himself and the human society of which he forms a part, such that any conduct which threatens the security of the society generally is threatening to his own, and calls forth his instinct (if instinct it be) of self-defense.

[5:116] The same superiority of intelligence, joined to the power of sympathizing with human beings generally, enables him to attach himself to the collective idea of his tribe, his country, or mankind in such a manner that any act hurtful to them raises his instinct of sympathy and urges him to resistance.

[5:117] The sentiment of justice, in that one of its elements which consists of the desire to punish, is thus, I conceive, the natural feeling of retaliation or vengeance, rendered by intellect and sympathy applicable to those injuries, that is, to those hurts, which wound us through, or in common with, society at large.

[5:118] This sentiment, in itself, has nothing moral in it; what is moral is the exclusive subordination of it to the social sympathies, so as to wait on and obey their call.

[5:119] For the natural feeling would make us resent indiscriminately whatever anyone does that is disagreeable to us; but, when moralized by the social feeling, it only acts in the directions conformable to the general good: just persons resenting a hurt to society, though not otherwise a hurt to themselves, and not resenting a hurt to themselves, however painful, unless it be of the kind which society has a common interest with them in the repression of.

[5:120] It is no objection against this doctrine to say that, when we feel our sentiment of justice outraged, we are not thinking of society at large or of any collective interest, but only of the individual case.

[5:121] It is common enough, certainly, though the reverse of commendable, to feel resentment merely because we have suffered pain; but a person whose resentment is really a moral feeling, that is, who considers whether an act is blamable before he allows himself to resent it—such a person, though he may not say expressly to himself that he is standing up for the interest of society, certainly does feel that he is asserting a rule which is for the benefit of others as well as for his own.

[5:122] If he is not feeling this, if he is regarding the act solely as it affects him individually, he is not consciously just; he is not concerning himself about the justice of his actions.

[5:123] This is admitted even by anti-utilitarian moralists.

[5:124] When Kant (as before remarked) propounds as the fundamental principle of morals, "So act that thy rule of conduct might be adopted as a law by all rational beings," he virtually acknowledges that the interest of mankind collectively, or at least of mankind indiscriminately, must be in the mind of the agent when conscientiously deciding on the morality of the act.

[5:125] Otherwise he uses words without a meaning; for that a rule even of utter selfishness could not *possibly* be adopted by all rational beings—that there is any insuperable obstacle in the nature of things to its adoption—cannot be even plausibly maintained.

[5:126] To give any meaning to Kant's principle, the sense put upon it must be that we ought to shape our conduct by a rule which all rational beings might adopt *with benefit to their collective interest.*

[5:127] To recapitulate: the idea of justice supposes two things—a rule of conduct and a sentiment which sanctions the rule.

[5:128] The first must be supposed common to all mankind and intended for their good.

[5:129] The other (the sentiment) is a desire that punishment may be suffered by those who infringe the rule.

[5:130] There is involved, in addition the conception of some definite person who suffers by the infringement, whose rights (to use the expression appropriated to the case) are violated by it.

[5:131] And the sentiment of justice appears to me to be the animal desire to repel or retaliate a hurt or damage to oneself or to those with whom one sympathizes, widened so as to include all persons, by the human capacity of enlarged sympathy and the human conception of intelligent self-interest.

[5:132] From the latter elements the feeling derives its morality; from the former, its peculiar impressiveness and energy of self-assertion.

[5:133] I have, throughout, treated the idea of a *right* residing in the injured person and violated by the injury, not as a separate element in the composition of the idea and sentiment, but as one of the forms in which the other two elements clothe themselves.

[5:134] These elements are a hurt to some assignable person or persons, on the one hand, and a demand for punishment, on the other.

[5:135] An examination of our own minds, I think, will show that these two things include all that we mean when we speak of violation of a right.

[5:136] When we call anything a person's right, we mean that he has a valid claim on society to protect him in the possession of it, either by the force of law or by that of education and opinion.

[5:137] If he has what we consider a sufficient claim, on whatever account, to have something guaranteed to him by society, we say that he has a right to it.

[5:138] If we desire to prove that anything does not belong to him by right, we think this done as soon as it is admitted that society ought not to take measure for securing it to him, but should leave him to chance or to his own exertions.

[5:139] Thus a person is said to have a right to what he can earn in fair professional competition, because society ought not to allow any other person to hinder him from endeavoring to earn in that manner as much as he can.

[5:140] But he has not a right to three hundred a year, though he may happen to be earning it; because society is not called on to provide that he shall earn that sum.

[5:141] On the contrary, if he owns ten thousand pounds three-per-cent stock, he *has* a right to three hundred a year because society has come under an obligation to provide him with an income of that amount.

[5:142] To have a right, then is, I conceive, to have something which society ought to defend me in the possession of.

[5:143] If the objector goes on to ask why it ought, I can give him no other reason than general utility.

[5:144] If that expression does not seem to convey a sufficient feeling of the strength of the obligation, nor to account for the peculiar energy of the feeling, it is because there goes to the composition of the sentiment, not a rational only but also an animal element—the thirst for retaliation; and this thirst derives its intensity, as well as its moral justification, from the extraordinarily important and impressive kind of utility which is concerned.

[5:145] The interest involved is that of security, to everyone's feelings the most vital of all interests.

[5:146] All other earthly benefits are needed by one person, not needed by another; and many of them can, if necessary, be cheerfully foregone or replaced by something else; but security no human being can possibly do without; on it we depend for all our immunity from evil and for the whole value of all and every good, beyond the passing moment, since nothing but the gratification of the instant could be of any worth to us if we could be deprived of everything the next instant by whoever was momentarily stronger than ourselves.

[5:147] Now this most indispensable of all necessaries, after physical nutriment, cannot be had unless the machinery for providing it is kept unintermittedly in active play.

[5:148] Our notion, therefore, of the claim we have on our fellow creatures to join in making safe for us the very groundwork of our existence gathers feelings around it so much more intense than those concerned in any of the more common cases of utility that the difference in degree (as is often the case in psychology) becomes a real difference in kind.

[5:149] The claim assumes that character of absoluteness, that apparent infinity and incommensurability with all other considerations which constitute the distinction between the feeling of right and wrong and that of ordinary expediency and inexpediency.

[5:150] The feelings concerned are so powerful, and we count so positively on finding a responsive feeling in others (all being alike interested) that *ought* and *should* grow into *must*, and recognized indispensability becomes a moral necessity, analogous to physical, and often not inferior to it in binding force.

[5:151] If the preceding analysis, or something resembling it, be not the correct account of the notion of justice—if justice be totally independent of utility, and be a standard *per se*, which the mind can recognize by simple introspection of itself—it is hard to understand why that internal oracle is so ambiguous, and why so many things appear either just or unjust, according to the light in which they are regarded.

[5:152] We are continually informed that utility is an uncertain standard, which every different person interprets differently, and that there is no safety but in the immutable, ineffaceable, and unmistakable dictates of justice, which carry their evidence in themselves and are independent of the fluctuations of opinion.

[5:153] One would suppose from this that on questions of justice there could be no controversy; that, if we take that for our rule, its application to any given case could leave us in as little doubt as a mathematical demonstration.

[5:154] So far is this from being the fact that there is as much difference of opinion, and as much discussion, about what is just as about what is useful to society.

[5:155] Not only have different nations and individuals different notions of justice, but in the mind of one and the same individual, justice is not some one rule, principle, or maxim, but many which do not always coincide in their dictates, and, in choosing between which, he is guided either by some extraneous standard or by his own personal predilections.

[5:156] For instance, there are some who say that it is unjust to punish anyone for the sake of example to others, that punishment is just only when intended for the good of the sufferer himself.

[5:157] Others maintain the extreme reverse, contending that to punish persons who have attained years of discretion, for their own benefit, is despotism and injustice, since, if the matter at issue is solely their own good, no one has a right to control their own judgment of it; but that they may justly be punished to prevent evil to others, this being the exercise of the legitimate right of self-defense.

[5:158] Mr. Owen, again, affirms that it is unjust to punish at all, for the criminal did not make his own character; his education and the circumstances which surrounded him have made him a criminal, and for these he is not responsible.

[5:159] All these opinions are extremely plausible; and so long as the question is argued as one of justice simply, without going down to the principles which lie under justice and are the source of its authority, I am unable to see how any of these reasoners can be refuted.

[5:160] For in truth every one of the three builds upon rules of justice confessedly true.

[5:161] The first appeals to the acknowledged injustice of singling out an individual and making him a sacrifice, without his consent, for other people's benefit.

[5:162] The second relies on the acknowledged justice of self-defense and the admitted injustice of forcing one person to conform to another's notions of what constitutes his good.

[5:163] The Owenite invokes the admitted principle that it is unjust to punish anyone for what he cannot help.

[5:164] Each is triumphant so long as he is not compelled to take into consideration any other maxims of justice than the one he has selected; but as soon as their several maxims are brought face to face, each disputant seems to have exactly as much to say for himself as the others.

[5:165] No one of them can carry out his own notion of justice without trampling upon another equally binding.

[5:166] These are difficulties; they have always been felt to be such; and many devices have been invented to turn rather than to overcome them.

[5:167] As a refuge from the last of the three, men imagined what they called the freedom of the will—fancying that they could not justify punishing a man whose will is in a thoroughly hateful state unless it be supposed to have come into that state through no influence of anterior circumstances.

[5:168] To escape from the other difficulties, a favorite contrivance has been the fiction of a contract whereby at some unknown period all the members of society engaged to obey the laws and consented to be punished for any disobedience to them, thereby giving to their legislators the right, which it is assume they would not otherwise have had, of punishing them, either for their own good or for that of society.

[5:169] This happy thought was considered to get rid of the whole difficulty and to legitimate the infliction of punishment, in virtue of another received maxim of justice, *volenti non fit injuria*—that is not unjust which is done with the consent of the person who is supposed to be hurt by it.

[5:170] I need hardly remark that, even if the consent were not a mere fiction, this maxim is not superior in authority to the others which it is brought in to supersede.

[5:171] It is, on the contrary, an instructive specimen of the loose and irregular manner in which supposed principles of justice grow up.

[5:172] This particular one evidently came into use as a help to the coarse exigencies of courts of law, which are sometimes obliged to be content with very uncertain presumptions, on account of the greater evils which would often arise from any attempt on their part to cut finer.

[5:173] But even courts of law are not able to adhere consistently to the maxim, for they allow voluntary engagements to be set aside on the ground of fraud, and sometimes on that of mere mistake or misinformation.

[5:174] Again, when the legitimacy of inflicting punishment is admitted, how many conflicting conceptions of justice come to light in discussing the proper apportionment of punishments to offenses.

[5:175] No rule on the subject recommends itself so strongly to the primitive and spontaneous sentiment of justice as the *lex talionis*, an eye for an eye and a tooth for a tooth.

[5:176] Though this principle of the Jewish and of the Mohammedan law has been generally abandoned in Europe as a practical maxim, there is, I suspect, in most minds, a secret hankering after it; and when retribution accidently falls on an offender in that precise shape, the general feeling of satisfaction evinced bears witness how natural is the sentiment to which this repayment in kind is acceptable.

[5:177] With many, the test of justice in penal infliction is that the punishment should be proportioned to the offense, meaning that it should be exactly measured by the moral guilt of the culprit (whatever be their standard for measuring moral guilt), the consideration what amount of punishment is necessary to deter from the offense having nothing to do with the question of justice, in their estimation; while there are others to whom that consideration is all in all, who maintain that it is not just, at least for man, to inflict on a fellow creature, whatever may be his offenses, any amount of suffering beyond the least that will suffice to prevent him from repeating, and others from imitating, his misconduct.

[5:178] To take another example from a subject already once referred to.

[5:179] In cooperative industrial association, is it just or not that talent or skill should give a title to superior remuneration?

[5:180] On the negative side of the question it is argued that whoever does the best he can deserves equally well, and ought not in justice to be put in a position of inferiority for no fault of his own; that superior abilities have already advantages more than enough, in the admiration they excite, the personal influence they command, and the internal sources of satisfaction attending them, without adding to these a superior share of the world's goods; and that society is bound in justice rather to make compensation to the less favored for this unmerited inequality of advantages than to aggravate it.

[5:181] On the contrary side it is contended that society receives more from the more efficient laborer; that, his services being more useful, society owes him a larger return for them; that a greater share of the joint result is actually his work, and not to allow his claim to it is a kind of robbery; that, if he is only to receive as much as others, he can only be justly required to produce as much, and to give a smaller amount of time and exertion, proportioned to his superior efficiency.

[5:182] Who shall decide between these appeals to conflicting principles of justice?

[5:183] Justice has in this case two sides to it, which it is impossible to bring into harmony, and the two disputants have chosen opposite sides; the one looks to what it is just that the individual should receive, the other to what it is just that the community should give.

[5:184] Each, from his own point of view, is unanswerable; and any choice between them, on grounds of justice, must be perfectly arbitrary.

[5:185] Social utility alone can decide the preference.

[5:186] How many, again, and how irreconcilable are the standards of justice to which reference is made in discussing the repartition of taxation.

[5:187] One opinion is that payment to the state should be in numerical proportion to pecuniary means.

[5:188] Others think that justice dictates what they term graduated taxation—taking a higher percentage from those who have more to spare.

[5:189] In point of natural justice a strong case might be made for disregarding means altogether, and taking the same absolute sum (whenever it could be got) from everyone; as the subscribers to a mess or to a club all pay the same sum for the same privileges, whether they can all equally afford it or not.

[5:190] Since the protection (it might be said) of law and government is afforded to and is equally required by all, there is no injustice in making all buy it at the same price.

[5:191] It is reckoned justice, not injustice, that a dealer should charge to all customers the same price for the same article, not a price varying according to their means of payment.

[5:192] This doctrine, as applied to taxation, finds no advocates because it conflicts so strongly with man's feelings of humanity and of social expediency; but the principle of justice which it invokes is as true and as binding as those which can be appealed to against it.

[5:193] Accordingly it exerts a tacit influence on the line of defense employed for other modes of assessing taxation.

[5:194] People feel obligated to argue that the state does more for the rich man than for the poor, as a justification for its taking more from them, though this is in reality not true, for the rich would be far better able to protect themselves, in the absence of law or government, than the poor, and indeed would probably be successful in converting the poor into their slaves.

[5:195] Others, again, so far defer to the same conception of justice as to maintain that all should pay an equal capitation tax for the protection of their persons (these being of equal value to all), and an unequal tax for the protection of their property, which is unequal.

[5:196] To this others reply that the all of one man is as valuable to him as the all of another.

[5:197] From these confusions there is no other mode of extrication than the utilitarian.

[5:198] Is, then, the difference between the just and the expedient a merely imaginary distinction?

[5:199] Have mankind been under a delusion in thinking that justice is a more sacred thing than policy, and that the latter ought only to be listened to after the former has been satisfied?

[5:200] By no means.

[5:201] The exposition we have given of the nature and origin of the sentiment recognizes a real distinction; and no one of those who profess the most sublime contempt for the consequences of actions as an element in their morality attaches more importance to the distinction than I do.

[5:202] While I dispute the pretensions of any theory which sets up an imaginary standard of justice not grounded on utility, I account the justice which is grounded on utility to be the chief part, and incomparably the most sacred and binding part, of all morality.

[5:203] Justice is a name for certain classes of moral rules which concern the essentials of human well-being more nearly, and are therefore of more absolute obligation, than any other rules for the guidance of life; and the notion which we have found to be of the essence of the idea of justice—that of a right residing in an individual—implies and testifies to this more binding obligation.

[5:204] The moral rules which forbid mankind to hurt one another (in which we must never forget to include a wrongful interference with each other's freedom) are more vital to human well-being than any maxims, however important, which only point out the best mode of managing some department of human affairs.

[5:205] They have also the peculiarity that they are the main element in determining the whole of the social feelings of mankind.

[5:206] It is their observance which alone preserves peace among human beings; if obedience to them were not the rule, and disobedience the exception, everyone would see in everyone else an enemy against whom he must be perpetually guarding himself.

[5:207] What is hardly less important, these are the precepts which mankind have the strongest and the most direct inducements for impressing upon one another.

[5:208] By merely giving to each other prudential instruction or exhortation, they may gain, or think they gain, nothing; in inculcating on each other the duty of positive beneficence, they have an unmistakable interest, but far less in degree; a person may possibly not need the benefits of others, but he always needs that they should not do him hurt.

[5:209] Thus the moralities which protect every individual from being harmed by others, either directly or by being hindered in his freedom of pursuing his own good, are at once those which he himself has most at heart and those which he has the strongest interest in publishing and enforcing by word and deed.

[5:210] It is by a person's observance of these that his fitness to exist as one of the fellowship of human beings is tested and decided; for on that depends his being a nuisance or not to those with whom he is in contact.

[5:211] Now it is these moralities primarily which compose the obligations of justice.

[5:212] The most marked cases of injustice, and those which give the tone to the feeling of repugnance which characterizes the sentiment, are acts of wrongful aggression or wrongful exercise of power over someone; the next are those which consist in wrongfully withholding from him something which is his due—in both cases inflicting on him a positive hurt, either in the form of direct suffering or of the privation of some good which he had reasonable ground, either of a physical or of a social kind, for counting upon.

[5:213] The same powerful motives which command the observance of these primary moralities enjoin the punishment of those who violate them; and as the impulses of self-defense, of defense of others, and of vengeance are all called forth against such persons, retribution, or evil for evil, becomes closely connected with the sentiment of justice, and is universally included in the idea.

[5:214] Good for good is also one of the dictates of justice; and this, though its social utility is evident, and though it carries with it a natural human feeling, has not at first sight that obvious connection with hurt or injury which, existing in the most elementary cases of just and unjust, is the source of the characteristic intensity of the sentiment.

[5:215] But the connection, though less obvious, is not less real.

[5:216] He who accepts benefits and denies a return of them when needed inflicts a real hurt by disappointing one of the most natural and reasonable of expectations, and one which he must at least tacitly have encouraged, otherwise the benefits would seldom have been conferred.

[5:217] The important rank, among human evils and wrongs, of the disappointment of expectation is shown in the fact that it constitutes the principal criminality of two such highly immoral acts as a breach of friendship and a breach of promise.

[5:218] Few hurts which human beings can sustain are greater, and none wound more, than when that on which they habitually and with full assurance relied fails them in the hour of need; and few wrongs are greater than this mere withholding of good; none excite more resentment, either in the person suffering or in a sympathizing spectator.

[5:219] The principle, therefore, of giving to each what they deserve, that is, good for good as well as evil for evil, is not only included within the idea of justice as we have defined it, but is a proper object of that intensity of sentiment which places the just human estimation above the simply expedient.

[5:220] Most of the maxims of justice current in the world, and commonly appealed to in its transactions, are simply instrumental to carrying in to effect the principles of justice which we have now spoken of.

[5:221] That a person is only responsible for what he has done voluntarily, or could voluntarily have avoided, that it is unjust to condemn any person unheard; that the punishment ought to be proportioned to the offense, and the like, are maxims intended to prevent the just principle of evil for evil from being perverted to the infliction of evil without that justification.

[5:222] The greater part of these common maxims have come into use from the practice of courts of justice, which have been naturally led to a more complete recognition and elaboration than was likely to suggest itself to others, of the rules necessary to enable them to fulfill their double function—of inflicting punishment when due, and of awarding to each person his right.

[5:223] That first of judicial virtues, impartiality, is an obligation of justice, partly for the reason last mentioned, as being a necessary condition of the fulfillment of other obligations of justice.

[5:224] But this is not the only source of the exalted rank, among human obligations, of those maxims of equality and impartiality, which, both in popular estimation and in that of the most enlightened, are included among the precepts of justice.

[5:225] In one point of view, they may be considered as corollaries from the principles already laid down.

[5:226] If it is a duty to do to each according to his deserts, returning good for good, as well as repressing evil by evil, it necessarily follows that we should treat all equally well (when no higher duty forbids) who have deserved equally well of *us*, and that society should treat all equally well who have deserved equally well of *it*, that is, who have deserved equally well absolutely.

[5:227] This is the highest abstract standard of social and distributive justice, toward which all institutions and the efforts of all virtuous citizens should be made in the utmost possible degree to converge.

[5:228] But this great moral duty rests upon a still deeper foundation, being a direct emanation from the first principle of morals, and not a mere logical corollary from secondary or derivative doctrines.

[5:229] It is involved in the very meaning of utility, or the greatest happiness principle.

[5:230] That principle is a mere form of words without rational signification unless one person's happiness, supposed equal in degree (with the proper allowance made for kind), is counted for exactly as much as another's.

[5:231] Those conditions being supplied, Bentham's dictum "everybody to count for one, nobody for more than one," might be written under the principle of utility as an explanatory commentary.[1]

[5:232] The equal claim of everybody to happiness, in the estimation of the moralist and of the legislator, involves an equal claim to all the means of happiness except in so far as the inevitable conditions of human life and the general interest in which that of

---

[1] This implication, in the first principle of the utilitarian scheme, of perfect impartiality between persons is regarded by Mr. Herbert Spencer (in his *Social Statics*) as a disproof of the pretensions of utility to be a sufficient guide to right; since (he says) the principle of utility presupposes the anterior principle that everybody has an equal right to happiness.

It may be more correctly described as supposing that equal amounts of happiness are equally desirable, whether felt by the same or different persons.

This, however, is not a *pre*supposition, not a premise needful to support the principle of utility, but the very principle itself for what is the principle of utility if it be not that "happiness" and "desirable" are synonymous terms? If there is any anterior principle implied, it can be no other than this, that the truths of arithmetic are applicable to the valuation of happiness, as of all other measurable quantities.

(Mr. Herbert Spencer, in a private communication on the subject of the preceding note, objects to being considered an opponent of utilitarianism and states that he regards happiness as the ultimate end of morality; but deems that end only partially attainable by empirical generalizations from the observed results of conduct, and completely attainable only by deducing, from the laws of life and the conditions of existence, what kinds of action necessarily tend to produce happiness, and what kinds to produce unhappiness.

With the exception of the word "necessarily," I have no dissent to express from this doctrine; and (omitting that word) I am not aware that any modern advocate of utilitarianism is of a different opinion.

Bentham, certainly to whom in the *Social Statics* Mr. Spencer particularly referred, is, least of all writers, chargeable with unwillingness to deduce the effect of actions on happiness from the laws of human nature and the universal conditions of human life.

The common charge against him is of relying too exclusively upon such deductions and declining altogether to be bound by the generalizations from specific experience which Mr. Spencer thinks that utilitarians generally confine themselves to.

My own opinion (and, as I collect, Mr. Spencer's) is that in ethics, as in all other branches of scientific study, the consilience of the results of both these processes, each corroborating and verifying the other, is requisite to give to any general proposition the kind and degree of evidence which constitutes scientific proof.)

every individual is included set limits to the maxim; and those limits ought to be strictly construed.

[5:233] As every other maxim of justice, so this is by no means applied or held applicable universally; on the contrary, as I have already remarked, it bends to every person's ideas of social expediency.

[5:234] But in whatever case it is deemed applicable at all, it is held to be the dictate of justice.

[5:235] All persons are deemed to have a *right* to equality of treatment, except when some recognized social expediency requires the reverse.

[5:236] And hence all social inequalities which have ceased to be considered expedient assume the character, not of simple inexpediency, but of injustice, and appear so tyrannical that people are apt to wonder how they ever could have been tolerated—forgetful that they themselves, perhaps, tolerate other inequalities under an equally mistaken notion of expediency, the correction of which would make that which they approve seem quite as monstrous as what they have at last learned to condemn.

[5:237] The entire history of social improvement has been a series of transitions by which one custom or institution after another, from being a supposed primary necessity of social existence, has passed into the rank of a universally stigmatized injustice and tyranny.

[5:238] So it has been with the distinctions of slaves and freemen, nobles and serfs, patricians and plebeians; and so it will be, and in part already is, with the aristocracies of color, race, and sex.

[5:239] It appears from what has been said that justice is a name for certain moral requirements which, regarded collectively, stand higher in the scale of social utility, and are therefore of more paramount obligation, than any others, though particular cases may occur in which some other social duty is so important as to overrule any one of the general maxims of justice.

[5:240] Thus, to save a life, it may not only be allowable, but a duty, to steal or take by force the necessary food or medicine, or to kidnap and compel to officiate the only qualified medical practitioner.

[5:241] In such cases, as we do not call anything justice which is not a virtue, we usually say, not that justice must give way to some other moral principle, but that what is just in ordinary cases is, by reason of that other principle, not just in the particular case.

[5:242] By this useful accommodation of language, the character of indefeasibility attributed to justice is kept up, and we are saved from the necessity of maintaining that there can be laudable injustice.

[5:243] The considerations which have now been adduced resolve, I conceive, the only real difficulty in the utilitarian theory of morals.

[5:244] It has always been evident that all cases of justice are also cases of expediency; the difference is in the peculiar sentiment which attaches to the former, as contradistinguished from the latter.

[5:245] If this characteristic sentiment has been sufficiently accounted for; if there is no necessity to assume for it any peculiarity of origin; if it is simply the natural feeling of resentment, moralized by being made co-extensive with the demands of social good; and if this feeling not only does but ought to exist in all the classes of cases to which the idea of justice corresponds—that idea no longer presents itself as a stumbling block to the utilitarian ethics.

[5:246] Justice remains the appropriate name for certain social utilities which are vastly more important, and therefore more absolute and imperative, than any others are as a class (though not more so than others may be in particular cases); and which, therefore, ought to be, as well as naturally are, guarded by **a sentiment, not only different in degree, but also in kind**; distinguished from the milder feeling which attaches to the mere idea of promoting human pleasure or convenience at once by the more definite nature of its commands and by the sterner character of its sanctions

***

GLOSSARY

Terminology

Absolute: No exceptions or qualifications.

Abstract: Thoughts that are not based on any type of sense data, i.e., sense perceptions.

Abstract Concepts: Concepts that are not based on any type of sense data, i.e., sense perceptions, or observations.

Abstract Ideas: Ideas that are not based on any type of sense data, i.e., sense perceptions, or observation.

Abstraction: Idea of a quality apart from its material accompaniments.

Absurd: Not logically consistent; foolish; ridiculous.

Accountable: Responsible, having to give an explanation for one's actions and/or thoughts.

Ad Infinitum: Continues without limits.

Adjudication: Come to a just or fair judgment between two or more options.

Aggregate: Total obtained by addition; mass or amount brought together.

Agnostic: No knowledge.

Amenable: Responsive; able to be guided or influenced.

Amendment: A change in the wording of a rule, or law usually done in order to improve or remove inadvertent faults and errors.

Analogy: The act of explaining by comparing something with another thing that has a partial likeness or similarity. Analogies are used to illustrate not to prove.

Analytical: Analysis that does not add any new information, e.g., all bachelors are unmarried. The predicate adds no new information to the subject. By definition bachelor means unmarried.

Analytic statements: Predicate is contained in the subject and therefore they do not provide new knowledge, i.e. tautological. True by definition and therefore categorically true as well.

Angstrom: Unit of length equal to one hundred-millionth of a centimeter, 10^{-10} meter, used mainly to express wavelengths and interatomic distances.

Animal Choice: Kant defines it as choice which can be determined only by *inclination* (sensible impulse, stimulus). Contrast with free choice and human choice.

Anthropologist: Literally means the study of the human race through the use of objective observations, i.e., descriptive sense data.

Apartheid: Separation of races in a particular country, e.g., in South Africa it was the policy of the white government to keep the blacks and the whites separated.

Appeal: To challenge a judgment by asking a higher authority to make a rejudgment.

Apprehend:

To understand (old use); To seize a person who breaks the law; Arrest

A Priori: That which does not depend on cause and effect and/or sense data.

A Posteriori: To have or come to have knowledge through the use of sense perception(s), i.e., sight, sound, smell, taste, and touch.

Arbitrary: Decided by or based on chance or personal sentiments rather than reason.

Architectonic: The division that practical reason lays out to establish a system of its concepts in ethics, i.e., matter and form. [6:411]

Aristocracies: Government by persons of highest social rank.

Arrogance: A kind of *ambition* in which we demand that others think little of themselves in comparison with us. A solicitation on the part of one seeking honor for followers, whom he thinks he is entitled to treat with contempt. Arrogance demands from others a respect it denies them. [6:465]

Ascertain: To find out; get to know.

Assent: Official agreement to a proposal.

Assertion: A forceful statement or claim.

Atheist: No god.

Attributes: Quality forming part of the nature of a person or thing.

Autonomy: Literally means self-rule, or self-governing. Often used to denote the concept of freedom.

Avenge: To take vengeance, meaning to inflict punishment in retaliation for an injury or bad treatment.

Axiom: Presupposition that is accepted without proof or argument. A statement or proposition that is regarded as being established, accepted, or self-evidently true.

Balancing: When two or more principles conflict, balancing tries to maximize each principle while minimizing the conflict between the principles.

Barbarian: Someone who did not speak Greek or was not a Greek citizen.

Basic Rights and Liberties: These are rights and liberties that are thought to belong to all rational and reasonable beings.

Basic Goods: Those things that are necessary in order to develop or exercise basic rights and liberties.

Beautiful: Adjective, giving pleasure of delight to the mind or senses.

Begging the Question: Justification of an argument by appealing to the argument that is being justified for its justification (see circular argument).

Belittling: To cause to seem unimportant or of small value.

Beneficence: To do good.

Benefits v. Burdens: Weighing and balancing the positive and negative elements of a decision.

Big Bang: Cosmological beginning.

Bottom-Up Reasoning: Reasoning from intuitions up to a theory(ies).

Break faith: To violate an engagement, either express or implied, or disappoint expectations raised by our own conduct.

Capital "T" Truth: An absolute truth with no exceptions or qualifications.

Casuistry: Is a practice in how *to seek* truth. It leads to questions that call upon judgment to decide how a maxim is to be applied to particular cases, and indeed in such a way that judgment provides another (subordinate) maxim (and one can always ask for yet another principle for applying this maxim to cases that may arise). [6:411]

Catechism (Moral): For the beginning pupil the first and most essential instrument for *teaching* the doctrine of virtue is a moral *catechism*. ... The formal principle of such instruction does not, however, permit Socratic *dialogue* as the way of teaching for this purpose, since the pupil has no idea what questions to ask; and so the teacher alone does the questioning. [6:478-479] The teacher elicits from his pupil's reason, by questioning, what he wants to teach him; and should the pupil not know how to answer the question, the teacher, guiding his reason, suggests the answer to him. ... It is the *shamefulness* of vice, not its *harmfulness* that must be emphasized above all. It is most important in this education not to present the moral catechism mixed with the religious one (to combine them into one) or, what is worse yet, to have it follow upon the religious catechism. ... For otherwise ... he will acknowledge duties out of fear and feign an interest in them that is not in his heart. [6:480]

Categorical: Universal. Of, affecting, or done by all people or things in the world or in a particular group; applicable to all cases.

Categorical Command: Unconditional; absolute.

Categorical Imperative: Determines which maxims are acceptable moral principles by their ability to serve as practical norms of conduct for everyone, that is, as laws within a civil community. The first formulation, called the Formula of Universality is a purely formal standard and so is analytically true. "Act only on that maxim through which you can at the same time will that it should become a universal law." or, alternatively, if its maxim can "coexist with the freedom of everyone in accordance with a universal law" of freedom. The second formula adds the moral matter, the notion of persons as ends, i.e., intrinsically valuable, and is a synthetic claim. "Act in accordance with a maxim of *ends* that it can be a universal law for everyone." All other imperatives are conditional. The moral *imperative* makes this constraint known through the categorical nature of its pronouncement (the unconditional ought). Such constraint, therefore, does not apply to rational beings as such (there could also be *holy* ones) but rather to *human beings*, rational *natural* beings, who are unholy enough that pleasure can induce them to break the moral law. Insofar as the categorical imperative provides criteria for determining what should be done by pointing out an end, a rule and an incentive, it is a practical principle.

Categories: Division or class in a complete system or grouping.

Chaos: In Physics it is behavior so unpredictable as to appear random, owing to great sensitivity to small changes in conditions.

Choice: Desire that is joined with one's consciousness of the ability to bring about its object by one's action. Contrast with wish.

Christian: A person who believes in the teachings of Jesus Christ.

Circular Argument: (See Begging the Question and Internal Justification).

Citizen: A person, who lives in a particular city or town, especially one who has voting rights.

Civil Disobedience: Organized citizens who refuse to obey certain laws as part of a political campaign.

Civil Law: Laws that relate to the rights of private citizens concerned with the judging of private quarrels between people rather than with criminal offenses.

Code Of Ethics: A set of rules, principles, and protocols that a profession adopts as a guide for moral actions, i.e., mid-level principles.

Coercion: Credible threat.

Cognitive: Mental.

Cognizance: Having knowledge, being fully aware.

Coherent: Logical and consistent.

Collective: When a number of parts or groups of parts act as one.

Compatible: When two or more thoughts or objects do not conflict with one another.

Compatibilism: Determinism and freedom can exist at the same time.

Compilation: Gathering together.

Comprehensive: Complete.

Compromise: Settlement of a dispute by which each side gives up something it has asked for and neither side gets all it has asked for.

Compulsion: To force or to have an irresistible urge to do something.

Conceited: Over-high opinion of, too much pride in, oneself or one's powers, abilities, etc.

Conceive: To form in the mind an idea, plan, etc.

Concepts: A general idea, thought, or understanding. The idea underlying a class of things.

Conceptual: Theoretical or abstract.

Conch shell: Shellfish with a large spiral shell.

Conducive: Promotes.

Conflict of duties: Would be a relation between duties in which one of them would cancel the other (wholly or in part). —But since duty and obligation are concepts that express the objective practical *necessity* of certain actions and two rules opposed to each other cannot be necessary at the same time, if its is a duty to act in accordance with one rule, to act in accordance with the opposite rule is not a duty but even contrary to duty; so a *collision of duties* and obligations is inconceivable. However, a subject may have, in a rule he prescribes to himself, two *grounds* of obligation one or the other of which is not sufficient to put him under obligation, so that one of them is not a duty. —When two such grounds conflict with each other, practical philosophy says, not that the stronger obligation takes precedence, but that the stronger *ground of obligation* prevails.

Conflict Resolution: Solving a problem.

Conform: To comply, harmonize or adjust one's belief or conduct with a differing belief or conduct.

Congruent: Identical or in agreement with something else.

Conjunction: In the vernacular, it means in combination with.

Conjunction—CJ is defined as follows:

1. p
2. q
3. **Therefore:** p and q (CJ 1 and 2)

Conscience: For Kant it is a kind of "second-order" reflection on how well we are making or have made our choices. We do not have a duty simply to *have* a conscience. We have a conscience whether we want one or not. However, since we can never be sure about the purity of our intentions, judgments of conscience apparently are limited to questions about the moral *legality* of our behavior and about whether we have tried or are trying as hard as possible to act dutifully. So holy are the judgments of our conscience that we cannot avoid thinking of them as if they were divine verdicts. It is also not possible to have an erring conscience as you cannot be mistaken in your subjective judgment as to whether you have submitted something to your practical reason.

To act in accordance with conscience cannot itself be a duty; for if it were, there would have to be yet a second conscience in order for one to become aware of the act of the first. The duty here is only to cultivate one's conscience. [6:400-401] Consciousness is an *internal court* in man. I, the prosecutor and yet the accused as well, am the same *human being*. But the human being as the subject of the moral lawgiving which proceeds from the concept of freedom and in which he is subject to a law that he gives himself (*noumenon*) is to be regarded as another from the human being as a sensible being endowed with reason, though only in a practical respect. But to think of a human being who is *accused* by his conscience as *one and the same person* as the judge is an absurd way of representing court. A human being's conscience will, accordingly, have to think of *someone other* than himself as the judge of his actions, if conscience is not to be in contradiction with itself. This other may be an actual person or a merely ideal person that reason creates for itself. Now since such a moral being must also have all power in order to give effect to his laws and since such an omnipotent moral being is call **God**, conscience must be thought of as the subjective principle of being accountable to God for all one's deeds. This is not to say that a human being is entitled, ... to *assume* that such a supreme being *actually exists* outside himself –still less that he is *bound* by his conscience to do so. For the idea is not given to him *objectively*, by theoretical reason, but only *subjectively*, by practical reason. ... The concept of religion is here for use only "a principle for estimating all our duties as divine commands." [6:437-440].

Consciousness: A moral feeling and/or self-awareness.

Consecration: To set apart as sacred or for a special purpose.

Consequential: That which has a cause and effect relationship.

Consequentialism: Moral philosophy that aims at a particular end or goal, i.e., consequence. A teleological, or ends oriented, moral philosophy.

Consistent: Conforming one's behavior, principles, etc., to a regular pattern or style.

Consonant: Agreement or harmony.

Constitution: The laws or principles according to which a country is governed.

Constitution: The laws or principles according to which a country is governed; The general condition of a person's body or mind.

Constitutional Stage: The part of Rawls's social political framework in which he establishes a constitution that guaranties the basic rights and liberties under the first principle of justice and also establishes what type of government a society is going to have.

Constraining: Binding or restricting.

Contradiction: To be opposite in nature or character. When two or more statements or events provide opposite assertions.

Contempt: Judging something to be worthless.

Contemporary: Belonging to the same time.

Convergence: To come together towards a common point.

Correct Argument: When the inference of an inductive argument is probable.

Cosmology: The science of the origin and development of the universe.

Counter-Example: An example that is opposed, opposite or contradicts another.

Covering-Precept Model: Justification is from the top-down perspective, i.e., it goes from the general to the particulars.

Creationism: God created the universe independent of evolution.

Creed: A system of beliefs or principles.

Criteria: Specification or standard of judgement.

Critical Analysis: The positive and negative judgements on something that is being evaluated.

Deduce: Logically derived (See deductive)

Deductive: To come to an absolute analytical conclusion through the use of premises that are assumed to be true.

Deliberate: To contemplate, reflect, or debate.

Democratic: Government by representation.

Deontological: Literally means the study of duty.

Derivable: Ability to come to a logical conclusion through the use of premises that are assumed or proven to be true.

Derivative: Derived from or part of something else.

Descriptive: As statement or account that describes.

Descriptive Approach: Presents only objective information available through the sense data, i.e., does not evaluate.

Desire: To wish or want.

Determinations: Judgment, decision, or diagnosis.

Determinator: Limits or establishes the meaning of a term or event.

Determined: As a result of cause and effect, i.e., no free choice.

Detract: To take away from.

Dialogue: When the teacher and pupil question and answer each other *in turn*. The teacher, by his questions, guides his young pupil's course of thought merely by presenting him with cases in which his predisposition for certain concepts will develop (the teacher is the midwife of the pupil's thoughts). The pupil, who thus sees that he himself can think, responds with questions of his own about obscurities in the propositions admitted or about his doubts regarding them, and so provides occasions for the *teacher* himself to *learn* how to question skillfully, according to the saying *by teaching we learn*. [6:478]

Dignity: Respect of a subject because of their intrinsic and inherent worth.

Dispassionate: Not to be affected by one's feelings and inclinations.

Dispute: Disagreement.

Distribution Principle: Rawls's second principal of justice that argues that if there is going to be any unequal distribution of basic goods then it must benefit all especially the least well off, i.e., maximin principle.

Distributive: To divide among several or many; to spread out.

Doctrine: A principle, or set of principles, that is taught.

Doctrine of duties: Kant says: "doctrine of duties in general is now divided into the system of the *doctrine of right* (ius), which deals with duties that can be given by external laws, and the system of the *doctrine of virtue* (ethica), which treats of duties that cannot be so given."

Doctrine of ends: Kant

Doctrine of right: For Kant the "doctrine of Right," is concerned only with "duties of outer freedom", i.e. narrow duties–the manner in which one person's behavior affects others, as in the fulfillment of contracts. External constraint is morally possible, i.e., duties the state coerces by using punitive prudential incentives. (Right behaviors are also moral duties that should all be done from an ethical motive.) Deals with the '*formal* condition of outer freedom (the consistency of outer freedom with itself if its maxim were made universal law.' One begins with the end and then seeks out the maxim of action in conformity with duty, i.e., to adopt maxims on empirical grounds. *p. xi,146, Metaphysics of Morals.*

Doctrine of virtue: Kant defines the "Doctrine of virtue" or "ethics," as "the science of how one is under obligation without regard for any possible external lawgiving." And "the part of the general doctrine of duties that brings inner, rather than outer, freedom under laws." 'the supreme principle of the doctrine of virtue is: act in accordance with a maxim of *ends* that it can be a universal law for everyone to have. – In accordance with this principle a human being is an end for himself as well as for others, and it is not enough that he is not authorized to use either himself or others merely as means; it is in itself his duty to make man as such his end.' Ethics 'provides a *matter* (an object of free choice), and **end** of pure reason which it represents as an end that is also objectively necessary, that is, an end that, as far as human beings are concerned, it is a duty to have. –For since the sensible inclinations of human beings tempt them to ends (the matter of choice) that can be contrary to duty, lawgiving reason can in turn check their influence only by a moral end setup against the ends of inclination, an end that must therefore be given *a priori*, independently of inclinations.' One begins with the maxim of actions in conformity with duty and then seeks out the end that is also a duty. Only *an end that is also a duty* can be called a **duty of virtue**. Duty of virtue is based on free self-constraint. (For finite holy beings, who could never be tempted to violate duty, there would be no doctrine of virtue but only a doctrine of morals. ... Thus human morality in its highest stage can still be nothing more than virtue.) The ends that are also duties are *one's own perfection* and *the happiness of others*. p. *xi, 146-8, Metaphysics of Morals.*

Dualist: Two distinct conceptual categories.

Durable: Long lasting.

Duty: Kant defines it as that action to which someone is bound. It is therefore the matter of obligation, and there can be one and the same duty (as to the action) although we can be bound to it in different ways. Duty also includes the concept of constraint to an end adopted reluctantly. All duties involve a concept of *constraint* through a law. *Ethical* duties involve a constraint for which only internal lawgiving is possible, whereas duties of right involve a constraint for which external lawgiving is also possible. *Metaphysics of Morals p. 156 [6:394]* See obligation.

Duty of Virtue: There are many duties of virtue; for there are many objects that it is our duty to have as ends. [6:410] (see obligation of virtue.

Egalitarian: The position that holds that all goods should be distributed equally.

Eleutheronomy: The principle of the freedom of internal lawgiving.

Emancipation: To make free socially, politically, and legally.

Empirical: Relying on observation and experiment, i.e., sense data, not by pure reason, which is independent of sense data.

Empirical knowledge: Knowledge based on verifiable and observational experience rather than theory or pure logic.

End: Object of free choice. Goal, consequence, towards which an activity is performed. Kant argued that every action has an end and is an act of freedom. Ends that are also duties are *one's own perfection* and *the happiness of others.* (see one's own perfection, and happiness of others) *Metaphysics of Morals p. 150.*

End that is in itself a duty: Belongs to the doctrine of virtue or ethics. 'If I am under obligation to make my end something that lies in concepts of practical reason, and so to have, besides the formal determining ground of choice (such as right contains), a material one as well, an end that could be set against the end arising from sensible impulses, this would be the concept of an *end that is in itself a duty.' Metaphysics of Morals, p. 146.*

Enfeeblement: To make feeble; weak, without energy; subnormal in intelligence.

Epistemology: Study of the origin, nature, limits, and justification of knowledge.

Equilibrate: To bring into a state of equilibrium.

Equilibrium: Balanced, stable, or symmetrical.

Ethereal: Abstract and nonobjective.

Ethics: Moral principles. For Kant it is the doctrine of virtue. Lawgiving which makes an action a duty and also makes this duty the incentive. (Lawgiving which does not include the incentive of duty and so admits an incentive other than the idea of duty itself is juridical.) Ethics is the science of one is under obligation without regard for any possible external lawgiving. [6:410] The doctrine of right has to do only with narrow duties, whereas ethics has to do with wide duties. Hence the doctrine of right, which by its nature must determine duties strictly (precisely), has no more need of general directions (a method) as to how to proceed in judging than does pure mathematics; instead, it certifies its method by what it does.–But ethics, because of the latitude it allows in its imperfect duties, unavoidably leads to questions that call upon judgment to decide how a maxim is to be applied in particular cases, and indeed in such a way that judgment provides another (subordinate)maxim (and one can always ask for yet another principle for applying this maxim to cases that may arise). So ethics falls into a casuistry, which has no place in the doctrine of right. [6:411]

Ethical Theory: A moral position in which right and wrong is deduced from the moral position, i.e., from the general to the particulars.

Etiquette: The formal rules of proper behavior.

Euclidian Geometry: Mathematics that deals with the geometric characteristics that are two-dimensional.

Euthanasia: Easy death.

Eudaemonism: The principle of happiness.

Evidence: Facts or information indicating whether a belief or proposition is true or valid.

Evolution: The gradual development of something.

Expedient: Likely to be useful or helpful for attaining an end or advantage.

Exposition: Explanation or interpretation.

External Justification: Justification that is independent of that which is being justified.

External Problem: In reference with cultural relativism it refers to the problem of not being able to judge other cultures.

Extrinsic value: Value that something has because of what it can do or accomplish outside of what it is, not existing within. Value because of its function as a means to an end. Antonym is intrinsic value.

External World: That which refers to the empirical or objective reality known through the use of sense data, i.e., perceptions.

Faculty: Power of mind; ability to do something.

Falsification: Facts that could be shown to be false.

Fantastic or Fanatical Virtue: Someone who allows *nothing to be morally indifferent* and strews all his steps with duties, as with mantraps; it is not indifferent to him whether I eat meat or fish, drink beer or wine, supposing that both agree with me. Fantastic virtue is concerned with petty details which, were it admitted into the doctrine of virtue, would turn the government of virtue into tyranny. *Metaphysics of Morals*, p. 167, [6:409].

Fetish: Object worshipped by pagan people because they believe a spirit lives in it; anything to which abnormal, excessive respect or attention is given.

First principles: For Mill it was utility or the greatest happiness principle: 'actions are right in proportion as they tend to promote happiness; wrong as they tend to produce the reverse of happiness.'

Flippant: Not showing deserved respect or seriousness.

Formal duties: (see Narrow duties)

Formula of autonomy: One should always act in such a way that his will can at the same time regard itself as legislating in its maxims universal laws.

Formula of end: One should always act in such a way that humanity either in oneself or in others is always treated as an end in itself and never as a means.

Formula of universal law: One such act only on that maxim that can at the same time be willed to become a universal law.

Fragmentation: The use of two or more approaches when trying to determine the nature of something.

Framework: Basic structure. An organizational structure.

Free Choice: Kant defines it as choice which can be determined by *pure reason*. Contrast with animal choice.

Free will: The power of acting without the constraint of necessity.

Freedom: The power or right to act, speak, or think as one wants without hindrance or restraint. Kant defines it as the independence from being constrained by another's choice,[or by one's own inclinations or any other sensible determining grounds]. Freedom insofar as it can coexist with the freedom of every other in accordance with a universal law, is the only original right belonging to every man by virtue of his humanity. Freedom is the ability to choose to follows one's internal lawgiving, not to oppose it. No theoretical deduction can be given for the possibility of the concept of freedom. It can only be inferred from the practical law of reason (the categorical imperative) as a fact of reason.

Freedom of choice: According to Kant; freedom is a pure rational concept, i.e., transcendent. The negative concept of freedom is the independence from being *determined* by sensible impulses. The positive concept of freedom is that of the ability of pure reason to be of itself practical by the subjection of the maxim of every action to the condition of its qualifying as universal law. Freedom proves its reality by practical principles, which are laws of a causality of pure reason for determining choice independently of any empirical conditions and prove a pure will in us, in which moral concepts and laws have their source.

Futile: Having no effect; unsuccessful; useless.

General Theory Of Relativity: Relationship between time, size, and mass are said to change in relation to speed.

General Theories: Theories that are complete or cover a broad range.

Genes: Unit of heredity that is transferred from a parent to offspring and determines some characteristic of the offspring.

Genocide: The deliberate killing of a large number of people from a particular nation or ethnic group with the aim of destroying that nation or group

Geocentric: Earth centered universe.

Good: This concept is defined differently for different moral theories but in general, it refers to that which is morally correct or right.

Good Samaritan: Provision that if you try to help someone you will not be held liable.

Greatest Happiness Principle: John Stuart Mill's principle that says that something is right in proportion to which it promotes happiness and wrong to the degree that it promotes the reverse of happiness.

Grey Areas: Those areas or issues in which a particular theory does not directly apply.

Hard determinism: Determinism and freedom cannot exist at the same time and only determinism exists.

Happiness of others: Kant says this is one of the ends that is also a duty, along with one's own perfection. 'When it comes to my promoting happiness as an end that is also a duty, this must therefore be the happiness of *other* human beings, whose (permitted) end I thus make my own end as well. It is for them to decide what they count as belonging to their happiness; but it is open to me to refuse them many things that they think will make them happy but that I do not, as long as they have no right to demand them from me as what is theirs.' (see one's own perfection) *Metaphysics of Morals p. 151.*

Heliocentric: Sun centered universe.

Hermeneutical Circle: To understand the whole you need to understand the parts and to understand the parts you need to understand the whole.

Heteronomy: That which is dependent on cause and effect.

Heuristic: Computing or proceeding to a solution by intuitional rules that are only loosely defined.

Hierarchical: Things need to be done chronologically so that the first is completed before the second and so on; it also means that things lower on the list cannot violate those that precede it.

Holistic: The comprehension of the parts of something as intimately interconnected and understood only by reference to the whole.

Holistically: To understand or comprehend something in its entirety and not just its parts.

Hologram: A type of three-dimensional pictures in which each part of the picture contains the whole picture.

Holy War: A war thought to be mandated by God.

Human choice: Kant defines it as a choice that can indeed be *affected* but not *determined* by impulses, and is therefore of itself (apart from an acquired proficiency of reason) not pure but can still be determined to actions by pure will. Contrast with animal choice.

Human Rights: Usually refers to inalienable rights that all human beings have by virtue of being a person, i.e., intrinsic rights.

Hypothetical: In relation to Rawls it refers to a society of ideally, rational and reasonable citizens that do not exist in reality which are used to construct a fair and just political system.

Idealistic: Perfect, to imagine or represent as perfect or better than in reality.

Illustrate: To show or explain the meaning of something by giving related examples, pictures, diagrams, etc.

Immanuel Kant: Born in Konigsberg, East Prussia (in what is now Kaliningrad, Russia), on April 22, 1724. Kant taught at the University of Konigsberg until his death on February 12, 1804. Kant is known in moral theory for his categorical imperatives and his emphasis on the autonomous good will and self-legislation. Kant has been classified as a deontologist.

Impede: To get in the way of, to make (something) difficult to do.

Imperative: Is a practical rule by which an action in itself contingent is *made* necessary. It is a directive to act in a certain way —it is not a statement of fact.

Impermissible: Not allowed or permitted.

Impenetrable: That which cannot be gone into or through.

Impulse: Sudden inclination, or feeling, to do something without thought.

In Concreto: Kant says that the typic of the moral law is "such a law as can be presented in concreto in objects of the senses and hence a law of nature" (5:69). ... For Kant, organisms are the actualization of an end. The ultimate end of nature is human beings themselves, and the highest end of humans is to be moral.

Inclinations: Impulses of nature, sentiments, feelings, and desires. Obstacles within man's mind to the fulfillment of duty and forces opposing it, which he must judge that he is capable of resisting and conquering by reason.

Incoherent: Not coherent; showing lack of suitable connection between ideas or words.

Incommunicable: Not able to be communicated to others.

Incompatiblist: Determinism and freedom cannot exist at the same time and only determinism exists.

Incomprehensible: Not able to be understood.

Inconceivable: That which cannot be thought of.

Inconsistency: Something that is illogical or contradicts itself.

Indefinable: Not able to be defined.

Indeterminable: Not able to determine the cause effect relationship.

Indeterminate duties: (see Wide duties)

Individual-Case Model: Intuition model in which justification is form a bottom-up-perspective, i.e., it goes from particulars to the general.

Inductive: Inductive reasoning uses probability reasoning, not analytic reasoning.

Inexorable Abandonment: Total and complete abandonment, which cannot be changed or prevented by one's effort.

Infallible: Not fallible; incapable of making mistakes or doing wrong; complete freedom from the possibility of being in error.

Inference: Evidence that is used towards coming to a conclusion.

Infinite Regress: Continuing on to infinity.

Infringe: To break transgress, or violate a rule, oath, copyright, etc.

Instrumental: Serving as a means to a particular end.

Integration: To combine parts to form a whole; to mix in order to obtain social, political, economic, etc. equality.

Intelligent design: Creationism.

Intelligible world: Aspect of the world in which you can have knowledge of.

Internal Problem: In reference with cultural relativism it refers to the problem of *not* being able to judge or criticize one's own culture, and thus promote any type of moral or cultural progress.

Intimate: Detailed, resulting from close study, or great familiarity.

Interrelated: That which is brought together in reciprocal relationship, e.g., politics, philosophy, and economics studied as a united group.

Internal Justification: A justification that appeals to what is being justified. It has often times been classified as "begging the question" or "circular argument".

Intersubjective: Existing between conscious minds; shared by more than one conscious mind.

Intolerant: Not able or willing to accept ways of thinking and behaving which are different from one's own?

Intractable: Difficult.

Intrinsic value: Value belonging naturally; existing within, not coming from outside. Value is because it is an end in itself, not a means to an end. Antonym is extrinsic value.

Intuition: The immediate understanding of something without conscious reasoning or study. Axiom or postulate that is presupposed without the use of sense data. Kant, however, used the term to represent *a posteriori* knowledge, which is necessary for Kant's phenomenal philosophy but not his neumenal philosophy.

Intuition Model: An individual-case model in which justification is from a bottom-up-perspective, i.e., it goes from the particulars to the general. Starting with what we know to be right or wrong we then develop moral theories.

Intuitive: Based on what one feels to be true even without conscious reasoning. That which uses intuition.

Invocation: To invoke; call upon the power of the law, God, etc., for help or protection.

Is-ought problem: From statements of facts it is impossible to derive statements of ought.

Ishihara plate: Colorblind test pictures.

Islam: (The people and countries that practice) the Muslim religion, started by Mohammed.

Jack Of All Trades And Master Of None: This is a slang term that refers to a person that is somewhat competent in many thing but is not fully competent in anything.

John Stuart Mill: Lived from 1806-1873. His books and essays are still studied for their insights concerning logic, epistemology, philosophy of science, social philosophy, and, of course, ethical theory.

John Rawls: (b. 1921, d. 2002) was an American political philosopher in the liberal tradition. His theory of justice as fairness describes a hypothetical free and equal democratic constitutional society. Citizens are ideally rational and reasonable with equal basic rights and liberties and fair distribution of basic social goods.

Judgement: To form or give an opinion or decision.

Judicial Stage: Part of John Rawls's social political framework in which the veil of ignorance disappears and individual situations are taken into account when implementing various laws.

Justice, Mill: Mill defines it as follows: 'Justice implies something which is not only right to do, and wrong not to do, but which some individual person can claim from us as his moral right.'

Justice: Rawls: Fair distribution of social goods that are necessary for the development of the rational and reasonable aspects of every citizen, especially the least well-off.

Kingdom of ends: This is the ideal of a moral community in which each member would act in such a way that if all other members acted in this way, then a community of free and equal members would result in which each member would, as he realizes his own purposes, also further the aims of his fellow members. In such a community each member freely disciplines himself under the very same rules that would be prescribed by him for others; the result would be that each member would act as a law unto himself (and hence autonomously) but yet would cooperate harmoniously with every other member. The Kingdom of ends has not only a for (the legality) but also a matter (its free and equal members and the aims or purposes, they pursue). To say that they are equally free means that any one of them has not the right either by coercion or deception to subject any of the others to his own private interests. *Grounding*, p. vi-vii.

Lackey: Someone who allows others to tread on their rights with impunity, i.e. without consequences.

Language: Means of communication.

Latter: The last one to be mentioned.

Least Well Off: Usually refers to those who are the poorest or lowest in social prestige.

Legislative Stage: Part of John Rawls's social political framework in which the veil of ignorance is starting to thicken but it is still thick enough so that laws can be legislated that are fair and impartial.

Libertarian: Believes in the existence of freedom. Not to be confused with political libertarian concepts.

Linguistic construct: Communication framework.

Logical: In accordance with formal rules of logic.

Logically Consistent: One thing necessarily follows another with no contradictions.

Love of Human Beings: Kant argues that a *Duty to love* is an absurdity. But *benevolence,* as conduct, can be subject to a law of duty. "You ought to *love* your neighbor as yourself" does not mean that you ought immediately (first) to love him and (afterwards) by mean of this love do good to him. It means, rather, *do good* to your fellow human beings, and your beneficence will produce love of them in you.

Marks: In reference to morality, it means the attachment of words to abstract moral concepts in the attempt to make the abstract moral concepts "perceivable".

Material duties: (see Wide duties)

Maxim: A subjective rule that the agent himself makes, by free choice. Hence, different agents can have very different maxims with regard to the same law; A rule that is followed in any deliberately intentional act. In any maxim the aim, means, and circumstances can always be identified.

Maxim of action: Kant argued that 'the law can prescribe only the maxim of action, not actions themselves, ... that is the law cannot specify precisely in what way one is to act and how much one is to do by the action for an end that is also a duty. ... [This] is not to be taken as permission to make exceptions to the maxim of actions but only as permission to limit one maxim of duty by another [maxim].'

Maximin: Usually refers to Rawls's second principal of justice, also known as the distribution principle, in which representatives try to maximize the minimal condition, of the least well off.

Maximize: To increase to the greatest degree possible.

Meddle: To take an interest or action in something (which is not to be of your concern).

Memes: An element of a culture or system of behavior that may be considered to be passed from one generation to another by nongenetic means, esp. imitation.

Memetic: Relating to memes.

Metaphysics: Deals with the questions of existence and the properties of that which does exist. A system of *a priori* cognition from concepts alone, i.e., independent of any sense data.

Metaphysical:

Above or beyond that which is physical, i.e., deals with the *a priori*—that which does not depend on cause and effect and/or sense data.

Merits:The quality of deserving praise, rewards or honor.

Mid-Level Principles: Principles that are compatible with, derivable from or at least not in logical contradiction with one's theories and/or intuitions.

Minimize: To decrease as much as possible.

Model: A thought out approach or protocol for accomplishing a particular task.

Modus Ponens: Modus Ponens—MP is defined as follows:

1. **If** p **then** q
2. p
3. **Therefore:** q (MP on 1 and 2)

Modus Tollens: Modus Tollens—MT is defined as follows **("~" means not, or it is not the case)**

1. **If** p **then** q
2. ~q
3. **Therefore:** ~p (MT on 1 and 2)

Morals: That which is considered to be ethically appropriate.

For Kant morals contains those maxims conforming to the ultimate moral norm and enunciating human moral obligations in very general "material" terms. *p. x, Metaphysics of Morals.*

Moral Apathy: Feeling arising form sensible impressions lose their influence of moral feeling only because respect of the law is more powerful than all such feelings together. *Metaphysics of Morals,* p. 167, [6:408]

Moral concepts: For Kant moral concepts require one to act *from* respect for the idea of conformity to law (incentive) *in accordance with* the capacity of one's maxim to be a universal law (rule) and *for the sake of* (end) a self-regulating community of free member (the kingdom of ends). Not one of these ideas (incentive, rule, end) can be adequately exemplified in experience, and they must therefore all be *a priori* conceptions. Insofar as the categorical imperative provides criteria for determining what should be done by pointing out an end, a rule and an incentive, it is a practical principle. *Grounding,* p. ix.

Moral Determinator: Limits or establishes the moral meaning of a term or event.

Moral Inquiry: To investigate an ethical situation, positions or model.

Moral Law: For Kant the moral law issues a double command: that we (1) act rightly and (2) do so because it is the right action. *p. x, Metaphysics of Morals.*

Moral Feeling: This is the susceptibility to feel pleasure or displeasure merely from being aware that our actions are consistent with or contrary to the law of duty. Respect for the law, which in its subjective aspect is called moral feeling, is identical with consciousness of one's duty. [6:464]

Moral Pluralism: Moral position that incorporates a number of differing moral approaches.

Moralist: Person who studies, practices and teaches morality.

Morality: Having to do with the rightness or wrongness of an action and/or intention. For Kant it is the conformity in which the ideal of duty arising from the law is also the incentive to the action. The mere conformity or nonconformity of an action with law, irrespective of the incentive to it, is called its legality.

Morose: Sullen; ill-tempered; unsocial.

Motive: The cause or reason for action.

Multi-Disciplinary: The coming together of several specialists in differing fields in order to come to a reasonable decision.

Multitude: Several.

Muslims: Also called Moslem, Mohammedan, Muhammadan, (a person) of the religion started by Mohammed—see also Islam.

Mutually Constraining: Two or more items, concepts or positions that set limits on each other.

Naive:

Implies a genuine, innocent simplicity or lack of artificiality but sometimes connotes an almost foolish lack of experience and wisdom.

Naïve realist: Holds to the position that secondary qualities are primary qualities.

Naïveté: Adjective is naïve; natural and innocent in speech and behavior (e.g., because young or inexperienced); amusingly simple.

Narrow duties: Kant explains that they are specific obligations of actions done for attaining particular consequences. They prescribe actions and how much one is to do by the action. They are limiting and negative formal duties. These perfect duties allow no exceptions for *any* reason whatsoever. "Doctrine of right has to do only narrow duties." See Wide obligations for comparison.

Natural Selection: Those beings that are most able to successfully reproduce will predominate and pass on their genetic traits. No purposes or ends are associated with it.

Naturalistic fallacy: Error in which a secondary quality is thought to be a primary quality, e.g., green grass.

Necessary Condition: In reference to morality, it is a condition that must be met in order for something to be even considered as being moral.

Necessity: The condition of being necessary, needed, or determined.

Nazis: A member of the German National Socialist Party (a fascist party) founded by Adolph Hitler (1889-1945).

Negative duties: *Forbid* a human being to act contrary to the **end** of his nature and so have to do merely with his oral *self-preservation.* Duty of virtue –duty of omission. (See Narrow duties) [6:419]

Neumenal: Knowledge that comes from pure *a priori* reasoning, i.e., no sense data. For Kant this is the only knowledge that is absolute.

Nonmaleficence: Do no harm.

Normative: Position or statement that tells us what actions is morally right or wrong or how we can determine if some action is right or wrong.

Norms: That which is considered to be morally right or wrong.

Notion: Speculative; not based on experiment or demonstration.

Noumenal world: Thing as it is in itself, as distinct from a thing as it is knowable by the senses through phenomenal attributes.

Objective Observer: One who relies solely on the perception of sense data, e.g., sight, sound, touch, smell, and taste. No influenced by subjective emotions, conflicts of interests, etc.

Objective: That which can be verified through the use of sense data.

Obligation: Kant defines it as the necessity of a free action under a categorical imperative of reason. (see duty)

Obligation of Virtue: There is only one obligation of virtue, i.e., respect for the law. [6:410] (see duty of virtue)

Obscure: Hard to understand; not clear. It may also refer to that which is not well known.

One's own perfection: Kant says that this is an end that is also a duty, along with the happiness of others. He argues that 'The word *perfection* is open to a good deal of misinterpretation. Perfection is sometimes understood as a concept belonging to transcendental philosophy, ... Then again, as a concept belonging to *teleology,* it is taken to mean the harmony of a thing's properties with an end. Perfection in the first sense could be called quantitative (material) perfection, and in the second, qualitative (formal) perfection. The quantitative perfection of a thing can be only one. But one thing can have several qualitative perfections, and it is really qualitative perfection that is under discussion here. The duty of one's own perfection is to cultivate one's faculties, the highest being understanding, the faculty of concepts and of one's will in which the law becomes also the incentive to his action that conform with duty and he obeys the law form duty. (see happiness of others) *Metaphysics of Morals p. 150.*

Original Position: That part of John Rawls's hypothetical game in which all the representatives are under the veil of ignorance and all they know is that they represent a citizen that is rational and reasonable and from this the representatives derive two basic principle of justice which enable the citizens to continue in their development as rational and reasonable citizens.

Ontology: A branch of metaphysics dealing with the nature of being.

Opposition: The act or state of being opposed to or fighting against.

Oppression: To rule or control in an unjust or cruel manner.

Partial: To favor.

Partialities: The quality or fact of being partial.

Patricians: Of noble birth.

Peculiarities: Belonging exclusively; used, adopted, practiced, only by something, or someone.

Pejorative: Derogatory or belittling.

Perceive: To have or come to have knowledge through one of the senses (*a posteriori*) or through the mind (*a priori*).

Perception: Process by which we become aware through the use of sense data, i.e., sight, sound, touch, taste, and smell.

Person: Person is not synonymous with human being. Person refers only to those who have autonomy and thus the capacity to act morally, i.e., a subject whose actions can be *imputed* to him. Contrast with thing.

Pervasive: Widespread.

Phenomenal: Knowledge that comes from *a posteriori* reasoning, i.e., cause and effect, sense data, etc. For Kant this knowledge can never be absolute.

Phenomenal world: The object of a person's perception.

Phenomenon: Something that is perceived through the use of sense data, i.e., sight, sound, smell, taste, touch.

Plebeians: Of the lower social classes.

Pluralistic: Form of society in which the members maintain their independent cultural traditions.

Pluralistic agents: Collective of people who hold to differing world-views.

Pluralistic Society: A society that is composed of a variety of races, religions, political, and moral persuasions.

Political Framework: Refers to the Constitutional, Legislative, and Judicial stages of John Rawls's theory.

Positive duties: *Command* a human being to make a certain object of choice his end, concerns his *perfecting* of himself. A duty of virtue –duty of commission. (See Wide duties) [6:419]

Postulate: Suggest or assume the existence, fact, or truth of something as a basis for reasoning, discussion, or belief.

Practical: That which deals with actions towards attaining a particular goal or end.

Practical law: A proposition that contains a categorical imperative which makes certain actions duties.

Practical Philosophy: Practical philosophy has two parts. One consists in the systematic study of practical metaphysics, that is, the *a priori* foundations of morally right conduct, as done in the *Groundwork*. The other involves what Kant called "moral anthropology," that is, an empirical examination of those features of the human condition that promote or impair how humans respond to their moral duties. pp. ix-x *Metaphysics of Morals*

Practical Reason: Insofar as the categorical imperative provides criteria for determining what should be done by pointing out an end, a rule and an incentive, it is a practical principle.

Pragmatic: A choice of action that most effectively accomplishes a particular goal or end. Dealing with matters in a way that seems best under the actual conditions, rather than following a rule. Concerned with practical results.

Pragmatism:

Mandates that we ought to do those actions that best and most effectively accomplishes a particular goal or end.

Precedence: The right to a particular place before others, especially because of importance.

Precept: A guiding rule on which behavior, a way of thought, or action, etc., is based.

Pre-Critical: Those writings of Kant that precede his *Critique of Pure Reason*, published in 1781.

Predicate: The part of a sentence or clause containing a verb and stating something about the subject.

Preference: Act of choosing one thing or action rather than another.

Premises: Parts of an argument that is used to establish a particular conclusion.

Presumption: That which is presupposed to be true without any proof.

Presuppose: To accept as true without proof.

Presuppositions: Those things that are presupposed.

Pretensions: A claim to possess a skill, quality, etc.

Prima facie: Principles you have to weigh and balance with other *prima facie* values.

Primary Qualities: That which exists independently of minds.

Primary Principle of Utility: (See the Greatest Happiness Principle)

Principles: General truth or belief that is used as a base for reasoning or action. Guiding rules for behavior.

Propounds: To put forward as a question or matter for consideration.

Provision: To provide or supply that which is needed. Condition or article.

Prudence: Acting only after careful thought or planning in regards to consequences.

Pure: Without the use of anything else.

Pure cognition: Knowledge using only *a priori* processes; based on logical consistence apart from any sense data or empirical observations.

Pure practical reason: Is Kant's moral reason that is a power of ends able to oppose and overcome the influence of any ends that are simply desired. There are two kinds of obligatory ends that can be identified in an *a priori* way. (1) respect for all of humanity and (2) love for all of humanity which means the adoption of other's ends as our own resulting in one's own perfection and the happiness of others. The highest, unconditional end of pure practical reason (which is still a duty) consists in this: that virtue be it s own end and, despite the benefits it confers on human beings, also its own reward.

Rabble: Disorderly crowd; a mob. A derogatory reference to ordinary people, especially when regarded as socially inferior or uncouth

Random: Made, done, happening, or chosen without method or conscious decision.

Rational: For John Rawls it means being able to form, revise or pursue one's good. Others think of it as being able to think in a logically consistent manner.

Rational Knowledge: Based on or in accordance with reason or logic.

Rationales: The reasons on which a system or practice is based.

Reality: The nature of being.

Realm: Literally means a kingdom. An area of activity.

Reasonable: For John Rawls it means being able to get along with others. Others think of it as being fair.

Rear: To care for until fully-grown and self-sufficient.

Reciprocal: Mutual obligation to respond in like fashion.

Requisite: Needed or required.

Reductio Ad Absurdum: This is a technique that is used to prove that a deductive argument is valid by assuming the opposite conclusion and showing that it results in a logical contradiction.

Reductive: Tending to present a subject or problem in a simplified form, esp. one viewed as crude.

Reflective: To mirror or compare back and forth.

Reflector: That which reflects.

Reflective-Equilibrium: Process in which individuals take their accepted intuitions, norms, and theories, mirror them back and forth, making appropriate changes, until an equilibrium or balance is achieved.

Relative: In reference to morality, it means that right or wrongs are never absolute; rather, what is right or wrong is determined by one's own evaluation or more popularly by one's culture. Term, thing, or concept that is dependent on something else.

Renounce: To give up; to declare formally that one will no longer have anything to do with somebody or something.

Representative: Someone who makes sure another person's interests are considered.

Representative heuristic: The psychological propensity to evaluate probabilities in such a way that to the degree to which "A" represents "B" is the degree towards which "A" comes from "B."

Reproach: To blame or find fault in someone, not angrily but sadly.

Respect: For Kant it is not correct to say that a human being has a *duty of self-esteem*; it must rather be said that the law within him unavoidably forces from him *respect* for his own being and this feeling is the basis of certain duties, that is, of certain actions that are consistent with his duty to himself.

Respectively: In the order that was presented.

Revelation: That which is made known.

Revolution: A great social change or a complete change in the way of thinking or acting.

Sanction: Permission or approval; an action taken against a person or country that has broken a law or rule.

Schema: For Kant that meant a general procedure of the imagination.

Scenario: Usually a hypothetical situation.

Secondary Principles: For John Stuart Mill it was those principles that have been determined to promote the greatest amount of happiness.

Secondary Qualities: That which exists only when a mind perceives it and only in the mind, e.g. color, sound, taste, feeling, smell.

Scope: The limit of a question, subject, or inquiry.

Self-Contradictory: To say or do something that is opposite in nature or character.

Sense Data: An immediate object of perception, which is not a material object; a sense impression, i.e., secondary quality. Information that we receive through our senses of perception, i.e., sight, sound, smell, tastes, and touches. Objective perception through the use of sight, sound, smell, touch, or taste.

Sensible: That which can be perceived through the use of sense data, i.e., sight, sound, smell, taste, and touch.

Sentiments: Thought or judgment arising from feeling.

Serfs: A person, not quite a slave, forced to stay and work on his/her master's land.

Social Goods: A Rawlsian term which denote those rights that are necessary for a citizen to develop both rationally and reasonably.

Soft Determinism: Holds to the position that determinism is compatible with freedom.

Solipsistic: The view or theory that the self, or subjective cognitive experiences, are all that can be known to exist.

Sophisticated: Cause (a person or their thoughts, attitudes, and expectations) to become less simple or straightforward through education or experience.

Sophisticated realist: Recognizes and is able to make the distinction between primary and secondary qualities.

Sophistry: Use of false reasoning or argument, intended to deceive.

Specific: Refers to something in particular as opposed to something in general.

Specification: In this paper it refers to theories and mid-level principles that are developed conceptually and shaped normatively so that they can be applied to particular circumstances, i.e., substantive development.

Speculative: Thought that is not based on facts or complete knowledge.

Standard: That which is recognized as being correct or acceptable.

Stark: Hard, bare, or severe in appearance.

Stigmatized: To be described scornfully, shame or disgrace.

Stimulus: A thing or event that evokes a specific functional reaction in an organ or tissue.

Straw-man argument: A straw-man argument is an Informal fallacy based on misrepresentation of an opponents position To "attack a straw man" is to create the illusion of having refuted a proposition by replacing it with a superficially similar yet unequivalent proposition (the "straw man"), and refuting it, without ever having actually refuted the original position.

Subject: A person or thing that is being discussed.

Subjective: Mind dependent. Moral values that are not objective are in some sense subjective, i.e., not based on any sensible or testable criteria.

Sublime:Of the greatest and highest sort; causing wonder or reverence; extreme; astounding; that which fills one with awe or reverence.

Subservient: Habitually will to do what other want; giving to much respect.

Substantive Development: (See specification)

Summum bonum: Ultimate good.

Sufficient Condition: If in reference to an action the action meets this sufficient condition then the action is not necessarily moral yet this action *may* be moral.

Supposition: The act of supposing or guessing, i.e., to consider as probable.

Survival of the fittest: Those that survive are the most fit. This term implies a purpose or end of fitness and is therefore a misnomer for natural selection which has no purposes or ends.

Sympathize: To share the feelings of others.

Syncretistic: When two or more "things" combine together so that the whole is greater than the sum of its parts.

Synergistic-Reflective-Equilibrium: A model of human decision-making that incorporates theories, intuitions, and mid-level principles into a coherent whole.

Synergy: When the whole is greater than the sum of the parts.

Synthesization: To synthesize, i.e., to combine several differing aspects of something into a whole.

Synthetic statements: The subject is not contained in the predicate and therefore the statement provides new knowledge at the expense of being only conditionally true.

Synthetical: Statement in which new knowledge is expressed, e.g., green light means go is a synthetical statement since the predicate gives new information about the predicate.

Systematically: Based on a regular plan or fixed method.

Teleology: Moral system in which the focus is on the end. *Telos*, meaning end, *ology* meaning study of. Kant defines it as the harmony of a thing's properties with an end. This is a qualitative (formal) perfection and one thing can have several qualitative perfections. (This is in contrast with perfection as belonging to transcendental philosophy, the concept of the totality of the manifold which taken together, constitutes a thing. This is called quantitative (material) perfection which can be only one.) *Metaphysics of Morals, p. 150,* (see Consequentialism)

Tautology: The saying of the same thing two time or more, using different forms, e.g., mathematics: 5+7=12, or definitional statements such as: "all bachelors are unmarried men." Bachelors = unmarried men.

Teleology: Study of ends or purposes.

Temper: To bring to the required condition by treatment.

Theoretical Development: Using intuitions and mid-level principles to develop a theory.

Theory: Covering-precept model which usually goes from the general to the particular.

Theory Model: Justification of what is right or wrong is done by reasoning down from a theory. From a theory, we deduce what action is logically consistent with the moral theory.

Thing: That to which nothing can be imputed. Any object of free choice which itself lacks freedom is therefore called a thing. Contrast with person.

Tiers: Subcategories that are usually arranged in hierarchical order.

Toleration: The practice of allowing opinions, beliefs, behavior, religion, culture, etc., different form one's own, to be held and practiced freely.

Top-Down Reasoning: Reasoning from covering-precepts or from a general theory down to individual cases.

Trifling: Thing, event, etc., of little value or importance.

Two Principles of Justice: Rawls's 1) basic rights and liberties and his 2) distribution principle.

Transcendent: To go beyond the range of human experience, reason, belief, powers of description, etc. In other words, no instance corresponding to it can be given in any possible experience, and of an object of which we cannot obtain any theoretical cognition.

Transcendental freedom: If an action can have both pure and empirical grounds, which grounds were the determining ones (pure or empirical)? Kant calls this a question of transcendental freedom, and much of the "analytic" of the *Critique of Practical reason* is devoted to it. His solution is to say that for practical purposes one can be sure that he is free, but one cannot fully grasp cognitively *how* transcendental freedom is possible. One knows that he can act autonomously, and thereby is the categorical imperative vindicated as a guide for action; but since knowledge (cognition) is a manifestation of the transcendental autonomy of intelligence, he cannot rise to a higher vantage point in order to attain a full cognitive grasp of ultimate grounds of both knowledge and action. *Grounding,* p. x.

Transference: The act of transferring to someone else the subjective cognitive experience or knowledge.

Treatise: A serious book or article that examines systematically a particular subject.

Tyrannical: Obtaining obedience by force or threats.

Ultimate ends: See Summum Bonum.

Unanimous: All agreeing.

Undetermined causation: When one cause can result in more than one possible result.

Unequivocal: Having only one possible meaning, totally clear in meaning.

Universal: Of, affecting, or done by all people or things in the world or in a particular group; applicable to all cases.

Unresolvable:Not resolvable; unable to settle or clear up a difficulty.

Utility: Usually refers to moral determination based on cause and effect.

Vain: Having too high an opinion of one's looks, abilities, etc.; conceited.

Valid Deductive Argument: An argument in which if the premises were in fact true it would be impossible for the conclusion to be false.

Values: The weighing and balancing of moral principles.

Veil Of Ignorance: Minimizes the amount of information that you know about the citizen that you represent so that you will not give him/her any unfair advantages.

Veneration: To regard with great respect and honor, and sometimes worship.

Veracity: Truthfulness.

Vicious circle: 1. A sequence of reciprocal cause and effect relationships in which two or more elements contradict each other.

2. In logic a definition or statement that begs the question, i.e., statements that assume the truth of an argument or proposition to be proved, without arguing it, e.g.

1. All intentional acts of killing human beings are morally wrong.
2. The death penalty is an intentional act of killing a human being.
3.Therefore the death penalty is wrong.

Violate or transgress:

Internal Justification: Justification that uses what it is trying to justify to justify itself (see begging the question).

Virtue: For Aristotle it was choosing the mean between the extremes. Kant argued that the well-known principle (Aristotle's) which locates virtue in the *mean* between two vices is false. What distinguishes *avarice* (as a vice) from thrift (as a virtue) is not that avarice carries thrift *too far* but that avarice has an *entirely different* principle (maxim), that of putting the end of economizing not in enjoyment of one's means but merely in possession of them, while denying oneself any enjoyment from them. In the same way, the vice of *prodigality* is not to be sought in an excessive enjoyment of one's means but in the bad maxim which makes the use of one's means the sole end, without regard for preserving them. Each of these vices has its distinctive maxim which necessarily contradicts the maxim of the other. *Metaphysics of Morals, p. 163, [6:404]*Virtue for Kant was the ability of the "will" to freely self-legislate one's maxim regardless of one's inclinations, i.e., the commitment to (1) right principles and (2) right intentions. But what it is virtuous to do may concern only *what is formal* in maxims, whereas as duty of virtue has to do with their matter, that is to say, with an end that is thought as also a duty. Like anything *formal,* virtue as the will's conformity with every duty, based on a firm disposition, is merely one and the same. But with respect to the *end* (what is material), there can be several virtues; and since obligation to the maxim of such an end is called a duty of virtue, there are many duties of virtue. The supreme principle of the doctrine of virtue is: act in accordance with a maxim of *ends* that it can be a universal law for everyone to have. –In accordance with this principle a human being is an end for himself as well as for others. … Pure reason can prescribe no ends *a priori* without setting them forth as duties, and such duties are then called duties of virtue. *Metaphysics of Morals, p. 157, [6:394-5]* Virtue so shines as an idea that it seems, by human standards, to eclipse *holiness* itself, which is never tempted to break the law. (Man with all his faults is better than a host of angels without a will) … The worth of virtue itself, as its own end, far exceeds the worth of any usefulness and any empirical ends and advantages that virtue may still bring in its wake. While the capacity to overcome all opposing sensible impulses can and must be simply *presupposed* in man on account of his freedom, yet this capacity as *strength* is something he must acquire; and the way to acquire it is to enhance the moral *incentive* both by contemplating the dignity of the pure rational law in us and by *practicing* virtue. [6:397] Virtue is the moral strength of a *human being's* will in fulfilling his *duty,* a moral *constraint* through his own lawgiving reason, insofar as this constitutes itself an authority *executing* the law. –Virtue itself, or possession of it, is not a duty rather, it commands and accompanies its command with a moral constraint. This moral strength as *courage,* also constitutes the greatest and the only true honor that man can win in war and is, moreover, called *wisdom* in the strict sense, namely practical wisdom, since it makes the *final end* of his existence on earth its own end. –Only in its possession is he "free," "healthy," "rich," "a king," and so forth and can suffer no loss by chance or fate, since he is in possession of himself and the virtuous man cannot lose his virtue. Virtue since it is its own end it must also be regarded as its own reward. Virtue is represented not as if a human being possesses virtue but rather as if virtue possesses him. *Ibid., p. 164-5, [6:405-406].* The true strength of virtue is a *tranquil mind* with a considered and firm resolution to put the law of virtue into practice. That is the state of *health* in the moral life, whereas an affect, even one aroused by the thought of *what is good,* is a momentary, sparkling phenomenon that leaves one exhausted. Ibid., p. 167, [6:409]. Virtue is always *in progress* and yet always starts *from the beginning.* –It is always in progress because, considered *objectively,* it is an ideal and unattainable, while yet constant approximation to it is a duty. That it always starts from the beginning has a *subjective* basis in human nature, which is affected by inclinations because of which virtue can never settle down in peace and quiet with its maxims adopted once and for all but, if it is not rising, is unavoidably sinking. For, moral maxims, unlike technical ones cannot be based on habit (since this belongs to the natural constitution of the will's determination); on the contrary, if the practice of virtue were to become a habit the subject would suffer loss to that *freedom* in adopting his maxims which distinguishes an action done from duty. Ibid., p. 167, [6:409]. Virtue must be acquired (that it is not innate). ... That virtue can and must be *taught* already follows from its not being innate. ... But one does not acquire the power to put the rules of virtue into practice merely by being taught how one ought to behave, ... but must be *exercised* and cultivated by efforts. ... But the *decision* to do this must be made all at once and completely. [6:477]

Vulgarest: The most: rude, low, or bad mannered; lack of fine feeling or good judgment in the choice of what is beautiful.

Vulnerable: Easily harmed, hurt, or attacked.

Weighing and Balancing: Maximizing as best as possible two or more mutually constraining principles.

Wide or indeterminate duties: When the categorical imperative requires us to adopt and act on *positive* maxims. These positive or material duties allow a latitude for free choice and personal judgment; imperfect duty. Ethics has to do with wide duties and unavoidably leads to questions that call upon judgment to decide how a maxim is to be applied in particular cases. "So ethics falls into a casuistry, which has no place in the doctrine of right." See narrow obligations.

Will: For Kant the will is the only thing that can be good in itself. The will legislates universal laws through the process of *a priori* knowledge. The will is not something that can be considered free or not free, since it is not directed to actions but immediately to giving laws which are the grounds determining the choice for the maxims of actions. The will itself, has no determining ground, it is instead practical reason itself. The will directs with absolute necessity and is itself subject to no necessitation. Only choice can therefore be called free.

Wish: Desire that is not joined with a consciousness of the ability to bring about its object by one's action. Contrast with choice.

World-View: How an individual interprets reality.

***

Author

Background

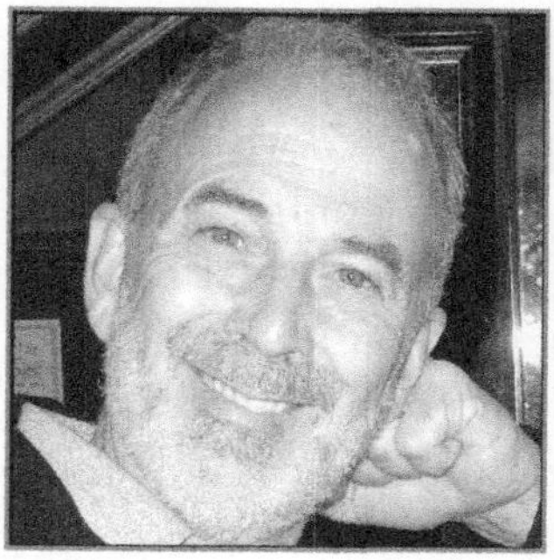

Education

Dr. Bulger has earned the rank of full Professor, at the Chicago Medical School, and is a nationally Certified Healthcare Ethics Consultant—HEC-C. His educational background includes a PhD in Philosophy from the University of Tennessee with a special concentration in Biomedical Ethics. Areas of study include Medical Ethics, Clinical Ethics, Policy Analysis, Human Rights, Social Political Philosophy, Healthcare Education, and Online Pedagogical Course Development.

He also holds a Master of Arts degree in Religious Studies from Western Seminary in Portland, OR, and a Bachelor of Science degree in Engineering from the University of North Dakota, Grand Forks.

Teaching

Professor Bulger has taught over 35 different philosophy courses face-to-face, blended, and online, including a range of lower-division and upper-division courses in Biomedical Ethics, Theoretical and Applied Ethics, Healthcare Issues, Public Policy, Professionalism, and Medical Ethics Research. He has demonstrated his pedagogical commitment as evidenced by Institutional Learning Outcomes and with 50 of his mentored students having successfully competed and presented academically peered reviewed papers at the National Conference of Undergraduate Studies—NCUR, documented exemplary Student Ratings of Instructor, and exceptionally high student satisfaction, success, and retention while holding to rigorous academic standards. In addition, he has years of clinical and teaching performance, computer and Learning Management System—LMS skills, and knowledge of the latest pedagogical theories and assessment strategies. Dr. Bulger's teaching expertise has been professionally and institutionally recognized with his induction into the Master Teacher Guild.

SERVICE

Professor Bulger has served on clinical, educational and research institutional governance committees, helping to coordinate and develop administrative policies which are in full compliance with the institutional mission and with federal, state, and institutional regulations and policies. He has actively served on hospital ethics committees, teaching and collaborating with interprofessional healthcare providers, staff and administration, for the advancement of advisory decision-making processes and outcomes.

He has successfully provided leadership in clinical, teaching and institutional environments with patient assisted decision-making, curriculum development and on department, division, institutional and district committees. These activities have assured the full articulation of various course offerings, the improvement of instructional programs, and the planning, implementation and teaching of special programs in order to support learning success as evidenced by the formulation of Learning Outcomes, their assessment cycles, and their results.

RESEARCH

Professor Bulger's research and publications have ranged from the writing of biomedical ethics course textbooks, courses, online course deliveries, and a variety of academic papers. Along with clinical ethics consultations, multi-disciplinary educational programs, and interdisciplinary and interprofessional collaborations, his current clinical and organizational ethics research focuses on:

"What are the necessary and sufficient conditions and responsibilities for categorizing shared decision-making as being a valid informed consent, and how do those necessary and sufficient conditions and responsibilities differ for the patient, profession, and public policy?"

Diversity

Professor Bulger is very sensitive to the socio-economic, academic, cultural, LGBTQ+ and ethnic diversity within the educational, healthcare, clinical, and patient population and has an understanding of physical and/or learning disabilities and differences in learning styles.

Life-Long Learning

Professor Bulger is passionate about professional growth and development and continues to strive towards exemplary excellence in teaching, scholarship and service.

❊❊❊

Made in the USA
Coppell, TX
05 November 2026

11307223R00360